Potato Salad No. 257

diabetes
FAMILY FRIENDLY COOKBOOK

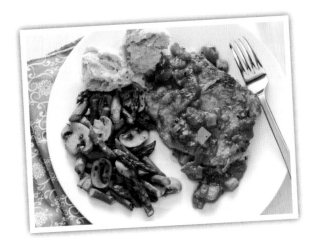

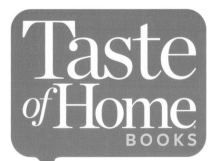

RDA ENTHUSIAST BRANDS, LLC
GREENDALE, WI

Taste of Home

Reader's Digest

A TASTE OF HOME/READER'S DIGEST BOOK

EDITORIAL

Editor-in-Chief: Catherine Cassidy
Creative Director: Howard Greenberg
Editorial Operations Director: Kerri Balliet

Managing Editor, Print & Digital Books: Mark Hagen
Associate Creative Director: Edwin Robles Jr.

Editors: Heather Ray, Janet Briggs
Associate Editor: Molly Jasinski
Contributing Layout Designer: Dit Rutland
Editorial Production Manager: Dena Ahlers
Copy Chief: Deb Warlaumont Mulvey
Copy Editor: Mary C. Hanson
Content Operations Manager: Colleen King
Content Operations Assisstant: Shannon Stroud
Executive Assistant: Marie Brannon

Chief Food Editor: Karen Berner
Food Editors: James Schend, Peggy Woodward, RD
Associate Food Editor: Krista Lanphier
Recipe Editors: Annie Rundle, Mary King, Jenni Sharp, RD; Irene Yeh

Test Kitchen & Food Styling Manager: Sarah Thompson
Test Cooks: Nicholas Iverson (lead), Matthew Hass, Lauren Knoelke
Food Stylists: Kathryn Conrad (senior), Shannon Roum, Leah Rekau
Prep Cooks: Megumi Garcia, Melissa Hansen, Nicole Spohrleder, Bethany Van Jacobson

Photography Director: Stephanie Marchese
Photographers: Dan Roberts, Jim Wieland
Photographer/Set Stylist: Grace Natoli Sheldon
Set Stylists: Stacey Genaw, Melissa Haberman, Dee Dee Jacq

Business Analyst: Kristy Martin
Billing Specialist: Mary Ann Koebernik

BUSINESS

General Manager, Taste of Home Cooking Schools: Erin Puariea

Vice President, Brand Marketing: Jennifer Smith
Vice President, Circulation & Continuity Marketing: Dave Fiegel

READER'S DIGEST NORTH AMERICA

Vice President, Business Development & Marketing: Alain Begun
President, Books & Home Entertainment: Harold Clarke
General Manager, Canada: Philippe Cloutier
Vice President, Operations: Mitch Cooper
Vice President, Chief Marketing Officer: Leslie Doty
Chief Operating Officer: Howard Halligan
Vice President, Chief Sales Officer: Mark Josephson
Vice President, Digital Sales: Steve Sottile
Vice President, Chief Content Officer: Liz Vaccariello
Vice President, Global Financial Planning & Analysis: Devin White

THE READER'S DIGEST ASSOCIATION, INC.

President and Chief Executive Officer: Robert E. Guth

For other Taste of Home books and products, visit us at **tasteofhome.com.**

For more Reader's Digest products and information, visit **rd.com** (in the United States) or see **rd.ca** (in Canada).

International Standard Book Number: 978-1-61765-306-3
Library of Congress Control Number: 2013919370

Cover Photography: Taste of Home Photo Studio

Pictured on front cover: Breezy Lemon-Berry Dessert, page 291; Thai Chicken Lettuce Wraps, page 69; Tuscan Portobello Stew, page 181
Pictured on back cover: Slow Cooker Turkey Breast, page 153; Dill Garden Salad, page 215; and Better-For-You-Buttermilk Pancakes, page 37

Printed in China.
1 3 5 7 9 10 8 6 4 2

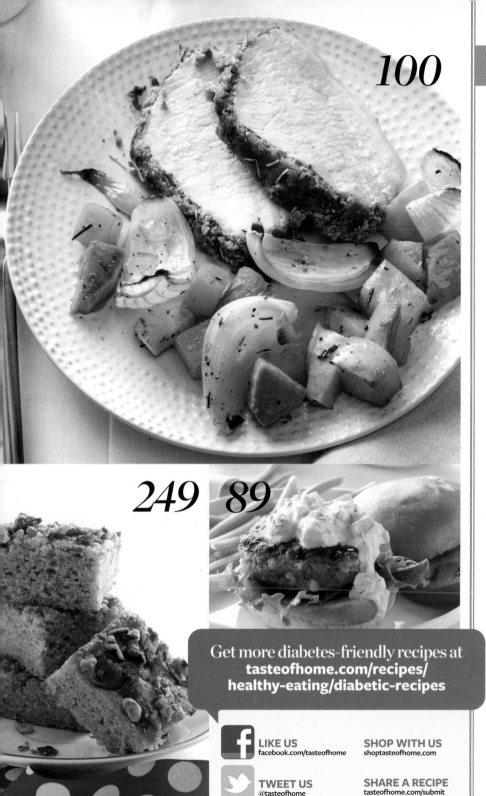

100

249 *89*

Contents

Get more diabetes-friendly recipes at
**tasteofhome.com/recipes/
healthy-eating/diabetic-recipes**

f **LIKE US**
facebook.com/tasteofhome

SHOP WITH US
shoptasteofhome.com

TWEET US
@tasteofhome

SHARE A RECIPE
tasteofhome.com/submit

FOLLOW US
pinterest.com/taste_of_home

UNDERSTANDING
DIABETES

What is it?

Our bodies require insulin **to help get glucose into our cells** for energy. When you have diabetes, your body is either **not producing enough insulin to feed your cells** or **cells are resisting the insulin.** When this happens, the level of glucose rises in the blood, leading to a variety of dangerous consequences.

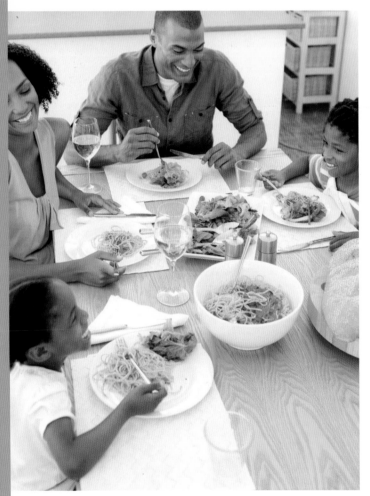

Different Types

Type 1 diabetes occurs when the body's immune system destroys the cells in the pancreas that produce insulin. That's why people with Type 1 diabetes take insulin shots or use an insulin pump.

Type 2 diabetes occurs when your cells begin to resist the insulin your pancreas produces. Healthy eating, physical activity and regular blood glucose testing are the main therapies for Type 2 diabetes.

Untreated, high blood glucose can cause nerve damage, kidney or eye problems, heart disease and stroke, so it's important to talk to your doctor about whether you should be actively checking your blood glucose levels.

The key to successfully managing diabetes is to control blood sugar while getting the right amount of nutrients. And that starts with a healthy diet. Each of the 514 recipes in this book has been analyzed to offer you Nutrition Facts and Diabetic Exchanges, so you can choose the best recipes for you and your family.

HOW WE CALCULATE
NUTRITION FACTS

- When a choice of ingredients is given in a recipe (such as ⅓ cup sour cream or plain yogurt), the first ingredient listed is always the one calculated in the Nutrition Facts.

- When a range is given for an ingredient (such as 2 to 3 teaspoons), we calculate the first amount given.

- Only the amount of marinade absorbed during preparation is calculated.

- Optional ingredients are not included in calculations.

DIABETIC EXCHANGES

A helpful tool in making smart food choices is the food-exchange system, which organizes foods into several groups—generally breads and starches, fruits, vegetables, milk, meat and protein-based substitutes, fats, and other carbohydrates such as sweets. The idea behind the exchange system is that every item within a category is nutritionally equivalent to every other item on that same list, providing roughly the same amount of carbohydrate, fat, protein and calories.

While Diabetic Exchanges are designed for people with diabetes, they can also be valuable for anyone trying to control calories, reduce fat and eat a balanced diet. Diabetic Exchanges are assigned to recipes in accordance with guidelines from the American Diabetic Association and the Academy of Nutrition and Dietetics. All the recipes in *Diabetes Family Friendly Cookbook* have been reviewed and approved by a registered dietitian as suitable for someone with diabetes to consider including in meal plans.

RANGES OF EXCHANGES

Some exchange lists are subdivided into groups that specify exchanges of, say, lean meats and substitutes (separate from high-fat meats), or fat-free milk products (separate from whole-milk products). Foods within each category are nutritionally equivalent in the exchange system.

STARCHES
1 slice bread
½ cup cooked lentils
⅓ cup cooked pasta
½ cup corn
1 small potato

VEGETABLES
½ cup cooked carrots
½ cup cooked green beans
1 cup raw radishes
1 cup raw salad greens
1 large tomato

FRUITS
1 small banana
½ large pear
17 small grapes
2 tablespoons raisins
½ cup fruit cocktail

FAT-FREE AND LOW-FAT MILKS
1 cup skim or 1% milk
1 cup plain nonfat yogurt
⅔ cup low-fat fruit-flavored yogurt
⅔ cup evaporated nonfat milk
1 cup low-fat buttermilk

LEAN MEATS AND SUBSTITUTES
1 ounce skinless chicken breast
1 ounce canned tuna (in water or oil, drained)
1 ounce cheese with 3 grams of fat or less per ounce
¼ cup low-fat cottage cheese
2 egg whites

FATS
1 teaspoon oil
1 teaspoon stick butter
1½ teaspoons peanut butter
1 tablespoon reduced-fat margarine spread
1 tablespoon reduced-fat mayonnaise
6 almonds
4½ teaspoons reduced fat cream cheese

HEY, THAT'S *NOT TRUE...*

3 Myths Worth Busting

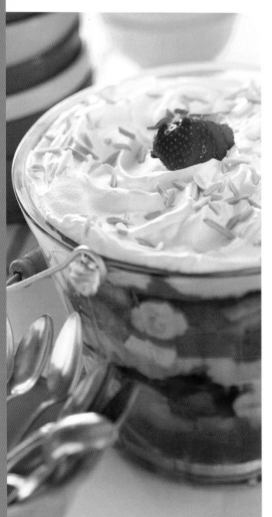

People with diabetes **have to eat different meals** and snacks from the rest of the family.

MYTH

It's true that family members with diabetes have to watch what they eat, but there's no need to cook separate dishes. Everyone will benefit from eating more leafy greens, high-fiber foods and lean proteins.

People with diabetes **can't eat sweets or desserts**.

MYTH

Almost everyone has a hankering for something sweet from time to time. A good way to deal with a food craving is to enjoy a little taste. Having a very small portion on special occasions will prevent you from feeling deprived so you can keep focusing on healthful foods.

People with diabetes **shouldn't eat starchy foods.**

MYTH

Everyone needs carbohydrates for energy. Whole grains and starchy vegetables like potatoes, yams, peas and corn can be included in meals and snacks, but portion size is key. According to the American Diabetes Association, a good place to start is to aim for 45-60 grams of carbohydrate per meal or 3-4 servings of carbohydrate-containing foods. Depending on your needs and how you manage your diabetes, you may need to adjust this amount. Your health care team can help you determine suitable portions.

QUICK FACTS FROM THE AMERICAN DIABETES ASSOCIATION

- Losing just 2 pounds **drops your diabetic risk** by 16 percent.
- According to the American Diabetes Association, Type 2 Diabetes accounts for **90 to 95 percent of all cases of diabetes,** approximately **90 percent of patients with Type 2 diabetes are overweight.**
- **26 million Americans have Type 2 diabete**s, and about **79 million have prediabetes.**

LIVE IT *UP!*

Three small changes that can improve health and happiness

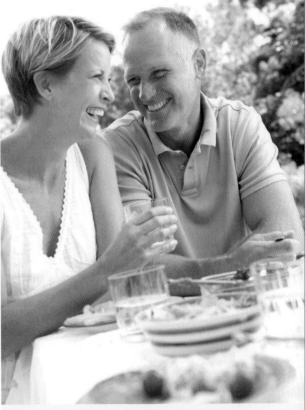

1 WALK IT OFF

Everybody gives in to temptation once in a while—the homemade biscuits, the mashed potatoes, the strawberry shortcake you just can't turn away. But that can make blood sugar rise too high later. While it's not a magic eraser, going for an after-meal stroll works wonders for the body. In one recent study, walking after eating controlled blood sugar better than hitting the pavement before the dinner bell rang.

TIP: *If foot problems make walking difficult, invest in an inexpensive "pedaler"—a set of bike pedals on a frame that you use while sitting in a chair.*

2 TALK IT OUT

Do a brief daily check-in with an online diabetes support group, or just post a comment or observation on a diabetes message board. It really can help you stay on track, blow off steam, and get much-needed encouragement from the real experts—people just like you who live with blood-sugar control challenges every day. Plus, you get the chance to reach out to someone else and share your own tips and experiences. The American Diabetes Association, the Joslin Diabetes Center, and the website Patients Like Me all host online groups.

TIP: *Load your smart phone with apps that help you track your blood sugar and remind you to take medications on time.*

3 LAUGH IT UP

Deciding between a silly comedy and an action flick for movie night? Go funny. Laughter helps your body process blood sugar more efficiently and relaxes your arteries. Indulging regularly even protects against heart attacks—good news for people with diabetes whose tickers are at higher risk for trouble.

ADDITIONAL RESOURCES:

American Diabetes Association
1-800-Diabetes (1-800-342-2383)
Diabetes.org

**American Association
of Diabetes Educators**
Diabeteseducator.org

Academy of Nutrition and Dietetics
Eatright.org

The Diabetic Newsletter
Diabeticnewsletter.com

SWAP & *DROP*

Losing just a few pounds can help with your diabetes and can reduce the risk for other health complications. With this in mind, **we rounded up some easy swaps** you can make. Pick a few and not only will the pounds start coming off, but your blood-sugar levels will stabilize as well.

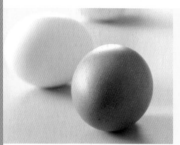

Cut just 1 yolk from meals that require 2 eggs (think omelets). A whole egg has 75 calories, but there are only 16 calories in the white and no fat.

▶ **Save 59 calories and 5 grams of fat.**

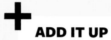 **ADD IT UP** Make this change twice a week and **cut out 6,136 calories a year,** which is approaching 2 pounds.

Replace a bagel (354 calories) or bran muffin (410 calories) with 2 slices of whole wheat toast (164 calories). Skip the butter (100 calories per tablespoon), and spread on ½ cup of fat-free cottage cheese (90 calories)—your calorie count is lowered, and you still get lots of creamy flavor without all that fat.

▶ **Save up to 246 calories.**

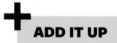 **ADD IT UP** Make this change once a week and you'll **cut almost 12,800 calories a year**—that's more than 3 pounds.

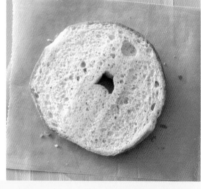

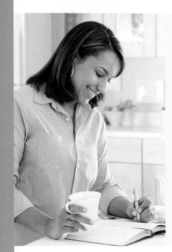

A "tall" cup (meaning the smallest size) of Grande Strawberries and Crème Frappuccino with whole milk and whipped cream is roughly 370 calories and 15 grams of fat. Instead, **choose a regular coffee.** Alone, coffee has no calories at all; add in two ounces of skim milk, and it still only contains 22 calories—and no fat! Need sweetening? Skip the sugar and go with a no-calorie sweetener.

▶ **Save 348 calories and 15 grams of fat.**

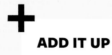 **ADD IT UP** Make this change once a week and you'll **cut 18,096 calories a year,** which adds up to more than 5 pounds. (Think of all the money you'll save, too!)

BUILD YOUR *PLATE*

Use these steps as a guide to **build an ideal meal.** Not only will this model help **keep portions in check**, it will help you make smart decisions for managing blood glucose levels.

1 **Draw a vertical line down the middle of your plate.**
On one of the halves, draw a horizontal line to cut one side in half. Now you should have 3 parts total.

2 **Fill the largest with non-starchy vegetables.**
Spinach, Brussels sprouts, lettuce, carrots, bell peppers, artichokes, celery, tomato, green beans, pea pods, cauliflower, asparagus, beets, broccoli and cucumber make great options.

3 **In one of the small sections, place starchy food.**
Whole grain breads, oats, barley, bulgur, polenta, pasta, rice, cooked beans, squash, sweet potatoes, corn, lima beans, peas, low-fat crackers, pretzels, fat-free popcorn are examples.

4 **In the other small section, put your protein.**
Try chicken, turkey, fish, shrimp, clams, crab, lean beef, pork loin, tofu, eggs, low-fat cheese.

5 **Add an 8-ounce glass of nonfat or low-fat milk.**
You can also add another small serving of carbohydrates like a small roll or 6 ounces of low-fat yogurt.

6 **Add a piece of fruit or ½ cup of fruit salad.**
Fresh fruit makes a great dessert after any meal!

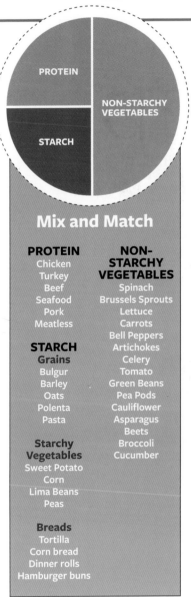

PROTEIN

NON-STARCHY VEGETABLES

STARCH

Mix and Match

PROTEIN
Chicken
Turkey
Beef
Seafood
Pork
Meatless

STARCH
Grains
Bulgur
Barley
Oats
Polenta
Pasta

Starchy Vegetables
Sweet Potato
Corn
Lima Beans
Peas

Breads
Tortilla
Corn bread
Dinner rolls
Hamburger buns

NON-STARCHY VEGETABLES
Spinach
Brussels Sprouts
Lettuce
Carrots
Bell Peppers
Artichokes
Celery
Tomato
Green Beans
Pea Pods
Cauliflower
Asparagus
Beets
Broccoli
Cucumber

For more tools and resources, visit **The American Diabetes Association** at *diabetes.org.*

appetizers, snacks & beverages

It's true! You can enjoy **savory bites**, refreshing beverages and other party-time favorites. Try these **no-fuss nibbles** the next time guests visit or whenever the munchies come calling.

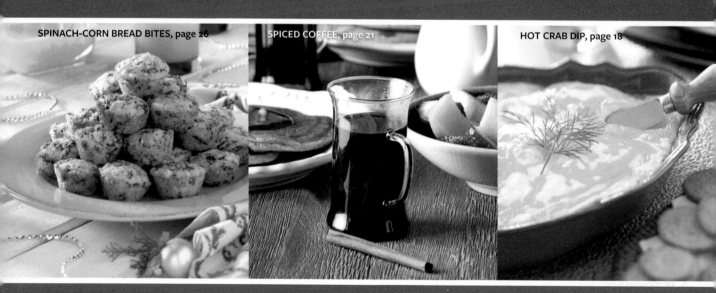

SPINACH-CORN BREAD BITES, page 26

SPICED COFFEE, page 21

HOT CRAB DIP, page 18

Turkey Wonton Cups

Convenient wonton wrappers make these hors d'oeuvres as fun to prepare as they are to eat. I sampled the cups at a get-together and couldn't believe how tasty they were. They disappeared quickly, and no one suspected they were light.

—**BARBARA RAFFERTY** PORTSMOUTH, RI

PREP: 30 MIN. • **BAKE:** 5 MIN./BATCH
MAKES: 4 DOZEN

- 48 **wonton wrappers**
- 1¼ **pounds lean ground turkey**
- 2 **cups (8 ounces) shredded reduced-fat cheddar cheese**
- 1 **cup fat-free ranch salad dressing**
- ½ **cup chopped green onions**
- ¼ **cup chopped ripe olives**

1. Press wonton wrappers into miniature muffin cups coated with cooking spray. (Keep wrappers covered with a damp paper towel until ready to bake.) Bake at 375° for 5 minutes or until lightly browned. Cool for about 2 minutes before removing from pans to wire racks.

2. In a large nonstick skillet coated with cooking spray, cook the turkey over medium heat until no longer pink; drain. In a large bowl, combine the turkey, cheese, ranch dressing, onions and olives. Spoon by rounded tablespoonfuls into wonton cups.

3. Place on an ungreased baking sheet. Bake at 375° for 5-6 minutes or until heated through. Serve warm.

PER SERVING *2 cups equals 154 cal., 7 g fat (3 g sat. fat), 34 mg chol., 366 mg sodium, 14 g carb., trace fiber, 11 g pro.* **Diabetic Exchanges:** *1 starch, 1 lean meat, ½ fat.*

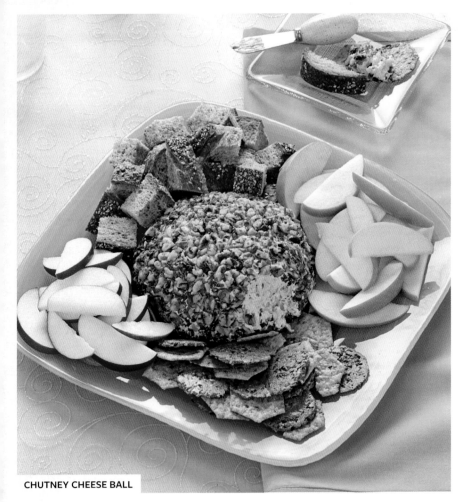

CHUTNEY CHEESE BALL

Chutney Cheese Ball

This classic party starter gets a tangy twist from mango chutney.

—**PATRICIA SCHNEIDER** ROLLINSFORD, NH

START TO FINISH: 15 MIN.
MAKES: 2½ CUPS

- 1 **package (8 ounces) reduced-fat cream cheese**
- 1 **package (8 ounces) fat-free cream cheese**
- 1 **cup (4 ounces) shredded reduced-fat Colby-Monterey Jack cheese**
- ½ **cup mango chutney**
- 2 **green onions, finely chopped**
- 1 **garlic clove, minced**
- ¼ **teaspoon salt**
- ¼ **teaspoon pepper**
- ½ **cup finely chopped walnuts**
- 2 **tablespoons minced fresh parsley Crackers, bread cubes and apples slices**

In a small bowl, combine the first eight ingredients. Shape into a ball and roll in walnuts. Press parsley into ball; cover and chill until serving. Serve with crackers, bread cubes and apple slices.

PER SERVING *2 tablespoons equals 99 cal., 5 g fat (3 g sat. fat), 12 mg chol., 254 mg sodium, 7 g carb., trace fiber, 5 g pro.* **Diabetic Exchanges:** *1 fat, ½ starch.*

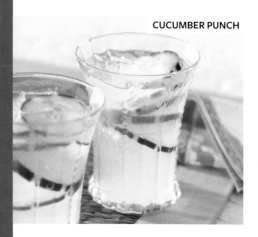

CUCUMBER PUNCH

Cucumber Punch

I first tried this wonderfully unique beverage at a ladies' luncheon and have since served it many times. Folks usually request copies of the recipe.
—RENEE OLSON KENDRICK, ID

PREP: 10 MIN. + CHILLING
MAKES: 25 SERVINGS (4¾ QUARTS)

- 2 medium cucumbers
- 3 cups water
- 1 can (12 ounces) frozen lemonade concentrate, thawed
- 2 liters diet ginger ale, chilled
- 4½ cups diet grapefruit or citrus soda, chilled

1. With a zester or fork, score cucumbers lengthwise; cut widthwise into thin slices. In a large pitcher, combine water and lemonade concentrate; add cucumbers. Cover and refrigerate overnight.
2. Just before serving, transfer cucumber mixture to a punch bowl; stir in ginger ale and grapefruit soda.
PER SERVING *¾ cup equals 29 cal., trace fat (trace sat. fat), 0 chol., 15 mg sodium, 7 g carb., trace fiber, trace pro.*
Diabetic Exchange: *½ starch.*

Sausage-Stuffed Red Potatoes

My husband and I have a large garden with red potatoes, so I am always trying to come up with creative ways to use them. My son calls these tasty noshes "potato poppers." As a bonus, they're low in calories.
—KAREN SULAK LAMPASAS, TX

PREP: 25 MIN. • **COOK:** 10 MIN.
MAKES: 16 APPETIZERS

- 8 small red potatoes
- 1 pound Italian turkey sausage links, casings removed
- ½ cup chopped sweet red pepper
- 4 green onions, chopped
- 9 teaspoons minced fresh parsley, divided
- ⅓ cup shredded reduced-fat cheddar cheese

1. Scrub and pierce potatoes; place on a microwave-safe plate. Microwave, uncovered, on high for 8-9 minutes or until tender, turning once.
2. Meanwhile, in a large skillet, cook sausage and pepper over medium heat until sausage is no longer pink. Add onions and 4½ teaspoons parsley; cook 1-2 minutes longer. Remove from the heat; stir in cheese. Cut each potato in half lengthwise. Scoop out 1 tablespoon pulp (save for another use).
3. Spoon about 2 tablespoons sausage mixture into each half. Place on a microwave-safe plate. Microwave on high for 1-2 minutes or until cheese is melted. Sprinkle with remaining parsley.
NOTE *This recipe was tested in a 1,100-watt microwave.*
PER SERVING *1 appetizer equals 63 cal., 3 g fat (1 g sat. fat), 19 mg chol., 186 mg sodium, 3 g carb., 1 g fiber, 5 g pro.*
Diabetic Exchange: *1 lean meat.*

SAUSAGE-STUFFED RED POTATOES

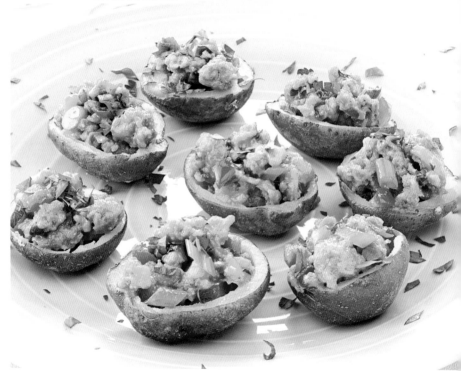

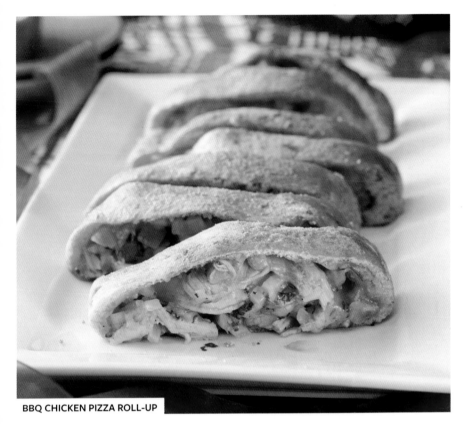

BBQ CHICKEN PIZZA ROLL-UP

Avocado Dip

I came up with this recipe in an attempt to create the perfect guacamole. Not only does it taste delicious seasoned with picante sauce, lime and garlic, but it's also a great low-fat alternative to higher-fat dips and spreads.

—**KAY DUNHAM** AMITY, MO

START TO FINISH: 15 MIN.
MAKES: 2½ CUPS

- 2 medium ripe avocados, peeled and pitted
- 1 package (8 ounces) fat-free cream cheese
- ⅓ cup plain yogurt
- ⅓ cup picante sauce
- 1 tablespoon lime juice
- ½ teaspoon salt
- ¼ teaspoon garlic powder
  Tortilla chips

In a small bowl, mash avocados and cream cheese until smooth. Stir in the yogurt, picante sauce, lime juice, salt and garlic powder. Serve with chips. Refrigerate leftovers.

PER SERVING *¼ cup equals 73 cal., 5 g fat (1 g sat. fat), 2 mg chol., 258 mg sodium, 5 g carb., 2 g fiber, 4 g pro.* **Diabetic Exchange:** *1 fat.*

AVOCADO DIP

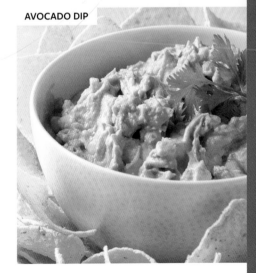

BBQ Chicken Pizza Roll-Up

Snack on this filling, flavorful appetizer without any guilt. Guests won't guess the slices are on the light side!

—**TRACEY BIRCH** QUEEN CREEK, AZ

PREP: 15 MIN. • **BAKE:** 15 MIN. + COOLING
MAKES: 2 DOZEN

- 1 tube (13.8 ounces) refrigerated pizza crust
- ¼ cup honey barbecue sauce
- 1½ cups (6 ounces) shredded part-skim mozzarella cheese
- 1½ cups shredded cooked chicken breast
- 1 small red onion, finely chopped
- ¼ cup minced fresh cilantro
- 1 teaspoon Italian seasoning, optional
- 1 egg white
- 1 tablespoon water
- ¼ teaspoon garlic powder

1. On a lightly floured surface, roll crust into a 12-in. x 9-in. rectangle; brush with barbecue sauce. Layer with cheese, chicken, onion, cilantro and Italian seasoning if desired.

2. Roll up jelly-roll style, starting with a long side; pinch seams to seal. Place seam side down on a baking sheet coated with cooking spray.

3. Beat egg white and water; brush over top. Sprinkle with garlic powder. Bake at 400° for 15-20 minutes or until lightly browned. Cool for 10 minutes before slicing.

PER SERVING *1 slice equals 81 cal., 2 g fat (1 g sat. fat), 11 mg chol., 177 mg sodium, 9 g carb., trace fiber, 6 g pro.* **Diabetic Exchanges:** *1 lean meat, ½ starch.*

Goat Cheese Crostini

My husband got this crostini recipe from a friend at work. I initially was skeptical about how it would taste, but now I love the bite-sized appetizers.

—REBECCA EBELING NEVADA CITY, CA

START TO FINISH: 10 MIN.
MAKES: 32 APPETIZERS

- 1 cup crumbled goat cheese
- 1 teaspoon minced fresh rosemary
- 1 French bread baguette (10½ ounces), cut into ½-inch slices and toasted
- 3 tablespoons honey
- ¼ cup slivered almonds, toasted

In a small bowl, combine cheese and rosemary; spoon over toast slices. Drizzle with honey; sprinkle with almonds.

BACON-ALMOND CROSTINI *Combine 2 cups shredded Monterey Jack cheese, ⅔ cup mayonnaise, ½ cup toasted sliced almonds, 6 slices crumbled cooked bacon, 1 chopped green onion and a dash of salt. Spread over toast. Bake for 5-7 minutes or until cheese is melted. Sprinkle with additional almonds if desired.*
PER SERVING *1 piece equals 76 cal., 4 g fat (2 g sat. fat), 6 mg chol., 92 mg sodium, 9 g carb., 1 g fiber, 3 g pro.*
Diabetic Exchanges: *½ starch, ½ fat.*

Fresh Summer Salsa

Spoon this salsa over baked tortilla chips, grilled salmon, chicken or pork chops for the ultimate healthy topping.

—LINDSAY ANDERSON INMAN, KS

START TO FINISH: 25 MIN.
MAKES: 4 CUPS

- 4 medium tomatoes, chopped
- 1 medium mango, peeled and chopped
- 1 medium ripe avocado, peeled and cubed
- ¾ cup fresh or frozen corn, thawed
- ½ cup minced fresh cilantro
- ½ cup canned black beans, rinsed and drained
- ¼ cup chopped red onion
- 1 jalapeno pepper, seeded and chopped
- 3 tablespoons lime juice
- 1 tablespoon olive oil
- 2 garlic cloves, minced
- ¼ teaspoon salt
  Baked tortilla chip scoops

In a large bowl, combine the first 12 ingredients. Chill until serving. Serve with tortilla chips.
NOTE *Wear disposable gloves when cutting hot peppers; the oils can burn skin. Avoid touching your face.*
PER SERVING *¼ cup equals 56 cal., 3 g fat (trace sat. fat), 0 chol., 56 mg sodium, 8 g carb., 2 g fiber, 1 g pro.*
Diabetic Exchange: *½ starch.*

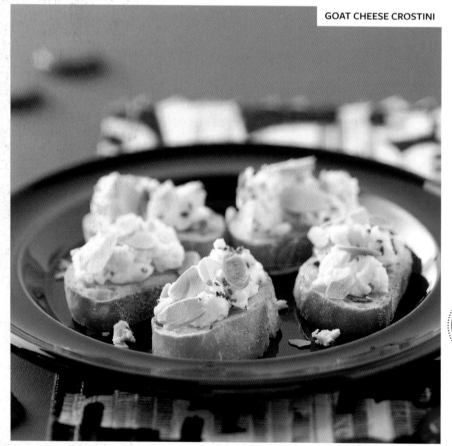

GOAT CHEESE CROSTINI

top tip — Pit Stop

To remove an avocado pit, cut the avocado in half, lengthwise, around the seed. Twist halves in opposite directions to separate. Spoon out the pit.

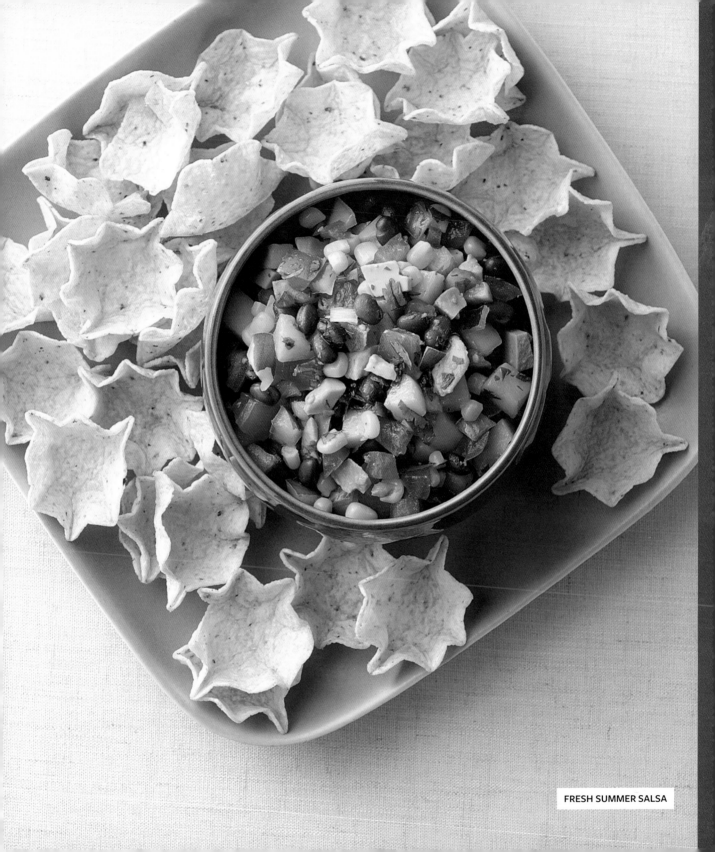

FRESH SUMMER SALSA

Easy Party Bruschetta

Fresh tomatoes are highlighted with this recipe. Adding jalapenos to the bruschetta adds a nice punch of heat.

—DEL MASON MARTENSVILLE, SK

START TO FINISH: 25 MIN.
MAKES: 2½ DOZEN

- 1½ cups chopped seeded tomatoes
- ⅔ cup finely chopped red onion
- 2 tablespoons minced seeded jalapeno pepper
- 2 garlic cloves, minced
- ½ teaspoon dried basil
- ¼ teaspoon salt
- ¼ teaspoon coarsely ground pepper
- 2 tablespoons olive oil
- 1 tablespoon cider vinegar
- 1 tablespoon red wine vinegar
- 3 dashes hot pepper sauce
- 1 loaf (8 ounces) French bread, cut into ¼-inch slices
- 2 tablespoons grated Parmesan cheese

1. In a small bowl, combine the first seven ingredients. In another bowl, whisk the oil, vinegars and pepper sauce; stir into tomato mixture.

2. Place bread slices on an ungreased baking sheet. Broil 3-4 in. from the heat for 1-2 minutes or until golden brown. With a slotted spoon, top each slice with tomato mixture. Sprinkle with cheese.

NOTE *Wear disposable gloves when cutting hot peppers; the oils can burn skin. Avoid touching your face.*

PER SERVING *1 piece equals 34 cal., 1 g fat (trace sat. fat), trace chol., 73 mg sodium, 5 g carb., trace fiber, 1 g pro. Diabetic Exchange: ½ starch.*

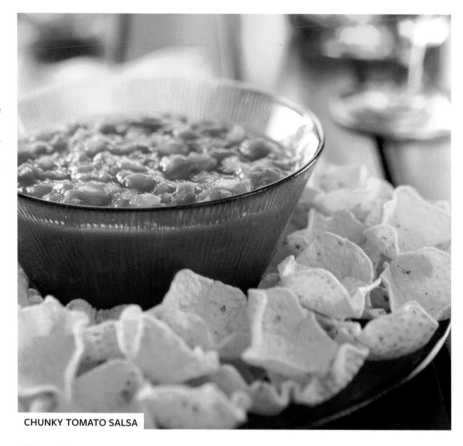

CHUNKY TOMATO SALSA

Chunky Tomato Salsa

Our college-age daughter, two of her friends and a nephew ate a quart of this salsa with chips in one sitting. They loved it so much that they each took another quart home with them!

—CAROL CARPENTER JANSEN, NE

PREP: 45 MIN. • **COOK:** 1¼ HOURS + CHILLING
MAKES: 4 CUPS

- 3½ cups peeled chopped tomatoes (about 4 large)
- 1 large green pepper, chopped
- 1 medium onion, chopped
- 1 serrano pepper, seeded and chopped
- 1 jalapeno pepper, seeded and chopped
- 1 tablespoon sugar
- 2¼ teaspoons salt
- 1 garlic clove, minced
- ¾ teaspoon ground cumin
- 1 can (6 ounces) tomato paste
- ¼ cup white vinegar
- 2 tablespoons lemon juice
  Baked tortilla chip scoops

In a large saucepan, combine the first nine ingredients. Stir in the tomato paste, vinegar and lemon juice. Bring to a boil. Reduce heat; simmer, uncovered, for 1 hour, stirring frequently. Cool to room temperature. Cover and refrigerate until chilled. Serve with chips.

NOTE *Wear disposable gloves when cutting hot peppers; the oils can burn skin. Avoid touching your face.*

PER SERVING *¼ cup equals 28 cal., trace fat (trace sat. fat), 0 chol., 344 mg sodium, 6 g carb., 1 g fiber, 1 g pro. Diabetic Exchange: 1 vegetable.*

Garlic Artichoke Dip

Not only is this chilled dip delicious and lower in fat, but it also offers make-ahead convenience for busy weekends.

—LISA VARNER EL PASO, TX

PREP: 25 MIN. + CHILLING
MAKES: 2½ CUPS

- 1 large onion, chopped
- ½ teaspoon dried oregano
- ½ teaspoon dried thyme
- 2 tablespoons olive oil
- 5 garlic cloves, minced
- 1 can (15 ounces) white kidney or cannellini beans, rinsed and drained
- 1 can (14 ounces) water-packed artichoke hearts, rinsed and drained
- 1 tablespoon lemon juice
- ½ teaspoon salt
- ⅛ teaspoon cayenne pepper
- Assorted fresh vegetables and/or baked pita chips

1. In a small nonstick skillet, saute the onion, oregano and thyme in oil until onions are tender. Add garlic; cook for 1 minute longer. Remove from the heat; cool slightly.

2. In a food processor, combine the beans, artichokes, lemon juice, salt, cayenne and onion mixture; cover and process until pureed.

3. Transfer to a small bowl. Cover and refrigerate at least 2 hours before serving. Serve with vegetables and/or pita chips.

PER SERVING *¼ cup equals 81 cal., 3 g fat (trace sat. fat), 0 chol., 271 mg sodium, 11 g carb., 2 g fiber, 3 g pro.* **Diabetic Exchanges:** *1 vegetable, ½ starch, ½ fat.*

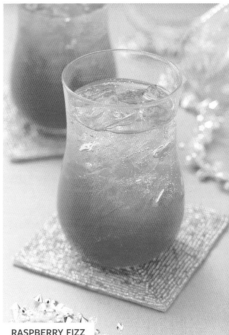

RASPBERRY FIZZ

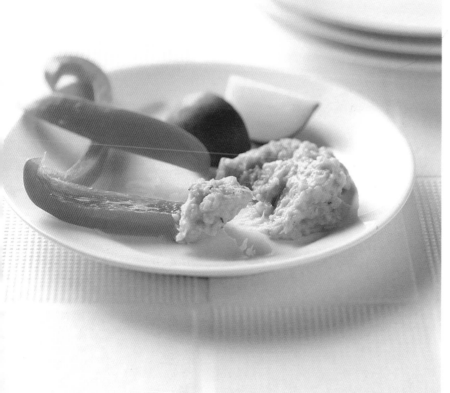

GARLIC ARTICHOKE DIP

Raspberry Fizz

Adults, especially, will enjoy this pretty pink beverage. It has a mild raspberry flavor and it isn't overly sweet.

—TASTE OF HOME TEST KITCHEN

START TO FINISH: 5 MIN.
MAKES: 1 SERVING

- 2 ounces ruby red grapefruit juice
- ½ to 1 ounce raspberry flavoring syrup
- ½ to ¾ cup ice cubes
- 6 ounces club soda, chilled

In a mixing glass or tumbler, combine grapefruit juice and syrup. Place ice in a highball glass; add juice mixture. Top with club soda.

NOTE *This recipe was tested with Torani brand flavoring syrup. Look for it in the coffee section.*

PER SERVING *70 cal., 0 fat (0 sat. fat), 0 chol., 37 mg sodium, 18 g carb., 0 fiber, trace pro.* **Diabetic Exchange:** *1 starch.*

Hot Crab Dip

I put a lighter spin on a traditional crab dip recipe by using reduced-fat and fat-free sour cream and cheeses. If you're hosting a party, make the recipe a day ahead and refrigerate it until guests arrive.

—**CAMMY BRITTINGHAM** CAMBRIDGE, MD

PREP: 15 MIN. • **BAKE:** 25 MIN.
MAKES: 2½ CUPS

- 1 **package (8 ounces) fat-free cream cheese**
- ½ **cup fat-free sour cream**
- 2 **tablespoons fat-free mayonnaise**
- 1 **teaspoon Worcestershire sauce**
- ½ **teaspoon seafood seasoning**
- ½ **teaspoon spicy brown mustard**
- ½ **teaspoon reduced-sodium soy sauce**
- ⅛ **teaspoon garlic salt**
- 2 **cans (6 ounces each) crabmeat, drained, flaked and cartilage removed or ½ pound imitation crabmeat, flaked**
- ⅓ **cup plus 2 tablespoons shredded reduced-fat cheddar cheese, divided**
- ⅓ **cup plus 2 tablespoons shredded part-skim mozzarella cheese, divided**
  Melba rounds or crackers

1. In a large bowl, beat cream cheese until smooth. Add the sour cream, mayonnaise, Worcestershire sauce, seafood seasoning, mustard, soy sauce and garlic salt. Stir in the crab, ⅓ cup cheddar cheese and ⅓ cup mozzarella cheese.

2. Transfer to a greased shallow 1-qt. baking dish. Sprinkle with remaining cheeses. Bake at 350° for 25-30 minutes or until bubbly around the edges. Serve warm with melba rounds or crackers.

PER SERVING *¼ cup equals 91 cal., 3 g fat (2 g sat. fat), 31 mg chol., 320 mg sodium, 5 g carb., trace fiber, 12 g pro.* ***Diabetic Exchange:*** *2 lean meat.*

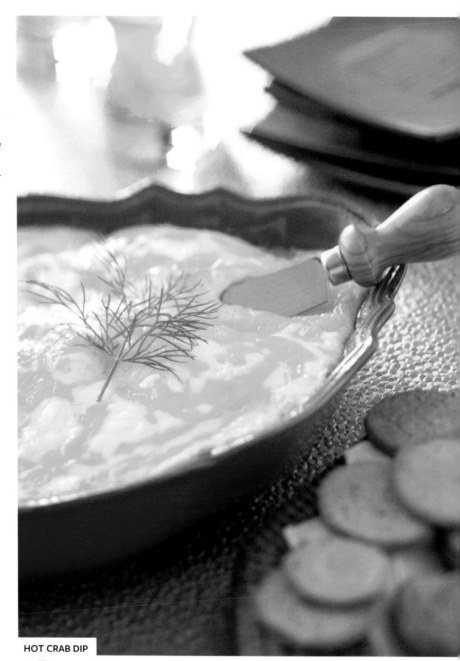

HOT CRAB DIP

top tip

The Greatest Form of Flattery

Imitation crabmeat is fish that is shaped and flavored to resemble crab. Often made from Alaskan pollock, it contains natural and artificial flavors.

Honey Barbecue Wings

Here is my family's all-time favorite way to eat chicken wings. My grown son and daughter always request them when they visit. We sometimes even eat the wings as a main dish.

—DIANE ACORD SAVAGE, MN

PREP: 40 MIN. + MARINATING • **BAKE:** 25 MIN.
MAKES: 3 DOZEN

- 2 garlic cloves, minced
- 1 tablespoon canola oil
- ½ cup honey
- ¼ cup ketchup
- 2 tablespoons orange juice
- 2 tablespoons lemon juice
- 2 tablespoons reduced-sodium soy sauce
- 2 teaspoons ground ginger
- 2 teaspoons cider vinegar
- 1 teaspoon Worcestershire sauce
- 1 teaspoon Dijon mustard
- ¼ teaspoon pepper
- ¼ teaspoon hot pepper sauce
- 18 whole chicken wings (about 3¾ pounds)

1. In a small saucepan, saute garlic in oil until for 1 minute. Stir in the honey, ketchup, juices, soy sauce, ginger, vinegar, Worcestershire sauce, mustard, pepper and hot pepper sauce. Bring to a boil. Reduce heat; simmer, uncovered, for 15 minutes. Remove from the heat; cool to room temperature.

2. Cut chicken wings into three sections; discard wing tip sections. Place wings in a large resealable heavy-duty plastic bag; add ¾ cup cooled honey mixture. Seal bag and turn to coat; refrigerate for 2 hours. Cover and refrigerate remaining honey mixture for basting.

3. Drain and discard marinade. Place chicken wings on a greased rack in a large baking pan. Bake at 400° for 10 minutes on each side, basting occasionally with honey mixture.

4. Broil 4-6 in. from the heat for 2-3 minutes or until browned and the juices run clear.

NOTE *Uncooked chicken wing sections (wingettes) may be substituted for whole chicken wings.*

PER SERVING *1 piece equals 69 cal., 4 g fat (1 g sat. fat), 15 mg chol., 73 mg sodium, 4 g carb., trace fiber, 5 g pro.* **Diabetic Exchange:** *1 medium-fat meat.*

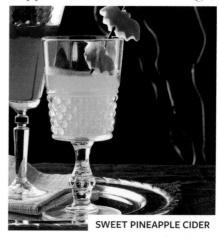

SWEET PINEAPPLE CIDER

Sweet Pineapple Cider

The best thing about this recipe? You can make it hours ahead, so you have more time to spend with your guests. And you can keep it warm on the stovetop or in a slow cooker throughout the party.

—MARY PRICE YOUNGSTOWN, OH

START TO FINISH: 30 MIN.
MAKES: 12 SERVINGS (¾ CUP EACH)

- 2 small apples, divided
- 10 whole cloves
- 1 bottle (48 ounces) unsweetened apple juice
- 4 cans (6 ounces each) unsweetened pineapple juice
- 2 cinnamon sticks (3 inches)

1. Core and cut one apple into 10 slices. Insert one clove into each slice. In a Dutch oven, combine juices. Add apple slices and cinnamon sticks. Bring to a boil. Reduce heat; simmer, uncovered, for 15-20 minutes or until flavors are blended.

2. Discard apple slices and cinnamon sticks. Core and cut remaining apple into 12 slices. Ladle cider into mugs; garnish with apple slices. Serve warm.

PER SERVING *¾ cup equals 93 cal., trace fat (trace sat. fat), 0 chol., 5 mg sodium, 23 g carb., trace fiber, trace pro.* **Diabetic Exchange:** *1½ fruit.*

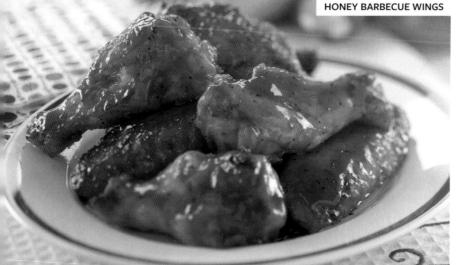

HONEY BARBECUE WINGS

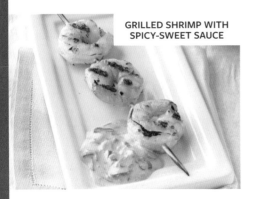

GRILLED SHRIMP WITH
SPICY-SWEET SAUCE

Grilled Shrimp with Spicy-Sweet Sauce

Just the right amount of spice adds a zip to this popular no-fuss appetizer.

—**SUSAN HARRISON** LAUREL, MD

START TO FINISH: 30 MIN.
MAKES: 15 SERVINGS (⅓ CUP SAUCE)

- 3 tablespoons reduced-fat mayonnaise
- 2 tablespoons sweet chili sauce
- 1 green onion, thinly sliced
- ¾ teaspoon Sriracha Asian hot chili sauce or ½ teaspoon hot pepper sauce
- 45 uncooked large shrimp (about 1½ pounds), peeled and deveined
- ¼ teaspoon salt
- ¼ teaspoon pepper

1. In a small bowl, mix mayonnaise, chili sauce, green onion and Sriracha. Sprinkle shrimp with salt and pepper. Thread three shrimp onto each of the 15 metal or soaked wooden skewers.
2. Moisten a paper towel with cooking oil; using long-handled tongs, rub on grill rack to coat lightly. Grill shrimp, covered, over medium heat or broil 4 in. from heat 3-4 minutes on each side or until the shrimp turn pink. Serve with the sauce.
PER SERVING *56 cal., 2 g fat (trace sat. fat), 61 mg chol., 156 mg sodium, 2 g carb., trace fiber, 8 g pro. **Diabetic Exchange:** ½ lean meat.*

Mini Sausage Bundles

These savory hors d'oeuvres cut fat as well as cleanup time by eliminating the need for a deep fryer.

—**TASTE OF HOME TEST KITCHEN**

START TO FINISH: 30 MIN.
MAKES: 1 DOZEN

- ½ pound turkey Italian sausage links, casings removed
- 1 small onion, finely chopped
- ¼ cup finely chopped sweet red pepper
- 1 garlic clove, minced
- ½ cup shredded cheddar cheese
- 8 sheets phyllo dough (14 inches x 9 inches)
- 12 whole chives, optional

1. Crumble the sausage into a large nonstick skillet; add onion, red pepper and garlic. Cook over medium heat until meat is no longer pink; drain. Stir in cheese; cool slightly.
2. Place one sheet of phyllo dough on a work surface; coat with cooking spray. Cover with a second sheet of phyllo; coat with cooking spray. (Until ready to use, keep remaining phyllo covered with plastic wrap and a damp towel to prevent drying out.) Cut widthwise into three 4-in. strips, discarding trimmings. Top each with 2 rounded tablespoons of sausage mixture; fold bottom and side edges over filling and roll up. Repeat with remaining phyllo and filling.
3. Place seam side down on an ungreased baking sheet. Bake at 425° for 5-6 minutes or until lightly browned. Tie a chive around each bundle if desired. Serve warm.
PER SERVING *1 bundle equals 67 cal., 3 g fat (2 g sat. fat), 15 mg chol., 168 mg sodium, 5 g carb., trace fiber, 5 g pro. **Diabetic Exchanges:** 1 lean meat, ½ fat.*

MINI SAUSAGE BUNDLES

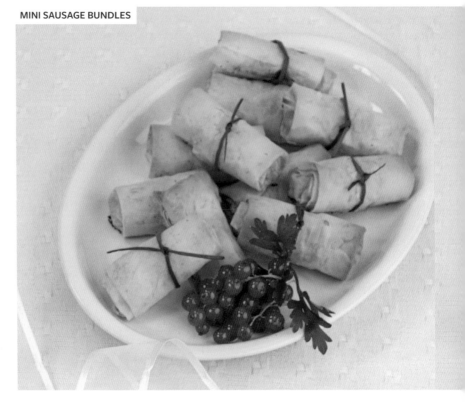

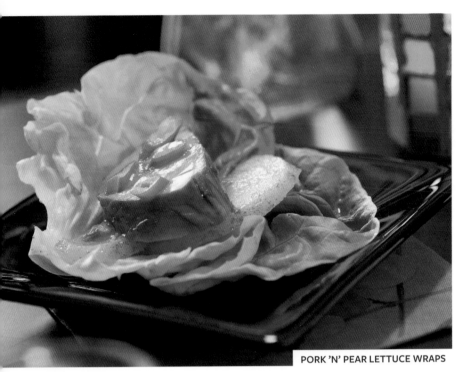

PORK 'N' PEAR LETTUCE WRAPS

Spiced Coffee

Use instant granules to quickly prepare this fall-flavored coffee. It's a great pick-me-up when you're tight on time.

—**JILL GARN** CHARLOTTE, MI

START TO FINISH: 20 MIN.
MAKES: 2 SERVINGS

- 2 **cups water**
- 5 **teaspoons instant coffee granules**
- ½ **cinnamon stick (3 inches)**
- 4 **whole cloves**
- 5 **teaspoons sugar**
  Whipped topping, optional

In a small saucepan, combine the water, coffee granules, cinnamon stick and cloves. Bring to a boil. Remove from the heat; cover and let stand for 5-8 minutes. Strain and discard spices. Stir in sugar until dissolved. Ladle into mugs. Serve with whipped topping if desired.

PER SERVING *46 cal., trace fat (trace sat. fat), 0 chol., 1 mg sodium, 11 g carb., 0 fiber, trace pro.* **Diabetic Exchange:** *½ starch.*

SPICED COFFEE

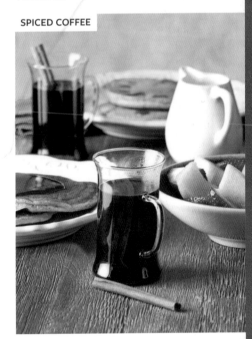

Pork 'n' Pear Lettuce Wraps

Depending on the weather, you can grill or broil the tenderloin for these wraps. No matter how you make it, this Asian-inspired appetizer is sure to please.

—**CHERYL PERRY** HERTFORD, NC

PREP: 20 MIN. • **BROIL:** 20 MIN.
MAKES: 10 WRAPS (1¼ CUPS SAUCE)

- 2 **cups pear nectar**
- 3 **tablespoons minced fresh gingerroot**
- 2 **tablespoons butter**
- ½ **teaspoon coriander seeds, crushed**
- ½ **teaspoon ground cumin**
- 1 **tablespoon brown sugar**
- ½ **teaspoon cayenne pepper**
- 2 **Asian pears, peeled, halved and cored**
- 4 **garlic cloves, minced**
- 1 **teaspoon salt**
- 1 **pork tenderloin (¾ pound)**
- 10 **green onions, cut into 1-inch pieces**
- 10 **Bibb or Boston lettuce leaves**

1. In a small saucepan, combine the first five ingredients. Bring to a boil; reduce heat. Simmer until sauce is reduced to 1¼ cups; keep warm.
2. Combine brown sugar and cayenne; sprinkle over pears. Place on a greased broiler pan. Rub garlic and salt over the tenderloin. Place on broiler pan with pears.
3. Broil 4-6 in. from the heat 9 minutes. Turn; broil 7-9 minutes longer or until a meat thermometer reads 160° and pears are lightly browned. Let stand for 5 minutes.
4. Cut each pear half into five slices. Cut pork into 10 slices. Place two slices of pear, a slice of pork and onions on each lettuce leaf. Top with sauce; wrap lettuce around filling. Serve immediately.
PER SERVING *141 cal., 4 g fat (2 g sat. fat), 25 mg chol., 272 mg sodium, 21 g carb., 3 g fiber, 8 g pro.* **Diabetic Exchanges:** *1 lean meat, ½ starch, ½ fruit, ½ fat.*

Strawberry Tofu Smoothies

Here is one sweet way to get more soy in your diet. It's light, tasty and portable. I take it with me every morning in an insulated mug for an energizing breakfast-on-the-go.

—DEBBIE STEPP OCALA, FL

START TO FINISH: 10 MIN.
MAKES: 2 SERVINGS

- 1 cup unsweetened apple juice
- 1½ cups frozen unsweetened strawberries
- 4 ounces silken firm tofu, cubed
- 1 teaspoon sugar

In a blender, combine all ingredients; cover and process for 45-60 seconds or until smooth. Pour into chilled glasses; serve immediately.

PER SERVING *136 cal., 2 g fat (trace sat. fat), 0 chol., 25 mg sodium, 26 g carb., 3 g fiber, 5 g pro.* **Diabetic Exchanges:** *1½ fruit, 1 lean meat.*

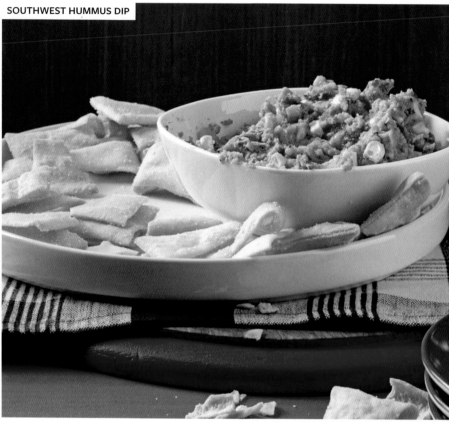

SOUTHWEST HUMMUS DIP

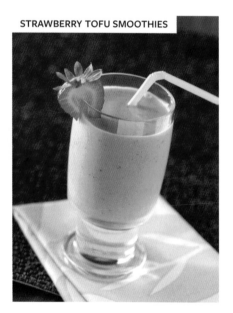

STRAWBERRY TOFU SMOOTHIES

Southwest Hummus Dip

Not your ordinary hummus, this dip is a combination of two things I love—chick peas and Southwestern flavors. You can substitute ¾ cup frozen corn, thawed, for the grilled corn.

—CHERAY BUCKALEW CUMBERLAND, MD

PREP: 15 MIN. • **GRILL:** 20 MIN.
MAKES: 2 CUPS

- 1 medium ear sweet corn, husk removed
- 1 can (15 ounces) garbanzo beans or chickpeas, rinsed and drained
- 2 tablespoons minced fresh cilantro
- 1 teaspoon ground cumin
- ½ teaspoon chili powder
- ¼ teaspoon salt
- ¼ teaspoon pepper
- ½ cup chopped roasted sweet red peppers
- ¼ cup fire-roasted diced tomatoes
  Baked pita chips or assorted fresh vegetables

1. Grill corn, covered, over medium heat for 10-12 minutes or until tender, turning occasionally. Meanwhile, in a food processor, combine the beans, cilantro, cumin, chili powder, salt and pepper. Cover and process 30 seconds or until blended. Transfer to a small bowl. Cover and refrigerate for at least 15 minutes.

2. Cut corn from cob. Add the corn, red peppers and tomatoes to bean mixture; mix well. Serve with pita chips or vegetables.

PER SERVING *¼ cup equals 68 cal., 1 g fat (trace sat. fat), 0 chol., 223 mg sodium, 12 g carb., 3 g fiber, 3 g pro.* **Diabetic Exchange:** *1 starch.*

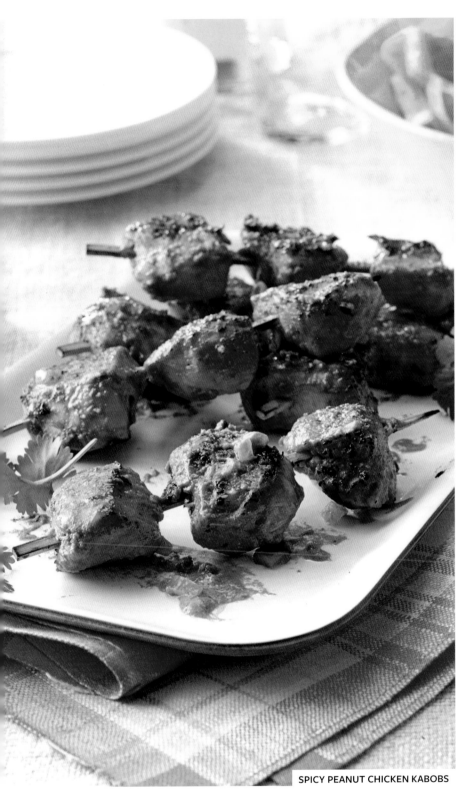

Spicy Peanut Chicken Kabobs

Serve up a little sweet, a little sour, and a whole lot of flavor when you present these tasty kabobs!

—NANCY ZIMMERMAN

CAPE MAY COURT HOUSE, NJ

PREP: 20 MIN. + MARINATING • **GRILL:** 10 MIN.
MAKES: 8 APPETIZERS

- ¼ cup reduced-fat creamy peanut butter
- 3 tablespoons reduced-sodium soy sauce
- 4½ teaspoons lemon juice
- 1 tablespoon brown sugar
- 1½ teaspoons ground coriander
- 1 teaspoon ground cumin
- ¾ teaspoon salt
- ¼ teaspoon pepper
- ¼ to ½ teaspoon cayenne pepper
- 1 garlic clove, minced
- 1 large onion, finely chopped
- 1 pound boneless skinless chicken breasts, cut into 1-inch cubes

1. In a small bowl, combine the first 10 ingredients. Set aside 3 tablespoons marinade for sauce. Pour remaining marinade into a large resealable plastic bag; add onion and chicken. Seal bag and turn to coat; refrigerate overnight. Cover and refrigerate reserved sauce.

2. Drain and discard marinade. Thread the chicken onto eight metal or soaked wooden skewers. Using long-handled tongs, moisten a paper towel with cooking oil and lightly coat the grill rack.

3. Grill chicken, covered, over medium heat or broil 4 in. from the heat for 4-5 minutes on each side or until no longer pink. Brush with the reserved sauce before serving.

PER SERVING *94 cal., 3 g fat (1 g sat. fat), 31 mg chol., 275 mg sodium, 4 g carb., 1 g fiber, 13 g pro.* **Diabetic Exchanges:** *2 lean meat, ½ fat.*

SPICY PEANUT CHICKEN KABOBS

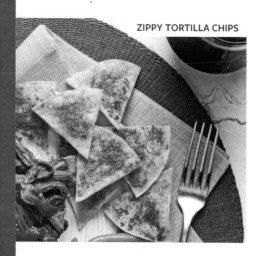

ZIPPY TORTILLA CHIPS

Zippy Tortilla Chips

If store-bought tortilla chips are too salty for you, give these homemade Southwestern chips a try. You'll be pleasantly surprised at how quick and easy they are to make, and you're sure to enjoy their spicy kick!

—KIM SUMRALL APTOS, CA

START TO FINISH: 20 MIN.
MAKES: 2 SERVINGS

- ½ teaspoon brown sugar
- ¼ teaspoon garlic powder
- ¼ teaspoon onion powder
- ¼ teaspoon ground cumin
- ¼ teaspoon paprika
- ⅛ teaspoon cayenne pepper
- 4 corn tortillas (6 inches)
  Cooking spray

1. In a small bowl, combine the first six ingredients. Stack the tortillas; cut into six wedges. Arrange in a single layer on a baking sheet coated with cooking spray.
2. Spritz the wedges with cooking spray; sprinkle with seasoning mixture. Bake at 375° for 9-10 minutes or until lightly browned. Cool for 5 minutes.
PER SERVING *12 chips equals 138 cal., 3 g fat (trace sat. fat), 0 chol., 85 mg sodium, 26 g carb., 3 g fiber, 3 g pro. Diabetic Exchanges: 1½ starch, ½ fat.*

Makeover Garlic Spinach Balls

These pop-in-your mouth bites not only taste wonderful, they're also a great way to get picky eaters to eat their spinach!

—AMY HORNBUCKLE PRATTVILLE, AL

PREP: 25 MIN. • **BAKE:** 15 MIN.
MAKES: 2 DOZEN

- 2 cups crushed seasoned stuffing
- 1 cup finely chopped onion
- ¾ cup egg substitute
- 1 egg, lightly beaten
- ¼ cup grated Parmesan cheese
- ¼ cup butter, melted
- 3 tablespoons reduced-sodium chicken broth or vegetable broth
- 1 garlic clove, minced
- 1½ teaspoons dried thyme
- ¼ teaspoon pepper
- ⅛ teaspoon salt
- 2 packages (10 ounces each) frozen chopped spinach, thawed and squeezed dry

1. In a large bowl, combine the first 11 ingredients. Stir in spinach until blended. Roll into 1-in. balls.
2. Place in a 15-in. x 10-in. x 1-in. baking pan coated with cooking spray. Bake at 350° for 15-20 minutes or until golden brown.
PER SERVING *1 appetizer equals 55 cal., 3 g fat (1 g sat. fat), 15 mg chol., 146 mg sodium, 6 g carb., 1 g fiber, 3 g pro. Diabetic Exchanges: ½ starch, ½ fat.*

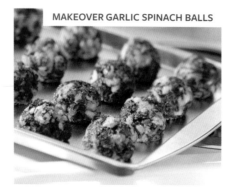

MAKEOVER GARLIC SPINACH BALLS

Tomato-Squash Appetizer Pizza

I grow herbs in my windowsill garden and needed new ideas to use them up. So I created this flatbread pizza, which is also ideal for a colorful main course.

—ANDREA TOVAR NEW YORK, NY

START TO FINISH: 30 MIN.
MAKES: 24 PIECES

- 1 loaf (1 pound) frozen bread dough, thawed
- ¼ teaspoon salt
- 1 tablespoon olive oil
- 1½ cups (6 ounces each) shredded part-skim mozzarella cheese
- 1 large yellow summer squash, sliced
- 1 large tomato, sliced
- 4 teaspoons shredded Parmesan cheese
- ¼ teaspoon pepper
- 1 teaspoon each minced fresh basil, oregano and chives

1. Roll dough into a 14-in. x 8-in. rectangle. Transfer to a greased baking sheet. Prick dough thoroughly with a fork. Sprinkle with salt. Bake at 425° for 8-10 minutes or until lightly browned.
2. Brush crust with oil. Top with mozzarella cheese, squash, tomato, Parmesan cheese, pepper and herbs. Bake 5-10 minutes longer or until the cheese is melted.
PER SERVING *81 cal., 3 g fat (1 g sat. fat), 4 mg chol., 169 mg sodium, 10 g carb., 1 g fiber, 4 g pro. Diabetic Exchanges: 1 fat, ½ starch.*

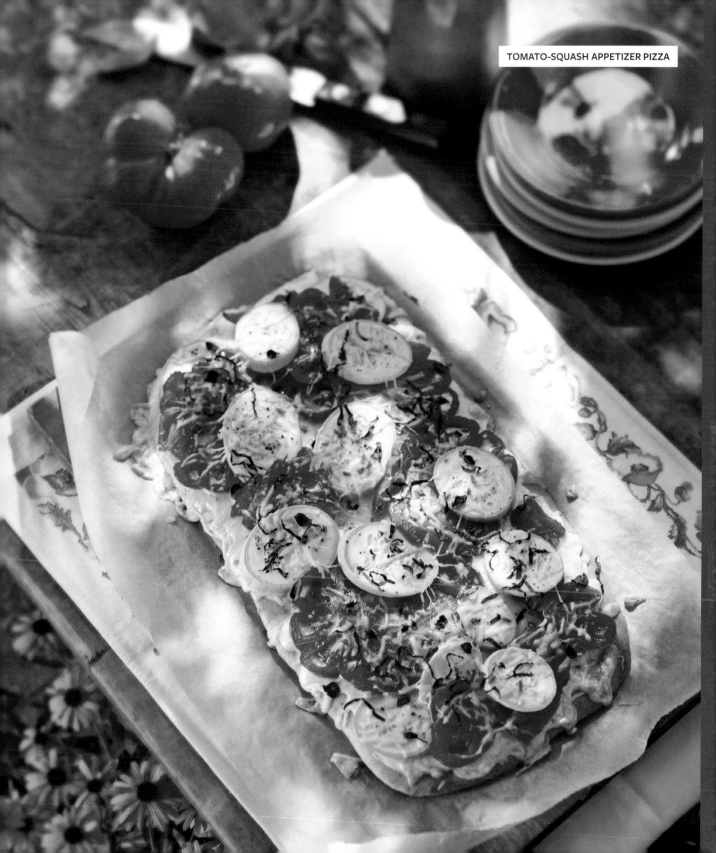

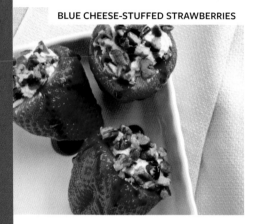

BLUE CHEESE-STUFFED STRAWBERRIES

Blue Cheese-Stuffed Strawberries

I was eating a strawberry and blue cheese salad when I realized I could also stuff the strawberries and serve them as an appetizer. It worked out great, and the flavors blend so nicely.

—**DIANE NEMITZ** LUDINGTON, MI

START TO FINISH: 25 MIN.
MAKES: 16 APPETIZERS

- ½ cup balsamic vinegar
- 3 ounces fat-free cream cheese
- 2 ounces crumbled blue cheese
- 16 fresh strawberries
- 3 tablespoons finely chopped pecans, toasted

1. Place vinegar in a small saucepan. Bring to a boil; cook until liquid is reduced by half. Cool to room temperature.

2. Meanwhile, in a small bowl, beat cream cheese until smooth. Beat in blue cheese. Remove stems and scoop out centers from strawberries; fill each with about 2 teaspoons cheese mixture. Sprinkle pecans over filling, pressing lightly. Chill until serving. Drizzle with balsamic vinegar.

PER SERVING *1 piece equals 36 cal., 2 g fat (1 g sat. fat), 3 mg chol., 80 mg sodium, 3 g carb., trace fiber, 2 g pro. Diabetic Exchange: ½ fat.*

Spinach-Corn Bread Bites

Although this recipe makes a big batch, I never have any leftovers. The appetizers are just that popular!

—**LAURA MAHAFFEY** ANNAPOLIS, MD

PREP: 25 MIN. • **BAKE:** 15 MIN./BATCH
MAKES: 4 DOZEN

- 1 package (8½ ounces) corn bread/ muffin mix
- ½ cup grated Parmesan cheese
- ⅛ teaspoon garlic powder
- 2 eggs
- ½ cup blue cheese salad dressing
- ¼ cup butter, melted
- 1 package (10 ounces) frozen chopped spinach, thawed and squeezed dry
- ½ cup shredded cheddar cheese
- ½ cup finely chopped onion

1. In a large bowl, combine the muffin mix, Parmesan cheese and garlic powder. In another bowl, whisk the eggs, salad dressing and butter; stir into dry ingredients just until moistened. Fold in the spinach, cheddar cheese and chopped onion.

2. Fill greased miniature muffin cups two-thirds full. Bake at 350° for 12-14 minutes or until a toothpick inserted near the center comes out clean. Cool for 5 minutes before removing from pans to wire racks. Serve warm. Refrigerate leftovers.

PER SERVING *1 bite equals 54 cal., 4 g fat (1 g sat. fat), 15 mg chol., 103 mg sodium, 4 g carb., trace fiber, 2 g pro. Diabetic Exchange: 1 fat.*

SPINACH-CORN BREAD BITES

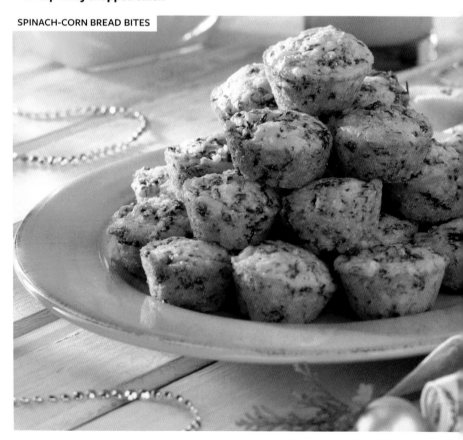

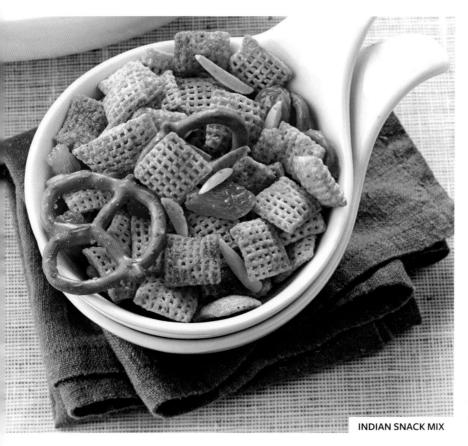

INDIAN SNACK MIX

Pineapple Iced Tea

This thirst-quenching tea is simple to mix up but most important, it has a sparkling citrus flavor we all enjoy.

—**K. KITTELL** LENEXA, KS

PREP: 10 MIN. + CHILLING
MAKES: 5 SERVINGS

- 4 **cups water**
- 7 **individual tea bags**
- 1 **cup unsweetened pineapple juice**
- ⅓ **cup lemon juice**
- 2 **tablespoons sugar**

1. In a large saucepan, bring water to a boil. Remove from the heat.
2. Add tea bags; cover and steep for 3-5 minutes. Discard tea bags. Stir in the pineapple juice, lemon juice and sugar until sugar is dissolved. Refrigerate overnight for the flavors to blend. Serve over ice.

PER SERVING *1 cup 51 cal., 0 fat (0 sat. fat), 0 chol., 1 mg sodium, 13 g carb., 0 fiber, 0 pro. **Diabetic Exchange:** 1 fruit.*

Indian Snack Mix

I love curry, so I added it to this crunchy snack mix. Since the recipe uses the microwave, prep work is a cinch. If you want to cut back on the spice, use only 1 teaspoon of curry and 1 teaspoon of the chipotle powder.

—**NOELLE MYERS** GRAND FORKS, ND

PREP: 15 MIN. • **BAKE:** 45 MIN. + COOLING
MAKES: ABOUT 3 QUARTS

- 4 **cups Corn Chex**
- 4 **cups Rice Chex**
- 3 **cups miniature pretzels**
- 1 **cup slivered almonds**
- ⅓ **cup butter, melted**
- 3 **tablespoons Louisiana-style hot sauce**
- 4½ **teaspoons Worcestershire sauce**
- 2½ **teaspoons curry powder**
- 1 **teaspoon onion powder**
- 1 **teaspoon seasoned salt**
- ¼ **teaspoon ground chipotle pepper**
- 1 **cup golden raisins**

1. In a large bowl, combine the cereals, pretzels and almonds. In a small bowl, combine the butter, hot sauce, Worcestershire sauce and seasonings. Drizzle over cereal mixture; toss to coat.
2. Transfer to two 15x10x1-in. baking pans coated with cooking spray. Bake at 250° for 45 minutes or until golden brown, stirring every 15 minutes. Stir in raisins. Cool completely on wire racks. Store in airtight containers.

PER SERVING *¾ cup equals 172 cal., 7 g fat (3 g sat. fat), 9 mg chol., 360 mg sodium, 26 g carb., 2 g fiber, 3 g pro. **Diabetic Exchanges:** 1½ starch, 1 fat.*

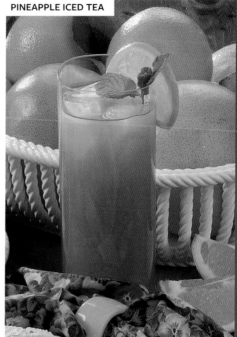

PINEAPPLE ICED TEA

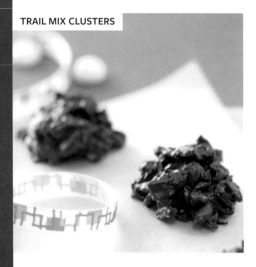

TRAIL MIX CLUSTERS

Trail Mix Clusters

They may look naughty, but these chocolaty clusters couldn't be nicer! The dried fruit and nuts are good for your heart and full of fiber, so you can always enjoy this treat guilt-free.

—**ALINA NIEMI** HONOLULU, HI

PREP: 25 MIN. + CHILLING
MAKES: 4 DOZEN

- 2 **cups (12 ounces) semisweet chocolate chips**
- ½ **cup unsalted sunflower kernels**
- ½ **cup salted pumpkin seeds or pepitas**
- ½ **cup coarsely chopped cashews**
- ½ **cup coarsely chopped pecans**
- ¼ **cup flaked coconut**
- ¼ **cup finely chopped dried apricots**
- ¼ **cup dried cranberries**
- ¼ **cup dried cherries or blueberries**

1. In a large microwave-safe bowl, melt chocolate chips; stir until smooth. Stir in the remaining ingredients.
2. Drop by tablespoonfuls onto waxed paper-lined baking sheets. Refrigerate until firm. Store in the refrigerator.
PER SERVING *1 piece equals 79 cal., 6 g fat (2 g sat. fat), 0 chol., 26 mg sodium, 8 g carb., 1 g fiber, 2 g pro.* **Diabetic Exchanges:** *1 fat, ½ starch.*

Iced Lemon Tea

Stir sugar-free lemonade drink mix into traditional iced tea. It not only tastes cool and refreshing, but it also cuts out some extra sugar.

—**DAWN LOWENSTEIN** HATBORO, PA

PREP: 15 MIN. • **COOK:** 10 MIN. + COOLING
MAKES: 12 SERVINGS (1 CUP EACH)

- 3½ **teaspoons sugar-free lemonade drink mix**
- 4 **cups cold water**
- 8 **cups water**
- 8 **individual decaffeinated tea bags**
- 1 **mint-flavored black tea bag**
  Ice cubes
  Fresh mint leaves and lemon slices, optional

1. In a 3-qt. pitcher, combine lemonade mix and cold water. Refrigerate until chilled.
2. Meanwhile, in a large saucepan, bring water to a boil. Remove from the heat; add tea bags. Cover and steep for 3-5 minutes. Discard tea bags. Cool; stir into lemonade mixture. Serve over ice with mint and lemon if desired.
PER SERVING *1 cup equals 3 cal., trace fat (0 sat. fat), 0 chol., 1 mg sodium, trace carb., trace fiber, trace pro.* **Diabetic Exchange:** *Free food.*

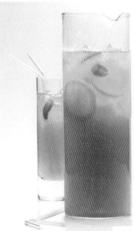

ICED LEMON TEA

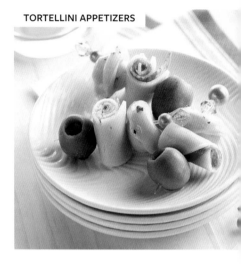

TORTELLINI APPETIZERS

Tortellini Appetizers

Lend a little Italian flavor to your next get-together with these kabobs. Cheese tortellini is marinated in salad dressing, then skewered onto toothpicks along with stuffed olives, salami and cheese.

—**PATRICIA SCHMIDT** STERLING HEIGHTS, MI

PREP: 25 MIN. + MARINATING
MAKES: 1½ DOZEN

- 18 **refrigerated cheese tortellini**
- ¼ **cup fat-free Italian salad dressing**
- 6 **thin slices (4 ounces) reduced-fat provolone cheese**
- 6 **thin slices (2 ounces) Genoa salami**
- 18 **large pimiento-stuffed olives**

1. Cook tortellini according to package directions; drain and rinse in cold water. In a resealable plastic bag, combine tortellini and salad dressing. Seal bag and refrigerate for 4 hours.
2. Place a slice of cheese on each slice of salami; roll up tightly. Cut into thirds. Drain tortellini and discard dressing. For each appetizer, thread a tortellini, salami roll-up and olive on a toothpick.
PER SERVING *2 appetizers equals 92 cal., 6 g fat (3 g sat. fat), 16 mg chol., 453 mg sodium, 5 g carb., trace fiber, 7 g pro.* **Diabetic Exchanges:** *1 lean meat, 1 fat.*

Hearty Poppers

For a potluck at our church, my husband and I came up with a healthy take on these popular bites.

—JANICE VERNON LAS CRUCES, NM

PREP: 35 MIN. • **BAKE:** 20 MIN.
MAKES: 2 DOZEN

- 12 jalapeno peppers
- ½ pound lean ground turkey
- ¼ cup finely chopped onion
- 4 ounces fat-free cream cheese
- 1⅓ cups shredded part-skim mozzarella cheese, divided
- 1 tablespoon minced fresh cilantro
- 1 teaspoon chili powder
- ½ teaspoon garlic powder
- ½ teaspoon ground cumin
- ⅛ teaspoon salt
- ⅛ teaspoon pepper

1. Cut jalapenos in half lengthwise, leaving stems intact; discard seeds. Set aside. In a small nonstick skillet over medium heat, cook turkey and onion until meat is no longer pink; drain.

2. In a small bowl, combine the cream cheese, ⅓ cup cheese, cilantro, chili powder, garlic powder, cumin, salt and pepper. Stir in turkey mixture. Spoon generously into pepper halves.

3. Place in a 15x10x1-in. baking pan coated with cooking spray; sprinkle with remaining cheese. Bake, uncovered, at 350° for 20 minutes for a spicy flavor, 30 minutes for medium and 40 minutes for mild.

NOTE *Wear disposable gloves when cutting hot peppers; the oils can burn skin. Avoid touching your face.*

PER SERVING *1 popper equals 38 cal., 2 g fat (1 g sat. fat), 11 mg chol., 78 mg sodium, 1 g carb., trace fiber, 4 g pro.* **Diabetic Exchange:** *1 lean meat.*

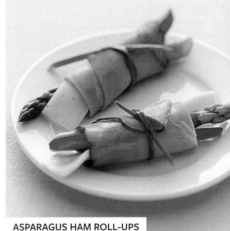

ASPARAGUS HAM ROLL-UPS

Asparagus Ham Roll-Ups

Havarti cheese, asparagus and red peppers make these tasty roll-ups ideal for a celebration. Fresh chive ties give them an extra special touch.

—RHONDA STRUTHERS OTTAWA, ON

START TO FINISH: 25 MIN.
MAKES: 16 SERVINGS

- 16 fresh asparagus spears, trimmed
- 1 medium sweet red pepper, cut into 16 strips
- 8 ounces Havarti cheese, cut into 16 strips
- 8 thin slices deli ham or prosciutto, cut in half lengthwise
- 16 whole chives

1. In a large skillet, bring 1 in. of water to a boil. Add asparagus; cover and cook for 3 minutes. Drain and immediately place asparagus in ice water. Drain and pat dry.

2. Place an asparagus spear, red pepper strip and cheese strip on each piece of ham. Roll up tightly; tie with a chive. Refrigerate until serving.

PER SERVING *1 appetizer equals 69 cal., 5 g fat (3 g sat. fat), 18 mg chol., 180 mg sodium, 2 g carb., trace fiber, 6 g pro.* **Diabetic Exchanges:** *1 fat, ½ vegetable.*

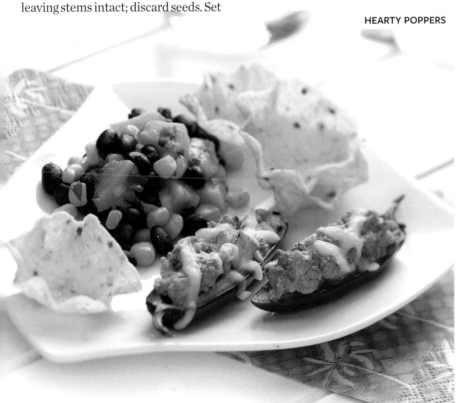

HEARTY POPPERS

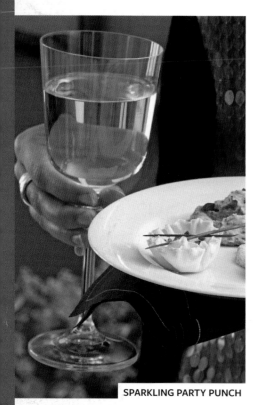

Spinach & Black Bean Egg Rolls

Black beans and spinach provide lots of healthy nutrients in these delicious baked egg rolls. Rolling them up is a cinch, too.

—**MELANIE SCOTT** AMARILLO, TX

START TO FINISH: 30 MIN.
MAKES: 20 EGG ROLLS

- 2 cups frozen corn, thawed
- 1 can (15 ounces) black beans, rinsed and drained
- 1 package (10 ounces) frozen chopped spinach, thawed and squeezed dry
- 1 cup (4 ounces) shredded reduced-fat Mexican cheese blend
- 1 can (4 ounces) chopped green chilies, drained
- 4 green onions, chopped
- 1 teaspoon ground cumin
- ½ teaspoon chili powder
- ½ teaspoon pepper
- 20 egg roll wrappers
  Cooking spray
  Salsa and reduced-fat ranch salad dressing, optional

1. In a large bowl, combine the first nine ingredients. Place ¼ cup mixture in the center of one egg roll wrapper. (Keep remaining wrappers covered with a damp paper towel until ready to use.) Fold bottom corner over filling. Fold sides toward center over filling. Moisten remaining corner with water; roll up tightly to seal. Repeat.

2. Place seam side down on baking sheets coated with cooking spray. Spray tops of egg rolls with cooking spray. Bake at 425° for 10-15 minutes or until lightly browned. Serve warm with the salsa and dressing if desired. Refrigerate leftovers.

FREEZE OPTION *Freeze cooled egg rolls in a freezer container, separating layers with waxed paper. To use, reheat rolls on a baking sheet in a preheated 350° oven until crisp and heated through.*

PER SERVING *1 egg roll equals 147 cal., 2 g fat (1 g sat. fat), 7 mg chol., 298 mg sodium, 26 g carb., 2 g fiber, 7 g pro. Diabetic Exchanges: 1½ starch, 1 lean meat.*

Sparkling Party Punch

This has been my go-to punch recipe for years. It's sparkly, fruity, frothy (if you add the sherbet) and so simple!

—**JAN WITTEVEEN** NORBORNE, MO

START TO FINISH: 5 MIN.
MAKES: 17 SERVINGS (¾ CUP EACH)

- 1 can (46 ounces) unsweetened pineapple juice, chilled
- 3 cups apricot nectar or juice, chilled
- 1 liter diet lemon-lime soda, chilled
  Pineapple sherbet, optional

In a punch bowl, combine the pineapple juice, apricot nectar and soda. Top with scoops of sherbet if desired. Serve immediately.

PER SERVING *¾ cup (without sherbet) equals 66 cal., trace fat (trace sat. fat), 0 chol., 9 mg sodium, 16 g carb., trace fiber, trace pro. Diabetic Exchange: 1 fruit.*

SPINACH & BLACK BEAN EGG ROLLS

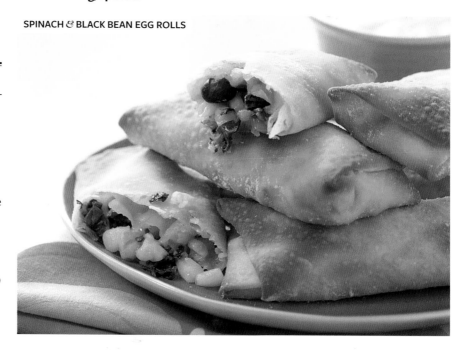

Crab-Stuffed Deviled Eggs

Filled with a creamy combination of crabmeat, hot pepper sauce and a dash of cayenne, these deviled eggs offer a unique flavor twist. Serve them as a good-for-you appetizer or alongside an entree.

—KAREN CONKLIN SUPPLY, NC

START TO FINISH: 20 MIN.
MAKES: 16 APPETIZERS

- 8 **hard-cooked eggs**
- 3 **tablespoons fat-free mayonnaise**
- 2 **tablespoons lemon juice**
- 4 **teaspoons minced fresh tarragon**
- 1 **tablespoon chopped green onion**
- ¼ **teaspoon salt**
- ¼ **teaspoon hot pepper sauce**
- ⅛ **teaspoon cayenne pepper**
- 1 **can (6 ounces) crabmeat, drained, flaked and cartilage removed**

1. Cut eggs in half lengthwise. Remove yolks; set aside egg whites and four yolks (discard remaining yolks or save for another use).

2. In a large bowl, mash reserved yolks. Stir in the mayonnaise, lemon juice, tarragon, onion, salt, hot pepper sauce and cayenne. Stir in crab until well combined. Stuff or pipe into egg whites. Refrigerate until serving.

PER SERVING *1 appetizer equals 36 cal., 1 g fat (trace sat. fat), 61 mg chol., 125 mg sodium, 1 g carb., trace fiber, 5 g pro.* **Diabetic Exchange:** *1 lean meat.*

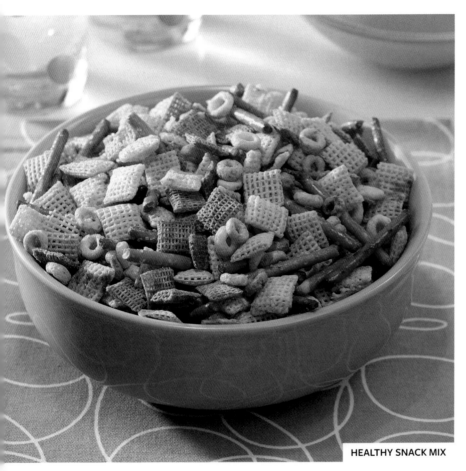

HEALTHY SNACK MIX

Healthy Snack Mix

Party mix has always been a tradition in our home. I lightened my mom's classic recipe, replacing margarine with heart-healthy olive oil. No one even noticed!

—MELISSA HANSEN ROCHESTER, MN

PREP: 15 MIN. • **BAKE:** 1 HOUR + COOLING
MAKES: 3½ QUARTS

- 3 **cups Corn Chex**
- 3 **cups Rice Chex**
- 3 **cups Wheat Chex**
- 3 **cups Multi Grain Cheerios**
- 1 **cup salted peanuts**
- 1½ **cups pretzel sticks**
- ⅓ **cup olive oil**
- 4 **teaspoons Worcestershire sauce**
- 1 **teaspoon seasoned salt**
- ⅛ **teaspoon garlic powder**

1. In a large bowl, combine the cereals, peanuts and pretzels. In a small bowl, combine remaining ingredients; pour over cereal mixture and toss to coat.

2. Transfer to two 15x10x1-in. baking pans coated with cooking spray. Bake at 250° for 1 hour, stirring every 15 minutes. Cool completely on wire racks. Store in an airtight container.

PER SERVING *¾ cup equals 150 cal., 8 g fat (1 g sat. fat), 0 chol., 310 mg sodium, 19 g carb., 2 g fiber, 4 g pro.* **Diabetic Exchanges:** *1½ starch, 1½ fat.*

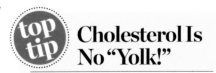

top tip

Cholesterol Is No "Yolk!"

If you have diabetes, it's important to watch your cholesterol for best heart health. Decreasing egg yolks in recipes is a great start!

Greek Pita Pizzas

Colorful, crunchy and loaded with fresh veggies, these quick pizzas taste just like a Greek salad. Whole wheat pitas were never more tasty!

—**TRISHA KRUSE** EAGLE, ID

START TO FINISH: 25 MIN.
MAKES: 6 SERVINGS

- 6 whole wheat pita breads (6 inches)
- 1½ cups meatless spaghetti sauce
- 1 can (14 ounces) water-packed artichoke hearts, rinsed, drained and quartered
- 2 cups fresh baby spinach, chopped
- 1½ cups sliced fresh mushrooms
- ½ cup crumbled feta cheese
- 1 small green pepper, thinly sliced
- ¼ cup thinly sliced red onion
- ¼ cup sliced ripe olives
- 3 tablespoons grated Parmesan cheese
- ¼ teaspoon pepper

1. Place pita breads on an ungreased baking sheet; spread with spaghetti sauce. Top with remaining ingredients.
2. Bake at 350° for 8-12 minutes or until cheese is melted. Serve immediately.
PER SERVING *273 cal., 5 g fat (2 g sat. fat), 7 mg chol., 969 mg sodium, 48 g carb., 7 g fiber, 13 g pro.* **Diabetic Exchanges:** *2 starch, 1 medium-fat meat, 1 vegetable.*

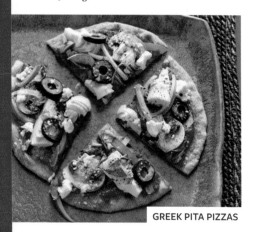

GREEK PITA PIZZAS

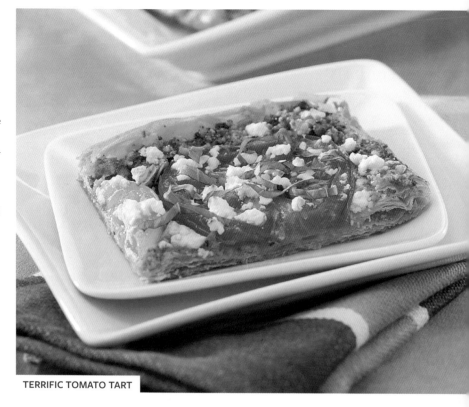

TERRIFIC TOMATO TART

Terrific Tomato Tart

Fresh, colorful tomatoes, feta cheese and prepared pesto perfectly complement my appetizer's crispy phyllo dough crust.

—**DIANE HALFERTY** CORPUS CHRISTI, TX

PREP: 15 MIN. • **BAKE:** 20 MIN.
MAKES: 8 SERVINGS

- 12 sheets phyllo dough (14 inches x 9 inches)
- 2 tablespoons olive oil
- 2 tablespoons dry bread crumbs
- 2 tablespoons prepared pesto
- ¾ cup crumbled feta cheese, divided
- 1 medium tomato, cut into ¼-inch slices
- 1 large yellow tomato, cut into ¼-inch slices
- ¼ teaspoon pepper
- 5 to 6 fresh basil leaves, thinly sliced

1. Place one sheet of phyllo dough on a baking sheet lined with parchment paper; brush with ½ teaspoon oil and sprinkle with ½ teaspoon bread crumbs. (Keep remaining phyllo covered with plastic wrap and a damp towel to prevent it from drying out.) Repeat layers, being careful to brush oil all the way to edges.
2. Fold each side ¾ in. toward center to form a rim. Spread with pesto and sprinkle with half of the feta cheese. Alternately arrange the red and yellow tomato slices over cheese. Sprinkle with pepper and remaining feta.
3. Bake at 400° for 20-25 minutes or until crust is golden brown and crispy. Cool on a wire rack for 5 minutes. Remove parchment paper before cutting. Garnish with basil.
PER SERVING *135 cal., 7 g fat (2 g sat. fat), 7 mg chol., 221 mg sodium, 13 g carb., 1 g fiber, 5 g pro.* **Diabetic Exchanges:** *1½ fat, 1 starch.*

Banana Mocha Cooler

Sip this thick milk shake-like drink for a pre-workout boost. You can also enjoy it for a cool, satisfying breakfast or snack.

—**CASSANDRA CORRIDON** FREDERICK, MD

START TO FINISH: 5 MIN.
MAKES: 3 SERVINGS

- 1 cup low-fat vanilla frozen yogurt
- ¾ cup fat-free milk
- 1 medium ripe banana, sliced
- 1 teaspoon instant coffee granules
- 1 cup ice cubes (7 to 8)

In a blender, combine all ingredients. Cover and process for 45-60 seconds or until frothy. Pour into glasses; serve immediately.

PER SERVING *122 cal., 1 g fat (1 g sat. fat), 5 mg chol., 72 mg sodium, 24 g carb., 1 g fiber, 6 g pro.* **Diabetic Exchanges:** *1 reduced-fat milk, ½ fruit.*

Ricotta Sausage Triangles

Stuffed with cheese, sausage and seasonings, these pockets are hard to put down! If you end up with leftovers, they freeze well for future get-togethers.

—**VIRGINIA ANTHONY** JACKSONVILLE, FL

PREP: 1 HOUR • **COOK:** 15 MIN./BATCH
MAKES: 12 DOZEN

- 1 carton (15 ounces) part-skim ricotta cheese
- 1 package (10 ounces) frozen chopped spinach, thawed and squeezed dry
- 1 jar (7 ounces) roasted sweet red peppers, drained and chopped
- ⅓ cup grated Parmesan cheese
- 3 tablespoons chopped ripe olives
- 1 egg
- 1 tablespoon minced fresh basil or 1 teaspoon dried basil
- 1 teaspoon Italian seasoning
- ¼ teaspoon salt
- ¼ teaspoon pepper
- 1 pound bulk Italian sausage
- 1 medium onion, chopped
- 96 sheets phyllo dough (14 inches x 9 inches)
  Olive oil-flavored cooking spray

1. In a large bowl, combine the first 10 ingredients. In a large skillet, cook sausage and onion over medium heat until meat is no longer pink; drain. Stir into cheese mixture.

2. Place one sheet of phyllo dough on a work surface with a short end facing you. (Keep remaining phyllo covered with plastic wrap and a damp towel to prevent it from drying out.) Spray sheet with cooking spray; repeat with one more sheet of phyllo, spraying the sheet with cooking spray. Cut into three 14-in. x 3-in. strips.

3. Place a rounded teaspoonful of filling on lower corner of each strip. Fold dough over filling, forming a triangle. Fold triangle up, then fold triangle over, forming another triangle. Continue folding, like a flag, until you come to the end of the strip.

4. Spritz end of dough with spray and press onto triangle to seal. Turn triangle and spritz top with spray. Repeat with the remaining phyllo and filling.

5. Place triangles on baking sheets coated with cooking spray. Bake at 375° for 15-20 minutes or until golden brown. Serve warm.

FREEZE OPTION *Freeze unbaked triangles in freezer containers, separating layers with waxed paper. Bake triangles as directed, increasing time as necessary until golden and heated through.*

PER SERVING *1 appetizer equals 42 cal., 2 g fat (trace sat. fat), 4 mg chol., 64 mg sodium, 5 g carb., trace fiber, 2 g pro.* **Diabetic Exchange:** *½ starch.*

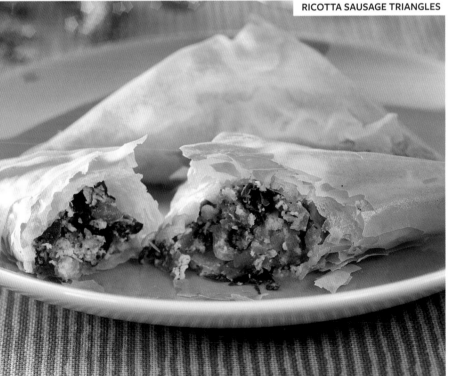

RICOTTA SAUSAGE TRIANGLES

Ginger Cardamom Tea

I like to add a little spice to my tea, which is why I mix in ginger and cardamom. Kick up your feet and relax with a steaming mugful.

—TRISHA KRUSE EAGLE, ID

START TO FINISH: 25 MIN.
MAKES: 4 SERVINGS

- 2 cups water
- 4 teaspoons honey
- 1 tablespoon minced fresh gingerroot
- ½ teaspoon ground cardamom
- 6 individual tea bags
- 1½ cups fat-free milk

1. In a small saucepan, combine water, honey, ginger and cardamom; bring to a boil. Reduce heat; simmer 10 minutes.
2. Pour over tea bags in a 2-cup glass measuring cup. Steep 3-5 minutes according to taste. Strain tea back into saucepan, discarding ginger and tea bags. Stir in milk; heat through.
PER SERVING 55 cal., trace fat (trace sat. fat), 2 mg chol., 39 mg sodium, 11 g carb., trace fiber, 3 g pro. **Diabetic Exchange:** ½ starch.

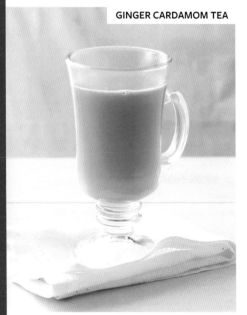
GINGER CARDAMOM TEA

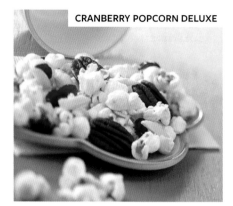
CRANBERRY POPCORN DELUXE

Cranberry Popcorn Deluxe

This recipe originally started as a holiday treat, but it became so popular that I now serve it year-round.

—CAROLYN SYKORA BLOOMER, WI

PREP: 15 MIN. • **BAKE:** 15 MIN. + COOLING
MAKES: 8 CUPS

- 8 cups air-popped popcorn
- ¾ cup dried cranberries
- ¼ cup slivered almonds
- ¼ cup pecan halves
- ¼ cup honey
- 3 tablespoons butter
- 2 tablespoons maple syrup
- ¼ teaspoon almond extract

1. In a shallow roasting pan, combine the popcorn, cranberries, almonds and pecans.
2. In a small saucepan, combine the honey, butter and syrup. Cook and stir over medium heat until butter is melted. Remove from the heat; stir in extract. Drizzle over popcorn mixture and toss to coat.
3. Bake at 325° for 15 minutes, stirring every 5 minutes. Cool on a wire rack, stirring occasionally. Store in an airtight container.
PER SERVING ½ cup equals 96 cal., 4 g fat (2 g sat. fat), 6 mg chol., 16 mg sodium, 14 g carb., 1 g fiber, 1 g pro. **Diabetic Exchanges:** 1 starch, 1 fat.

Makeover Creamy Artichoke Dip

Folks are sure to gather around this cheesy dip whenever it's placed on the buffet table. It's a better-for-you take on a treasured family recipe.

—MARY SPENCER GREENDALE, WI

PREP: 20 MIN. • **COOK:** 1 HOUR
MAKES: 5 CUPS

- 2 cans (14 ounces each) water-packed artichoke hearts, rinsed, drained and coarsely chopped
- 1 package (8 ounces) reduced-fat cream cheese, cubed
- ¾ cup (6 ounces) plain yogurt
- 1 cup (4 ounces) shredded part-skim mozzarella cheese
- 1 cup reduced-fat ricotta cheese
- ¾ cup shredded Parmesan cheese, divided
- ½ cup shredded reduced-fat Swiss cheese
- ¼ cup reduced-fat mayonnaise
- 2 tablespoons lemon juice
- 1 tablespoon chopped seeded jalapeno pepper
- 1 teaspoon garlic powder
- 1 teaspoon seasoned salt
  Tortilla chips

1. In a 3-qt. slow cooker, combine the artichokes, cream cheese, yogurt, mozzarella cheese, ricotta cheese, ½ cup Parmesan cheese, Swiss cheese, mayonnaise, lemon juice, jalapeno, garlic powder and seasoned salt. Cover and cook on low for 1 hour or until heated through.
2. Sprinkle with remaining Parmesan cheese. Serve with tortilla chips.
NOTE Wear disposable gloves when cutting hot peppers; the oils can burn skin. Avoid touching your face.
PER SERVING ¼ cup equals 104 cal., 6 g fat (3 g sat. fat), 20 mg chol., 348 mg sodium, 5 g carb., trace fiber, 7 g pro. **Diabetic Exchanges:** 1 fat, ½ starch.

Little Mexican Pizzas

Bite into these pizzas for fast snacks or appetizers. Whole wheat English muffins offer more fiber than regular pizza crust.
—**LINDA EGGERS** ALBANY, CA

START TO FINISH: 25 MIN.
MAKES: 1 DOZEN

- 1 package (13 ounces) whole wheat English muffins, split
- ¾ cup fat-free refried beans
- ¾ cup salsa
- ⅓ cup sliced ripe olives
- 2 green onions, chopped
- 2 tablespoons canned chopped green chilies
- 1½ cups (6 ounces) shredded part-skim mozzarella cheese

1. Spread cut sides of muffins with refried beans; top with salsa, olives, onions, chilies and cheese.
2. Place on baking sheets; broil 4-6 in. from the heat for 2-3 minutes or until cheese is melted.
PER SERVING *129 cal., 3 g fat (2 g sat. fat), 8 mg chol., 368 mg sodium, 17 g carb., 2 g fiber, 7 g pro.* **Diabetic Exchanges:** *1 starch, 1 lean meat.*

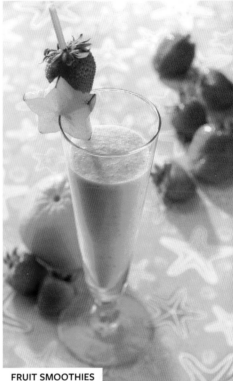

FRUIT SMOOTHIES

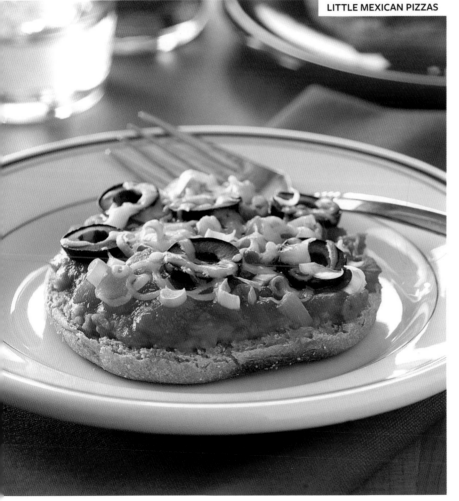

LITTLE MEXICAN PIZZAS

Fruit Smoothies

Instead of pouring a glass of ordinary orange juice, blend up this refreshing smoothie in just a few minutes.
—**TASTE OF HOME TEST KITCHEN**

START TO FINISH: 10 MIN.
MAKES: 4 SERVINGS

- 2 cups 2% milk
- 1 cup frozen unsweetened sliced peaches
- 1 cup frozen unsweetened strawberries
- ¼ cup orange juice
- 2 tablespoons honey

In a blender, combine all ingredients. Cover and process until smooth. Pour into chilled glasses; serve immediately.
PER SERVING *128 cal., 2 g fat (1 g sat. fat), 9 mg chol., 62 mg sodium, 23 g carb., 1 g fiber, 5 g pro.* **Diabetic Exchanges:** *1 fruit, ½ reduced-fat milk.*

breakfast & brunch

Rise and shine and **dig into a great day** with the stick-to-your-ribs dishes found in this section. Low on sugar and carbohydrates yet **big on flavor**, these eye-openers start the day off right!

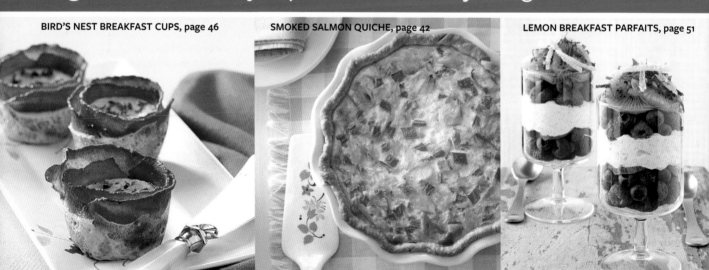

BIRD'S NEST BREAKFAST CUPS, page 46

SMOKED SALMON QUICHE, page 42

LEMON BREAKFAST PARFAITS, page 51

Moist Bran Muffins

My husband requests these hearty bran muffins for breakfast often. They prove that healthy food doesn't have to be boring.

—ELIZABETH PROBELSKI
PORT WASHINGTON, WI

PREP: 15 MIN. + STANDING
BAKE: 15 MIN. + COOLING
MAKES: ABOUT 1½ DOZEN

- 2 **cups All-Bran**
- 1 **cup fat-free plain yogurt**
- ⅔ **cup unsweetened applesauce**
- ½ **cup fat-free milk**
- 1½ **cups all-purpose flour**
- ⅓ **cup packed brown sugar**
- 1 **teaspoon baking powder**
- 1 **teaspoon baking soda**
- 1 **teaspoon ground cinnamon**
- ¼ **teaspoon salt**
- ½ **cup egg substitute**
- 2 **tablespoons molasses**
- 1 **tablespoon canola oil**
- 1 **teaspoon vanilla extract**

1. In a large bowl, combine the bran, yogurt, applesauce and milk; let stand for 5 minutes.
2. Meanwhile, in a large bowl, combine the flour, brown sugar, baking powder, baking soda, cinnamon and salt. In another bowl, combine the egg substitute, molasses, oil, vanilla and bran mixture. Stir into dry ingredients just until moistened.
3. Fill muffin cups coated with cooking spray two-thirds full. Bake at 400° for 15-20 minutes or until a toothpick inserted near the center comes out clean. Cool for 5 minutes before removing from pans to wire racks.
PER SERVING *105 cal., 1 g fat (trace sat. fat), trace chol., 158 mg sodium, 21 g carb., 3 g fiber, 4 g pro.* **Diabetic Exchange:** *1½ starch.*

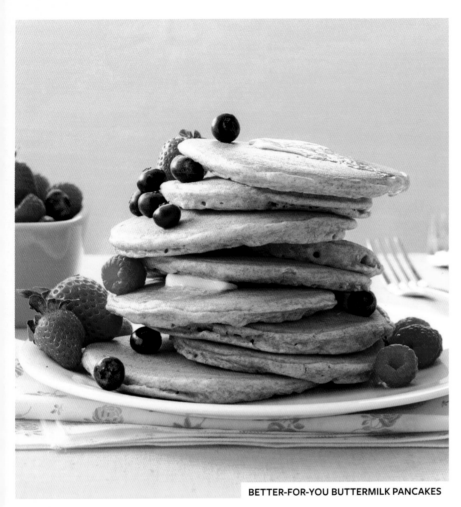

BETTER-FOR-YOU BUTTERMILK PANCAKES

Better-For-You Buttermilk Pancakes

Add whatever fruits you might have on hand to this recipe. My family's favorite version always includes blueberries.

—JANET SCHUBERT RIB LAKE, WI

PREP: 15 MIN. • **COOK:** 10 MIN./BATCH
MAKES: 16 PANCAKES

- 1 **cup all-purpose flour**
- 1 **cup whole wheat flour**
- 2 **tablespoons sugar**
- 2 **teaspoons baking powder**
- 1 **teaspoon baking soda**
- 2 **egg whites**
- 1 **egg**
- 2 **cups buttermilk**
- 2 **tablespoons canola oil**
  Fresh mixed berries, optional

1. In a large bowl, combine the first five ingredients. Combine the egg whites, egg, buttermilk and oil; stir into dry ingredients just until moistened.
2. Pour batter by ¼ cupfuls onto a hot griddle coated with cooking spray. Turn when bubbles just form on top; cook until second side is golden brown. Serve with berries if desired.
PER SERVING *2 pancakes equals 189 cal., 5 g fat (1 g sat. fat), 29 mg chol., 345 mg sodium, 29 g carb., 2 g fiber, 7 g pro.* **Diabetic Exchanges:** *2 starch, 1 fat.*

Oatmeal Cranberry Breakfast Bake

Even though it comes together in just 10 minutes, I like to prepare this baked oatmeal on weekend mornings when I have a little extra time. Even guests who typically don't like oatmeal fill their bowls, since I mix in dried cranberries, brown sugar and cinnamon. It's great for cool-weather mornings.

—ANGELA HIGINBOTHAM WILLITS, CA

PREP: 10 MIN. • **BAKE:** 50 MIN.
MAKES: 12 SERVINGS

- 3 cups old-fashioned oats
- 1 cup dried cranberries
- ¾ cup packed brown sugar
- 2 teaspoons ground cinnamon
- 1 teaspoon salt
- 4 egg whites, lightly beaten
- 3 cups fat-free milk
- ¼ cup canola oil
- 1 tablespoon vanilla extract
  Additional milk, optional

1. In a large bowl, combine the first five ingredients. In another bowl, whisk together the egg whites, milk, oil and vanilla. Stir into the oat mixture just until moistened.

2. Place in a 13x9-in. baking dish coated with cooking spray. Bake at 350° for 50-55 minutes or until oats are tender and liquid is absorbed.

3. Cut into bars. Serve in bowls with milk if desired.

PER SERVING *230 cal., 6 g fat (1 g sat. fat), 1 mg chol., 253 mg sodium, 36 g carb., 3 g fiber, 7 g pro.* **Diabetic Exchanges:** *2½ starch, 1 fat.*

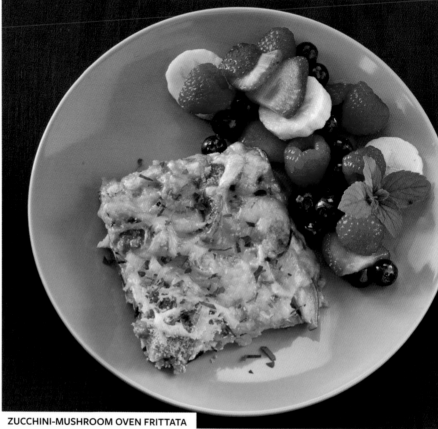

ZUCCHINI-MUSHROOM OVEN FRITTATA

Zucchini-Mushroom Oven Frittata

With a fresh veggie flavor as big as its serving size, this cheesy frittata makes for a nice lunch option, too.

—MICHELLE SANDOVAL ESCALON, CA

PREP: 20 MIN. • **BAKE:** 20 MIN.
MAKES: 4 SERVINGS

- 1 large onion, chopped
- 2 medium zucchini, halved and thinly sliced
- 1 cup thinly sliced fresh mushrooms
- 4½ teaspoons butter
- 3 eggs
- ⅓ cup fat-free milk
- 1 teaspoon Dijon mustard
- ½ teaspoon ground mustard
- ¼ teaspoon salt
- ¼ teaspoon pepper
- 1 cup (4 ounces) shredded reduced-fat Swiss cheese
- 2 tablespoons dry bread crumbs

1. In a large skillet, saute the onion, zucchini and mushrooms in butter until tender; drain. Transfer to an 8-in. square baking dish coated with cooking spray.

2. In a large bowl, whisk the eggs, milk, mustards, salt and pepper; pour over vegetable mixture. Sprinkle with cheese and bread crumbs. Bake, uncovered, at 375° for 18-22 minutes or until set. Let stand for 5 minutes.

PER SERVING *209 cal., 10 g fat (5 g sat. fat), 182 mg chol., 391 mg sodium, 13 g carb., 2 g fiber, 17 g pro.* **Diabetic Exchanges:** *2 medium-fat meat, 1 vegetable, 1 fat.*

Potato Basil Scramble

This potato dish is so popular at our house, we argue over who gets the leftovers! I grow my own herbs, so I toss in fresh basil, but dried works just as well.

—**TERRI ZOBEL** RALEIGH, NC

START TO FINISH: 30 MIN.
MAKES: 4 SERVINGS

- 2 **cups cubed potatoes**
- ½ **cup chopped onion**
- ½ **chopped green pepper**
- 1 **tablespoon vegetable oil**
- 2 **cups egg substitute**
- 2 **tablespoons minced fresh basil**
- ½ **teaspoon salt**
- ⅛ **teaspoon cayenne pepper**

1. Place potatoes in a microwave-safe bowl; add 1 in. of water. Cover and microwave on high for 7 minutes; drain.

2. In a large nonstick skillet coated with cooking spray, saute the onion, green pepper and potatoes in oil until tender. Add the egg substitute, basil, salt and pepper. Cook and stir over medium heat until the eggs are completely set.

NOTE *This recipe was tested in a 1,100-watt microwave.*

PER SERVING *163 cal., 4 g fat (0.55 g sat. fat), 0 chol., 549 mg sodium, 19 g carb., 2 g fiber, 14 g pro.* **Diabetic Exchanges:** *2 lean meat, 1 starch.*

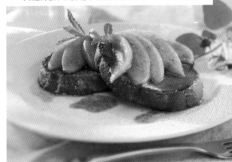

FRENCH TOAST WITH APPLE TOPPING

POTATO BASIL SCRAMBLE

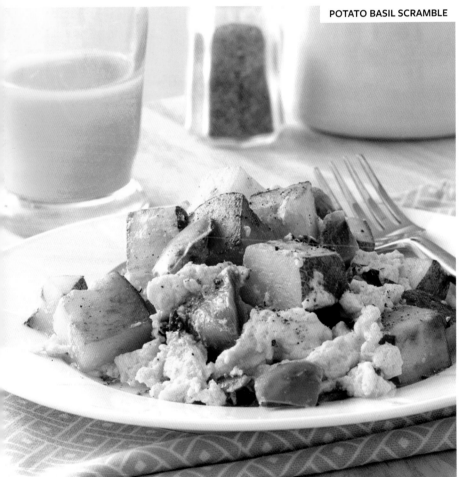

French Toast with Apple Topping

You can't top this impressive dish for breakfast or brunch. Warm sweet apples and a hint of cinnamon add a unique twist to French toast.

—**JANIS SCHARNOTT** FONTANA, WI

START TO FINISH: 20 MIN.
MAKES: 2 SERVINGS

- 1 **medium apple, peeled and thinly sliced**
- 1 **tablespoon brown sugar**
- ¼ **teaspoon ground cinnamon**
- 2 **tablespoons butter, divided**
- 1 **egg**
- ¼ **cup 2% milk**
- 1 **teaspoon vanilla extract**
- 4 **slices French bread (½ inch thick)**
  Maple syrup, optional

1. In a large skillet, saute apple, brown sugar and cinnamon in 1 tablespoon butter until apple is tender.

2. In a shallow bowl, whisk the egg, milk and vanilla. Dip both sides of bread in egg mixture.

3. In a large skillet, melt remaining butter over medium heat. Cook bread on both sides until golden brown. Serve with the apple mixture and maple syrup if desired.

PER SERVING *219 cal., 10 g fat (5 g sat. fat), 113 mg chol., 279 mg sodium, 29 g carb., 2 g fiber, 6 g pro.* **Diabetic Exchanges:** *1½ starch, 1½ fat, ½ fruit.*

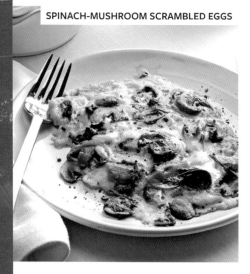

SPINACH-MUSHROOM SCRAMBLED EGGS

Berry Best Smoothies

Have over-ripened bananas you need to use up? Get blending! This sweet treat gives my family five daily servings of fruit and veggies.

—**PAMELA KLIM** BETTENDORF, IA

START TO FINISH: 10 MIN.
MAKES: 3 SERVINGS

- 3 **tablespoons orange juice concentrate**
- 3 **tablespoons fat-free half-and-half**
- 12 **ice cubes**
- 1 **cup fresh strawberries, hulled**
- 1 **medium ripe banana, cut into chunks**
- ½ **cup fresh or frozen blueberries**
- ½ **cup fresh or frozen raspberries**

In a blender, combine all ingredients; cover and process for 30-45 seconds or until smooth. Stir if necessary. Pour into chilled glasses; serve immediately.
PER SERVING *1 cup equals 108 cal., 1 g fat (trace sat. fat), 0 chol., 14 mg sodium, 26 g carb., 4 g fiber, 2 g pro. Diabetic Exchange: 1½ fruit.*

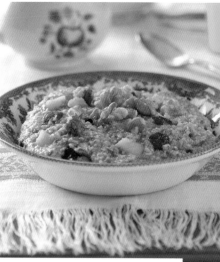

WARM 'N' FRUITY BREAKFAST CEREAL

Spinach-Mushroom Scrambled Eggs

My husband and I enjoyed an amazing mushroom dish at a hotel restaurant. As soon as I got home, I made my own rendition. Here's the tasty result!

—**RACHELLE MCCALLA** WAYNE, NE

START TO FINISH: 15 MIN.
MAKES: 2 SERVINGS

- ½ **cup thinly sliced fresh mushrooms**
- ½ **cup fresh baby spinach, chopped**
- 1 **teaspoon butter**
- 2 **eggs, lightly beaten**
- 2 **egg whites, lightly beaten**
- ⅛ **teaspoon salt**
- ⅛ **teaspoon pepper**
- 2 **tablespoons shredded provolone cheese**

1. In a small nonstick skillet, saute mushrooms and spinach in butter until tender. Whisk the eggs, egg whites, salt and pepper. Add egg mixture to skillet; cook and stir until almost set. Stir in the cheese. Cook and stir until completely set.
PER SERVING *162 cal., 11 g fat (5 g sat. fat), 226 mg chol., 417 mg sodium, 2 g carb., trace fiber, 14 g pro. Diabetic Exchange: 2 medium-fat meat.*

Warm 'n' Fruity Breakfast Cereal

We pile yogurt and sliced bananas over this wholesome dish. Try it with berries, too!

—**JOHN VALE** HARDIN, MT

PREP: 10 MIN. • **COOK:** 6 HOURS
MAKES: 10 SERVINGS

- 2 **cups seven-grain cereal**
- 1 **medium apple, peeled and chopped**
- ¼ **cup dried apricots, chopped**
- ¼ **cup dried cranberries**
- ¼ **cup raisins**
- ¼ **cup chopped dates**
- 5 **cups water**
- 1 **cup unsweetened apple juice**
- ¼ **cup maple syrup**
- 1 **teaspoon ground cinnamon**
- ½ **teaspoon salt**
  Chopped walnuts, optional

In a 4- or 5-qt. slow cooker, combine the first 11 ingredients. Cook, covered, on low 6-7 hours or until cereal and fruit are tender. If desired, top with walnuts.
PER SERVING *1 cup equals 185 cal., 3 g fat (trace sat. fat), 0 chol., 120 mg sodium, 37 g carb., 5 g fiber, 5 g pro. Diabetic Exchanges: 1 starch, 1 fruit, ½ fat.*

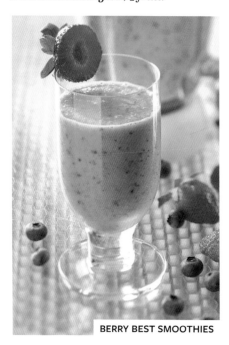

BERRY BEST SMOOTHIES

Yogurt Pancakes

Whip up a quick batch of these pancakes on the weekend, then pop them in your freezer for later. They taste just as good thawed as they do right from the pan. You might not even need syrup!

—CHERYLL BABER HOMEDALE, ID

PREP: 15 MIN. • **COOK:** 5 MIN./BATCH
MAKES: 12 PANCAKES

- 2 cups all-purpose flour
- 2 tablespoons sugar
- 2 teaspoons baking powder
- 1 teaspoon baking soda
- 2 eggs, lightly beaten
- 2 cups (16 ounces) plain yogurt
- ¼ cup water
  Semisweet chocolate chips, dried cranberries, sliced ripe bananas and coarsely chopped pecans, optional

1. In a small bowl, combine the flour, sugar, baking powder and baking soda. In another bowl, whisk the eggs, yogurt and water. Stir into dry ingredients just until moistened.

2. Pour batter by ¼ cupfuls onto a hot griddle coated with cooking spray. Sprinkle with optional ingredients if desired. Turn when bubbles form on top; cook until the second side is golden brown.

3. To freeze, arrange cooled pancakes in a single layer on baking sheets. Freeze overnight or until frozen. Transfer to a resealable plastic freezer bag. May be frozen for up to 2 months.

TO USE FROZEN PANCAKES *Place pancakes on a microwave-safe plate; microwave on high for 40-50 seconds or until heated through.*

PER SERVING *2 pancakes equals 242 cal., 5 g fat (2 g sat. fat), 81 mg chol., 403 mg sodium, 40 g carb., 1 g fiber, 9 g pro.* **Diabetic Exchange:** *3 starch.*

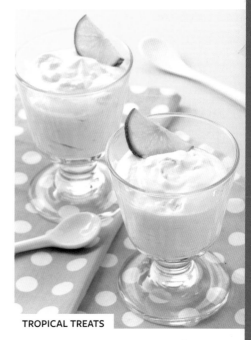

TROPICAL TREATS

Tropical Treats

Plain yogurt becomes a full-flavored delight with a little help from coconut extract, pineapple and a hint of lime.

—TASTE OF HOME TEST KITCHEN

START TO FINISH: 5 MIN.
MAKES: 4 SERVINGS

- 2 cups (16 ounces) reduced-fat plain yogurt
- 1 can (8 ounces) unsweetened crushed pineapple, drained
- 2 teaspoons sugar
- ¼ teaspoon coconut extract
- ¼ teaspoon grated lime peel

In a small bowl, combine all ingredients. Chill until serving.

PER SERVING *½ cup equals 121 cal., 2 g fat (1 g sat. fat), 7 mg chol., 86 mg sodium, 20 g carb., trace fiber, 7 g pro.* **Diabetic Exchanges:** *1 reduced-fat milk, ½ fruit.*

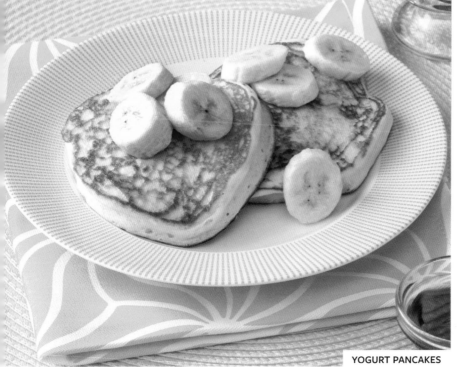

YOGURT PANCAKES

Waffle Sandwich

Keep 'em going until lunchtime with this quick and hearty breakfast sandwich.

—MICHELE MCHENRY BELLINGHAM, WA

START TO FINISH: 20 MIN.
MAKES: 1 SERVING.

- 1 **slice Canadian bacon**
- 1 **egg**
- 1 **green onion, chopped**
- 2 **frozen low-fat multigrain waffles**
- 1 **tablespoon shredded reduced-fat cheddar cheese**
  Sliced tomato, optional

1. In a nonstick skillet coated with cooking spray, cook Canadian bacon over medium-high heat 1-2 minutes on each side or until lightly browned. Remove and keep warm.

2. In a small bowl, whisk egg and green onion; add to the same pan. Cook and stir until egg is thickened and no liquid egg remains.

3. Meanwhile, prepare waffles according to package directions. Place one waffle on a plate. Top with Canadian bacon, scrambled egg, cheese and, if desired, tomato. Top with remaining waffle.

PER SERVING *261 cal., 10 g fat (3 g sat. fat), 223 mg chol., 733 mg sodium, 30 g carb., 3 g fiber, 16 g pro.* **Diabetic Exchanges:** *2 starch, 2 medium-fat meat.*

WAFFLE SANDWICH

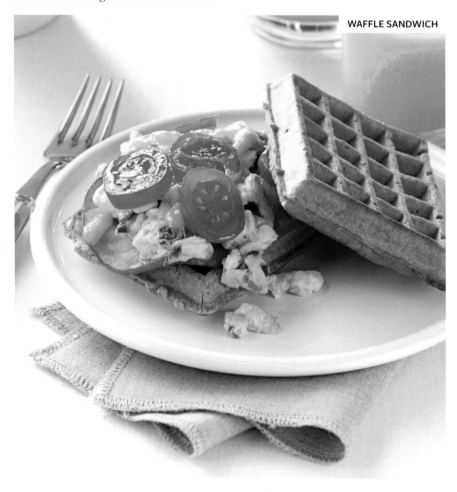

Smoked Salmon Quiche

My son fishes for salmon on the Kenai River in Alaska, and he smokes much of what he catches. My mother passed this recipe on to me since I'm always looking for new ways to cook with salmon. You can use regular salmon, but if you ask me, the smoked flavor can't be beat.

—ROSE MARIE CHERVEN ANCHORAGE, AK

PREP: 30 MIN. • **BAKE:** 35 MIN. + STANDING
MAKES: 8 SERVINGS

- 1 **sheet refrigerated pie pastry**
- 1 **cup (4 ounces) shredded reduced-fat Swiss cheese**
- 1 **tablespoon all-purpose flour**
- 3 **plum tomatoes, seeded and chopped**
- 2 **tablespoons finely chopped onion**
- 2 **teaspoons canola oil**
- 3 **ounces smoked salmon fillet, flaked (about ½ cup)**
- 4 **eggs**
- 1 **cup whole milk**
- ¼ **teaspoon salt**

1. On a lightly floured surface, unroll pastry. Transfer to a 9-in. pie plate. Trim pastry to ½ in. beyond edge of plate; flute edges.

2. In a small bowl, combine cheese and flour. Transfer to pastry.

3. In a large skillet, saute tomatoes and onion in oil just until tender. Remove from the heat; stir in salmon. Spoon over cheese mixture.

4. In a small bowl, whisk the eggs, milk and salt. Pour into pastry. Bake at 350° for 35-40 minutes or until a knife inserted near the center comes out clean. Let stand for 15 minutes before cutting.

PER SERVING *235 cal., 13 g fat (5 g sat. fat), 122 mg chol., 348 mg sodium, 17 g carb., trace fiber, 12 g pro.* **Diabetic Exchanges:** *2 medium-fat meat, 1 starch.*

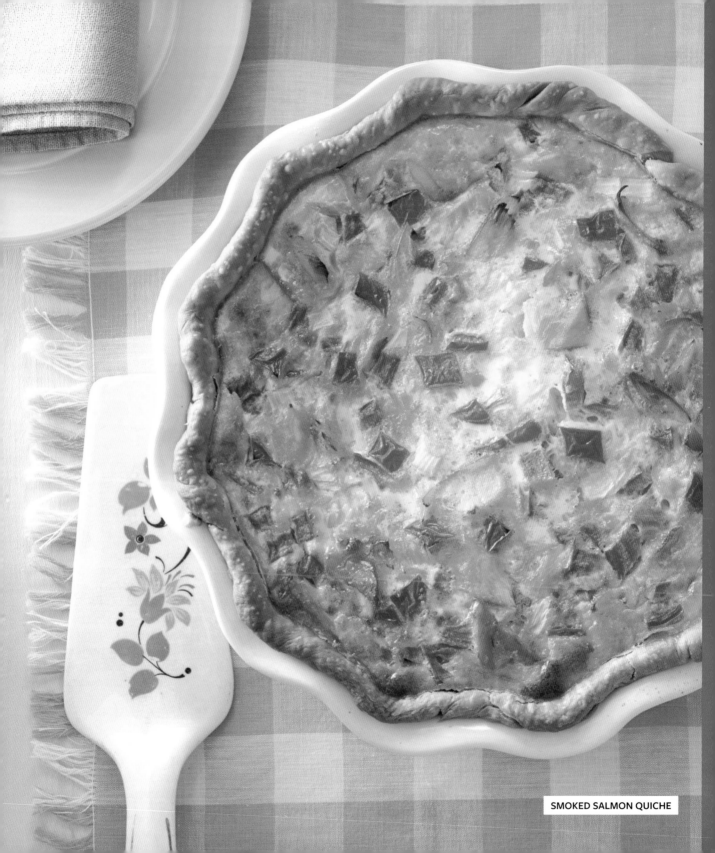

SMOKED SALMON QUICHE

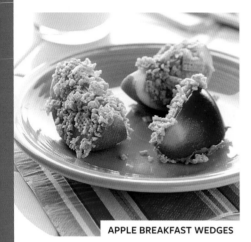

APPLE BREAKFAST WEDGES

Apple Breakfast Wedges

Break out these easy, fun apple wedges before you head out the door. The protein in the peanut butter will fill you up.

—**JACQUIE BERG** ST. CLOUD, WI

START TO FINISH: 10 MIN.
MAKES: 1 DOZEN

- 2 **medium apples**
- 1 **cup Rice Chex, crushed**
- 1½ **teaspoons packed brown sugar**
- 2 **tablespoons reduced-fat creamy peanut butter**

1. Core apples; cut each into six wedges. Pat dry with paper towels.
2. In a small shallow bowl, combine the cereal and brown sugar. Spread cut sides of apples with peanut butter; roll in cereal mixture. Serve immediately.
PER SERVING *1 piece equals 36 cal., 1 g fat (trace sat. fat), 0 chol., 33 mg sodium, 6 g carb., 1 g fiber, 1 g pro. Diabetic Exchange: ½ starch.*

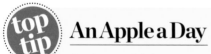

An Apple a Day

Apples are rich in vitamins A, B1, B2 and C. They also contain calcium, phosphorous, magnesium and potassium.

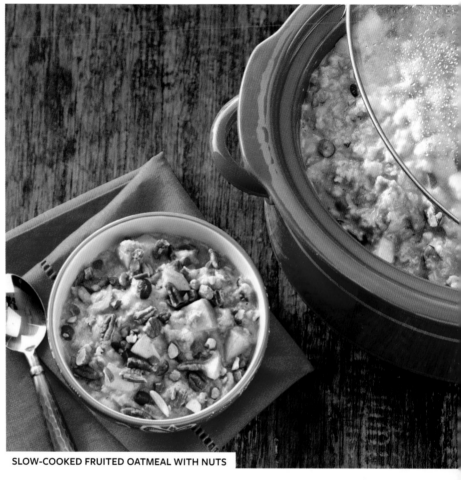

SLOW-COOKED FRUITED OATMEAL WITH NUTS

Slow-Cooked Fruited Oatmeal with Nuts

Let this bubble away in the slow cooker overnight, then just pull out a ladle, spoons and bowls in the morning. Breakfast will be such a breeze!

—**TRISHA KRUSE** EAGLE, ID

PREP: 15 MIN. • **COOK:** 6 HOURS
MAKES: 6 SERVINGS

- 3 **cups water**
- 2 **cups old-fashioned oats**
- 2 **cups chopped apples**
- 1 **cup dried cranberries**
- 1 **cup fat-free milk**
- 2 **teaspoons butter, melted**
- 1 **teaspoon pumpkin pie spice**
- 1 **teaspoon ground cinnamon**
- 6 **tablespoons chopped almonds, toasted**
- 6 **tablespoons chopped pecans, toasted**
  Additional fat-free milk

1. In a 3-qt. slow cooker coated with cooking spray, combine the first eight ingredients. Cover and cook on low for 6-8 hours or until liquid is absorbed.
2. Spoon oatmeal into bowls. Sprinkle with almonds and pecans; drizzle with additional milk if desired.
PER SERVING *1 cup equals 306 cal., 13 g fat (2 g sat. fat), 4 mg chol., 28 mg sodium, 45 g carb., 6 g fiber, 8 g pro. Diabetic Exchanges: 3 starch, 2 fat.*

Sage Turkey Sausage Patties

Turkey sausage is a good option when you want to cut down on salt and saturated fat. You'll love the aroma of this recipe when it's sizzling in the pan.

—**SHARMAN SCHUBERT** SEATTLE, WA

START TO FINISH: 30 MIN.
MAKES: 12 SERVINGS

- ¼ cup grated Parmesan cheese
- 3 tablespoons minced fresh parsley or 1 tablespoon dried parsley flakes
- 2 tablespoons fresh sage or 2 teaspoons dried sage leaves
- 2 garlic cloves, minced
- 1 teaspoon fennel seed, crushed
- ¾ teaspoon salt
- ½ teaspoon pepper
- 1½ pounds lean ground turkey
- 1 tablespoon olive oil

1. In a large bowl, combine the first seven ingredients. Crumble turkey over mixture and mix well. Shape into twelve 3-in. patties.
2. In a large skillet coated with cooking spray, cook patties in oil in batches over medium heat for 3-5 minutes on each side or until meat is no longer pink. Drain on paper towels if necessary.
3. To freeze, wrap each patty in plastic wrap; transfer to a resealable plastic freezer bag. May be frozen for up to 3 months.
TO USE FROZEN PATTIES *Unwrap patties and place on a baking sheet coated with cooking spray. Bake at 350° for 15 minutes on each side or until heated through.*
PER SERVING *1 patty equals 104 cal., 6 g fat (2 g sat. fat), 46 mg chol., 227 mg sodium, trace carb., trace fiber, 11 g pro.* **Diabetic Exchanges:** *1 lean meat, 1 fat.*

SAGE TURKEY SAUSAGE PATTIES

Apple Butter French Toast

Here, I give a special treatment to my baked French toast slices by topping them with cinnamony apple butter and toasted slivered almonds for a pleasant crunch.

—**MAVIS DIMENT** MARCUS, IA

PREP: 10 MIN. + CHILLING • **BAKE:** 30 MIN.
MAKES: 6 SERVINGS

- 6 slices French bread (1 inch thick)
- ¾ cup egg substitute
- ⅔ cup fat-free milk
- 2 tablespoons thawed apple juice concentrate
- ½ teaspoon vanilla extract
- 2 tablespoons slivered almonds, toasted
- ¼ cup apple butter
- ⅛ teaspoon ground cinnamon

1. Place bread in a 9-in. square baking dish that has been coated with cooking spray. In a large bowl, combine egg substitute, milk, apple juice concentrate and vanilla. Pour over bread and turn to coat. Cover and refrigerate for 2 hours or overnight.
2. Remove from the refrigerator 30 minutes before baking. Bake, uncovered, at 350° for 30-35 minutes or until a knife inserted near the center comes out clean and the edges are golden brown.
3. Sprinkle with almonds. Combine apple butter and cinnamon; serve with French toast.
NOTE *This recipe was tested with commercially prepared apple butter.*
PER SERVING *154 cal., 3 g fat (0 sat. fat), 0.55 mg chol., 224 mg sodium, 23 g carb., 0 fiber, 8 g pro.* **Diabetic Exchanges:** *1½ starch, ½ fat.*

Bird's Nest Breakfast Cups

This is a lightened-up version of an original recipe that called for regular bacon and eggs. Everyone loves it and thinks I really fussed, but it's so simple!

—ARIS GONZALEZ DELTONA, FL

START TO FINISH: 30 MIN.
MAKES: 6 SERVINGS

- 12 turkey bacon strips
- 1½ cups egg substitute
- 6 tablespoons shredded reduced-fat Mexican cheese blend
- 1 tablespoon minced fresh parsley

1. In a large skillet, cook bacon over medium heat for 2 minutes on each side or until partially set but not crisp. Coat six muffin cups with cooking spray; wrap two bacon strips around the inside of each cup. Fill each with ¼ cup egg substitute; top with cheese.

2. Bake at 350° for 18-20 minutes or until set. Cool for 5 minutes before removing from pan. Sprinkle with the parsley.

PER SERVING *120 cal., 7 g fat (2 g sat. fat), 30 mg chol., 515 mg sodium, 2 g carb., trace fiber, 12 g pro.* **Diabetic Exchange:** *2 lean meat.*

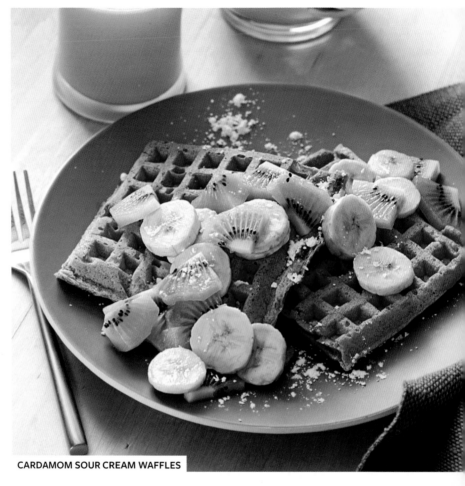

CARDAMOM SOUR CREAM WAFFLES

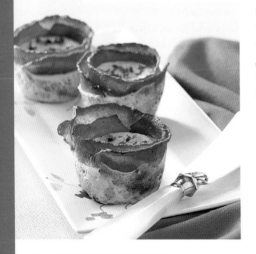

BIRD'S NEST BREAKFAST CUPS

Cardamom Sour Cream Waffles

Sweet with just the right amount of spice, these easy waffles make it nearly impossible to skip your morning meal.

—BARB MILLER OAKDALE, MN

PREP: 15 MIN. • **COOK:** 5 MIN./BATCH
MAKES: 14 WAFFLES

- ¾ cup all-purpose flour
- ¾ cup whole wheat flour
- 1½ teaspoons baking powder
- 1 teaspoon ground cardamom
- ¾ teaspoon baking soda
- ½ teaspoon ground cinnamon
- ¼ teaspoon salt
- 2 eggs
- 1 cup fat-free milk
- ¾ cup reduced-fat sour cream
- ½ cup packed brown sugar
- 1 tablespoon butter, melted
- 1 teaspoon vanilla extract

1. In a large bowl, combine the first seven ingredients. In another bowl, whisk the eggs, milk, sour cream, brown sugar, butter and vanilla. Stir into dry ingredients just until combined.

2. Bake in a preheated waffle iron according to manufacturer's directions until golden brown.

PER SERVING *2 waffles equals 235 cal., 6 g fat (3 g sat. fat), 74 mg chol., 375 mg sodium, 39 g carb., 2 g fiber, 8 g pro.* **Diabetic Exchanges:** *2½ starch, 1 fat.*

Asparagus Tart

This light egg bake features asparagus spears and Gruyere cheese. You can serve it for breakfast or as an impressive side dish.

—**MARY RELYEA** CANASTOTA, NY

PREP: 20 MIN. • **BAKE:** 25 MIN. + STANDING
MAKES: 8 SERVINGS

- 1 **pound fresh asparagus, trimmed**
- 3 **cups water**
  Pastry for single-crust pie
     (9 inches)
- ⅔ **cup shredded Gruyere or Swiss cheese, divided**
- ½ **cup minced fresh flat-leaf parsley**
- 4 **eggs, lightly beaten**
- ¾ **cup half-and-half cream**
- ½ **teaspoon salt**
- ⅛ **teaspoon cayenne pepper**
- ⅛ **teaspoon ground nutmeg**

1. Cut 2 in. from the top of each asparagus spear; set tops aside. Cut stem ends into ¾-in. pieces. In a small saucepan, bring water to a boil. Add the ¾-in. asparagus pieces; cover and boil for 3-4 minutes. Drain and immediately place asparagus in ice water. Drain and pat dry.

2. On a lightly floured surface, roll out pastry into a 13-in. circle. Press onto the bottom and up the sides of an ungreased 11-in. fluted tart pan with removable bottom; trim edges. Place the blanched asparagus, ⅓ cup cheese and parsley in crust.

3. In a small bowl, combine the eggs, cream, salt, cayenne and nutmeg; pour into crust. Arrange asparagus tops over egg mixture. Sprinkle with remaining cheese.

4. Place pan on a baking sheet. Bake at 400° for 25-30 minutes or until a knife inserted near the center comes out clean. Let stand for 10 minutes before cutting.

PER SERVING *233 cal., 15 g fat (7 g sat. fat), 132 mg chol., 326 mg sodium, 16 g carb., 1 g fiber, 8 g pro.* **Diabetic Exchanges:** *2½ fat, 1 starch, 1 lean meat.*

Cream Cheese Ham Omelet

My husband and I are watching our cholesterol, so I use an egg substitute for this rich, hearty recipe. It only takes 15 minutes to whip up...start to finish!

—**MICHELLE REVELLE** GUYTON, GA

START TO FINISH: 15 MIN.
MAKES: 2 SERVINGS

- ½ **cup chopped sweet onion**
- 2 **teaspoons olive oil**
- 1 **cup egg substitute**
- ½ **cup diced fully cooked lean ham**
- ¼ **teaspoon seasoned salt**
- ⅛ **teaspoon pepper**
- ⅛ **teaspoon paprika**
- 3 **tablespoons reduced-fat cream cheese, cubed**

In a 10-in. nonstick skillet, saute onion in oil until tender. Reduce heat to medium; add egg substitute. As eggs set, lift edges, letting uncooked portion flow underneath. When the eggs are set, sprinkle ham and seasonings over one side. Top with cream cheese cubes. Fold omelet over filling. Cover and let stand for 1-2 minutes or until the cream cheese is melted.

PER SERVING *215 cal., 10 g fat (4 g sat. fat), 23 mg chol., 905 mg sodium, 7 g carb., 1 g fiber, 22 g pro.* **Diabetic Exchanges:** *2 lean meat, 1 fat, ½ fat-free milk.*

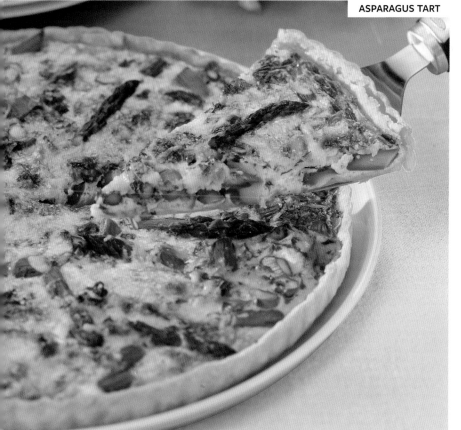
ASPARAGUS TART

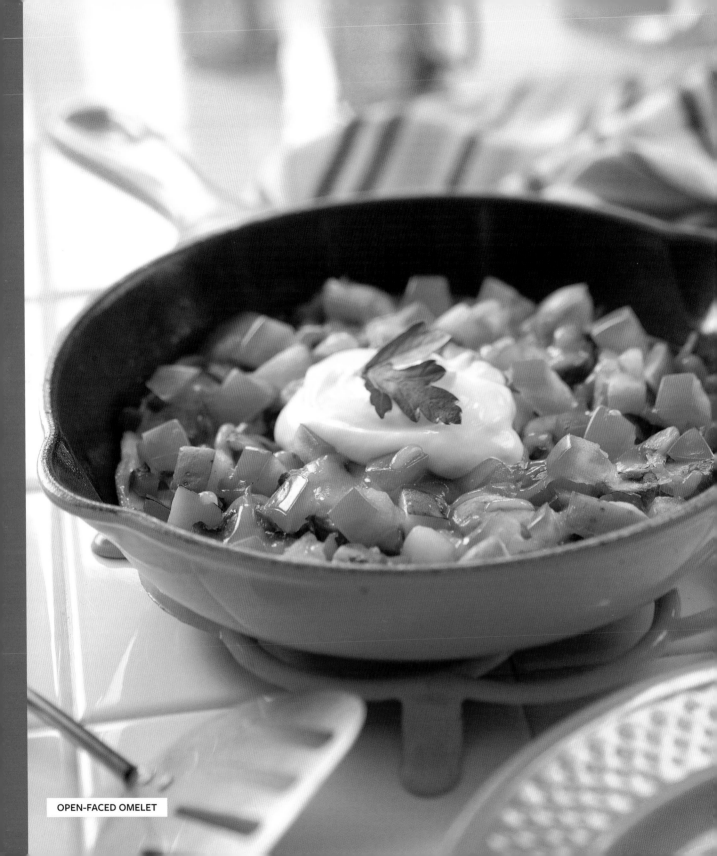

OPEN-FACED OMELET

Open-Faced Omelet

I used to make this recipe with bacon, ham and regular cheese, but now I enjoy it with low-fat and fat-free ingredients.
—**PAMELA SHANK** PARKERSBURG, WV

START TO FINISH: 20 MIN.
MAKES: 2 SERVINGS

- 2 **small red potatoes, diced**
- ¼ **cup sliced fresh mushrooms**
- 1 **tablespoon chopped green pepper**
- 1 **tablespoon chopped sweet red pepper**
- 1 **green onion, chopped**
- 1 **tablespoon olive oil**
- ⅔ **cup egg substitute**
- ¼ **cup shredded reduced-fat cheddar cheese, divided**
- 2 **tablespoons fat-free sour cream**
- ¼ **cup chopped tomatoes**

1. Place potatoes in a small saucepan and cover with water. Bring to a boil. Reduce heat; cover and cook for 5-7 minutes or until tender. Drain.
2. In a small skillet, saute the mushrooms, peppers, onion and potatoes in oil until tender. Coat a nonstick skillet with cooking spray and place over medium heat. Add egg substitute. As eggs set, push cooked edges toward the center, letting uncooked portion flow underneath. When the eggs are set, spoon vegetable mixture over egg; sprinkle with 2 tablespoons cheese.
3. Transfer to a serving plate. Top with sour cream, tomatoes and the remaining cheese.
PER SERVING *202 cal., 10 g fat (3 g sat. fat), 13 mg chol., 276 mg sodium, 15 g carb., 2 g fiber, 14 g pro.* **Diabetic Exchanges:** *2 lean meat, 1 starch, 1 fat.*

Gluten-Free Breakfast Blintzes

These cheese-filled, berry-topped blintzes taste just as mouthwatering and special as they look. They're also friendly to those with gluten allergies.
—**LAURA FALL-SUTTON** BUHL, ID

PREP: 30 MIN. + CHILLING • **BAKE:** 10 MIN.
MAKES: 9 SERVINGS

- 1½ **cups fat-free milk**
- 3 **eggs**
- 2 **tablespoons butter, melted**
- ⅔ **cup gluten-free all-purpose baking flour**
- ½ **teaspoon salt**

FILLING

- 1 **cup (8 ounces) 2% cottage cheese**
- 3 **ounces reduced-fat cream cheese**
- 2 **tablespoons sugar**
- ¼ **teaspoon almond extract**
- 2¼ **cups each fresh blueberries and raspberries**
  Confectioners' sugar, optional

1. In a small bowl, combine the milk, eggs and butter. Combine the flour and salt; add to milk mixture and mix well. Cover and refrigerate for 1 hour.

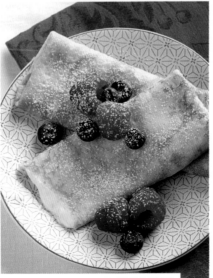

GLUTEN-FREE BREAKFAST BLINTZES

2. Coat an 8-in. nonstick skillet with cooking spray; heat over medium heat. Stir crepe batter; pour 2 tablespoons into center of skillet. Lift and tilt pan to coat bottom evenly. Cook until top appears dry; turn and cook 15-20 seconds longer. Remove to a wire rack. Repeat with remaining batter, coating skillet with cooking spray as needed. When cool, stack crepes with waxed paper or paper towels in between.
3. In a blender, cover and process cheeses until smooth. Add sugar and extract; pulse until combined. Spread a scant 1 tablespoonful onto each crepe. Fold opposite sides of crepe over filling, forming a little bundle.
4. Place seam side down in 15x10x1-in. baking pan coated with cooking spray. Bake, uncovered, at 350° for 10-12 minutes or until heated through. Serve topped with berries and dust with confectioners' sugar if desired.
NOTE *Read all ingredient labels for possible gluten content prior to use. Ingredient formulas can change, and production facilities vary among brands. If you're concerned that your brand may contain gluten, contact the company.*
PER SERVING *2 blintzes equals 180 cal., 7 g fat (4 g sat. fat), 88 mg chol., 319 mg sodium, 22 g carb., 4 g fiber, 9 g pro.* **Diabetic Exchanges:** *1 starch, 1 lean meat, ½ fruit, ½ fat.*

top tip

Quick Clean

To clean my blender, I fill it halfway with hot water, add a drop of dishwashing liquid, cover it and blend on high for 10-15 seconds. Then I rinse it with hot water and air-dry.
—**KATHY H.**, RAYLAND, OH

Start-Right Strata

I reworked this recipe to fit my diet without losing any of the taste. Served with melon on the side, it's ideal for overnight guests.
—CECILE BROWN CHILLICOTHE, TX

PREP: 15 MIN. + CHILLING
BAKE: 35 MIN. + STANDING
MAKES: 4 SERVINGS

- 4 slices white bread, torn into pieces
- 4 breakfast turkey sausage links, casings removed, crumbled
- ⅓ cup chopped onion
- 1 cup fat-free milk
- ¾ cup egg substitute
- ½ cup reduced-fat sour cream
- ¼ cup shredded reduced-fat cheddar cheese
- ¼ cup salsa

1. Place bread in an 8-in. square baking dish coated with cooking spray; set aside.
2. In a small nonstick skillet, cook the sausage and onion over medium heat until meat is no longer pink; drain. Spoon over bread. In a small bowl, combine the milk, egg substitute and sour cream. Stir in the cheese. Pour over the meat mixture. Cover and refrigerate overnight.
3. Remove from the refrigerator 30 minutes before baking. Bake, uncovered, at 325° for 35-40 minutes or until a knife inserted near the center comes out clean. Let stand for 10 minutes before cutting. Serve with salsa.
4. Or before refrigerating, cover and freeze strata for up to 3 months.
TO USE FROZEN STRATA *Thaw in the refrigerator overnight. Remove from the refrigerator 30 minutes before baking. Cover and bake according to directions.*
PER SERVING *247 cal., 10 g fat (4 g sat. fat), 39 mg chol., 580 mg sodium, 21 g carb., 1 g fiber, 17 g pro.* **Diabetic Exchanges:** *2 lean meat, 1½ starch, 1 fat.*

START-RIGHT STRATA

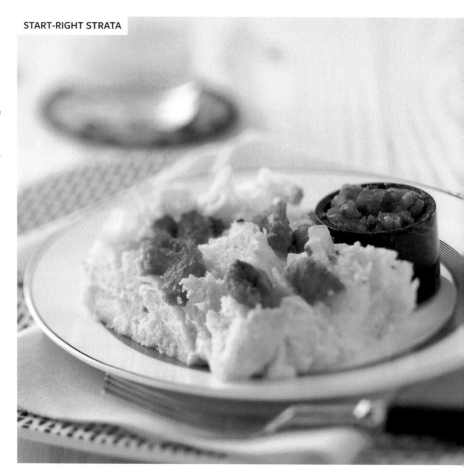

Sausage Egg Pitas

When I was growing up, my mom made these sausage and egg sandwiches for us on Sundays. Now that I'm a mom, I share the same tradition with my own kids.
—MELANIE LOVE PITTSBURGH, PA

START TO FINISH: 30 MIN.
MAKES: 6 SERVINGS

- 1 package (7 ounces) reduced-fat brown-and-serve sausage links
- 1 cup egg substitute
- ½ cup chopped green onions
- 2 tablespoons fat-free milk
- ⅛ teaspoon dried oregano
- ⅛ teaspoon pepper
- 2 tablespoons fat-free mayonnaise
- 6 pita pocket halves
- ⅓ cup chopped lettuce
- ⅓ cup chopped fresh tomato
- 2 tablespoons sliced ripe olives

1. In a large skillet, cook the sausage until heated through; remove from the pan. Cut into ¼-in. slices; keep warm.
2. In a small bowl, beat the egg substitute, onions, milk, oregano and pepper. Lightly coat another large skillet with cooking spray. Add egg mixture; cook and stir over medium heat until the eggs are set. Spread 1 teaspoon mayonnaise inside each pita half. Fill with the egg mixture, sausage, lettuce, tomato and olives.
PER SERVING *198 cal., 7 g fat (2 g sat. fat), 26 mg chol., 531 mg sodium, 21 g carb., 1 g fiber, 13 g pro.* **Diabetic Exchanges:** *2 lean meat, 1 starch, ½ fat.*

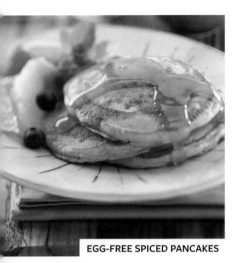

EGG-FREE SPICED PANCAKES

Egg-Free Spiced Pancakes

Golden brown and fluffy, these pancakes are so nice served with syrup or berries. You'll never guess the eggs are missing!

—TASTE OF HOME TEST KITCHEN

PREP: 10 MIN. • **COOK:** 10 MIN./BATCH
MAKES: 8 PANCAKES

- 1 **cup all-purpose flour**
- 2 **tablespoons brown sugar**
- 2½ **teaspoons baking powder**
- ½ **teaspoon pumpkin pie spice**
- ¼ **teaspoon salt**
- 1 **cup fat-free milk**
- 2 **tablespoons canola oil**
  Maple syrup, optional

1. In a large bowl, combine the flour, brown sugar, baking powder, pie spice and salt. In another bowl, combine milk and oil; stir into dry ingredients just until moistened.

2. Pour batter by ¼ cupfuls onto a hot griddle coated with cooking spray; turn when bubbles form on top. Cook until the second side is golden brown. Serve with syrup if desired.

PER SERVING *2 pancakes equals 223 cal., 7 g fat (1 g sat. fat), 1 mg chol., 427 mg sodium, 34 g carb., 1 g fiber, 5 g pro.* **Diabetic Exchanges:** *2 starch, 1½ fat.*

Lemon Breakfast Parfaits

I serve these lovely, layered parfaits as a refreshing start to a busy day. You can make the couscous mixture ahead, then cover and chill until you're ready to eat.

—JANELLE LEE APPLETON, WI

PREP: 25 MIN. + COOLING
MAKES: 6 SERVINGS

- ¾ **cup fat-free milk**
  Dash salt
- ⅓ **cup uncooked couscous**
- ½ **cup reduced-fat sour cream**
- ½ **cup lemon yogurt**
- 1 **tablespoon honey**
- ¼ **teaspoon grated lemon peel**
- 1 **cup sliced peeled kiwifruit**
- 1 **cup fresh blueberries**
- 1 **cup fresh raspberries**
  Chopped crystallized ginger and minced fresh mint

1. In a small saucepan, bring milk and salt to a boil. Stir in couscous. Remove from the heat; cover and let stand for 5-10 minutes or until milk is absorbed. Fluff with a fork; cool.

2. In a small bowl, combine the sour cream, yogurt, honey and lemon peel. Stir in couscous.

3. Combine the kiwi, blueberries and raspberries; spoon ¼ cup into each of six parfait glasses. Layer with couscous mixture and remaining fruit. Garnish with ginger and mint.

PER SERVING *146 cal., 2 g fat (1 g sat. fat), 8 mg chol., 64 mg sodium, 27 g carb., 3 g fiber, 5 g pro.* **Diabetic Exchanges:** *1 starch, ½ fruit.*

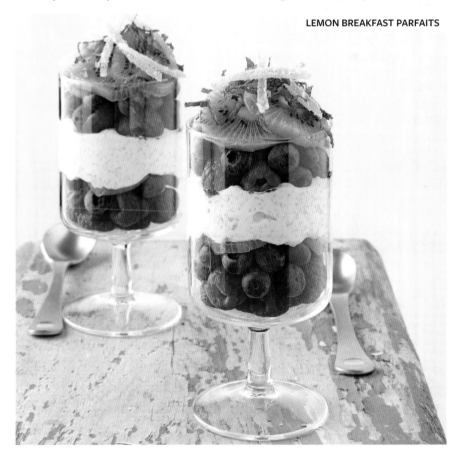

LEMON BREAKFAST PARFAITS

Ultimate Breakfast Burritos

I recently started eating healthier foods, and this is one of my favorite items for breakfast. The peppery eggs and crunchy veggies are sure to wake you up!

—PAMELA SHANK PARKERSBURG, WV

START TO FINISH: 20 MIN.
MAKES: 2 SERVINGS

- ½ cup chopped fresh mushrooms
- ¼ cup chopped green pepper
- ¼ cup chopped sweet red pepper
- 1 teaspoon olive oil
- 1 cup egg substitute
- ¼ teaspoon pepper
- 2 whole wheat tortillas (8 inches), warmed
- ¼ cup shredded reduced-fat cheddar cheese
- 2 tablespoons salsa
- 2 tablespoons fat-free sour cream

1. In a small nonstick skillet coated with cooking spray, saute mushrooms and peppers in oil until tender. Transfer to a small bowl; keep warm.
2. Add egg substitute and pepper to the pan; cook and stir over medium heat until eggs are set.
3. Spoon vegetable mixture and eggs off-center on each tortilla; top with cheese, salsa and sour cream. Fold sides and ends over filling and roll up.
PER SERVING *294 cal., 8 g fat (2 g sat. fat), 13 mg chol., 585 mg sodium, 31 g carb., 3 g fiber, 21 g pro.* **Diabetic Exchanges:** *2 starch, 2 lean meat, 1 vegetable, 1 fat.*

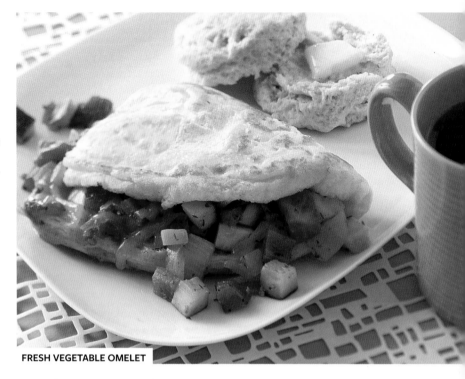

FRESH VEGETABLE OMELET

Fresh Vegetable Omelet

You'll be proud to serve this tasty main dish at breakfast, and guests will have no problem making their way to the table!

—EDIE DESPAIN LOGAN, UT

PREP: 30 MIN. • **BAKE:** 10 MIN.
MAKES: 2 SERVINGS

- 4 egg whites
- ¼ cup water
- ¼ teaspoon cream of tartar
- 2 eggs
- ¼ teaspoon salt
- 1 teaspoon butter
- 1 medium tomato, chopped
- 1 small zucchini, chopped
- 1 small onion, chopped
- ¼ cup chopped green pepper
- ½ teaspoon Italian seasoning
- ⅓ cup shredded reduced-fat cheddar cheese

1. In a small bowl, beat the egg whites, water and cream of tartar until stiff peaks form. In a large bowl, beat eggs and salt until thick and lemon-colored, about 5 minutes. Fold in the whites.
2. In a 10-in. ovenproof skillet coated with cooking spray, melt butter. Pour egg mixture into skillet. Cook for 5 minutes over medium heat or until puffed and lightly browned on the bottom. Bake, uncovered, at 350° for 10-12 minutes or until a knife inserted 2 in. from edge comes out clean.
3. Meanwhile, in a large skillet, saute the tomato, zucchini, onion, green pepper and Italian seasoning until tender. Carefully run a knife around edge of ovenproof skillet to loosen omelet. With a knife, score center of omelet. Place vegetables on one side and sprinkle with cheese; fold other side over filling. Slide onto a serving plate; cut in half.
PER SERVING *222 cal., 11 g fat (5 g sat. fat), 231 mg chol., 617 mg sodium, 12 g carb., 3 g fiber, 20 g pro.* **Diabetic Exchanges:** *3 lean meat, 2 vegetable, ½ fat.*

Strawberry Breakfast Shortcakes

I don't let a busy schedule stop me from eating healthy. Here, protein, fruit, dairy and whole grains come together in a flash for a delectable start to the day.

—**PAULA WHARTON** EL PASO, TX

START TO FINISH: 10 MIN.
MAKES: 2 SERVINGS

- 4 frozen low-fat multigrain waffles
- 1 cup fresh strawberries, sliced
- ½ cup plain Greek yogurt
  Maple syrup

1. Prepare waffles according to package directions. Divide among two serving plates. Top with strawberries and yogurt. Serve with syrup.
NOTE *If Greek yogurt is not available in your area, line a strainer with a coffee filter and place over a bowl. Place 1 cup plain yogurt in prepared strainer; refrigerate overnight. Discard liquid from bowl; proceed as directed.*
PER SERVING *230 cal., 8 g fat (4 g sat. fat), 15 mg chol., 466 mg sodium, 36 g carb., 4 g fiber, 7 g pro.* **Diabetic Exchanges:** *2 starch, 1 fat, ½ fruit.*

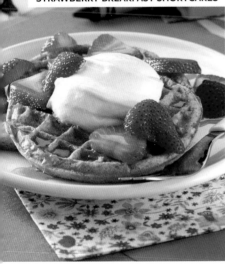

STRAWBERRY BREAKFAST SHORTCAKES

Zucchini Frittata

This frittata hits the spot without being too heavy. I like to prepare it with sharp cheddar cheese for an extra flavor punch.

—**AMY CRANE** SWARTZ CREEK, MI

PREP: 25 MIN. • **BAKE:** 25 MIN.
MAKES: 4 SERVINGS

- 3 medium zucchini, thinly sliced
- 3 tablespoons whole wheat flour
- 2 teaspoons olive oil
- 6 egg whites
- 3 eggs
- ½ cup reduced-fat ricotta cheese
- ½ cup shredded cheddar cheese, divided
- ⅓ cup plain yogurt
- 1 tablespoon dried parsley flakes
- 2 garlic cloves, minced
- ½ teaspoon salt
- ¼ teaspoon white pepper
- ½ teaspoon poppy seeds

1. Toss zucchini with flour. In a large nonstick skillet coated with cooking spray, saute zucchini in oil until crisp-tender and lightly browned. Remove from the heat.
2. In a large bowl, whisk the egg whites, eggs, ricotta cheese, ¼ cup cheddar cheese, yogurt, parsley, garlic, salt and pepper. Stir in zucchini. Transfer to a 9-in. pie plate coated with cooking spray. Sprinkle with poppy seeds and remaining cheddar cheese.
3. Bake at 350° for 25-30 minutes or until a knife inserted near the center comes out clean. Let stand 5 minutes before cutting.
PER SERVING *238 cal., 12 g fat (6 g sat. fat), 185 mg chol., 552 mg sodium, 13 g carb., 3 g fiber, 19 g pro.* **Diabetic Exchanges:** *2 lean meat, 2 fat, 1 vegetable, ½ starch.*

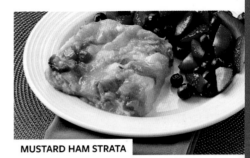

MUSTARD HAM STRATA

Mustard Ham Strata

Years ago, I adored this dish at a bed-and-breakfast. I was able to get a copy of the recipe, and I've made it many times since.

—**DOLORES ZORNOW** POYNETTE, WI

PREP: 15 MIN. + CHILLING • **BAKE:** 45 MIN.
MAKES: 12 SERVINGS

- 12 slices day-old bread, crusts removed and cubed
- 1½ cups cubed fully cooked ham
- 1 cup chopped green pepper
- ¾ cup shredded cheddar cheese
- ¾ cup shredded Monterey Jack cheese
- ⅓ cup chopped onion
- 7 eggs
- 3 cups whole milk
- 3 teaspoons ground mustard
- 1 teaspoon salt

1. In a 13x9-in. baking dish coated with cooking spray, layer the bread cubes, ham, green pepper, cheeses and onion. In a large bowl, combine the eggs, milk, mustard and salt. Pour over top. Cover and refrigerate overnight.
2. Remove from the refrigerator 30 minutes before baking. Bake, uncovered, at 325° for 45-50 minutes or until a knife inserted near the center comes out clean. Let stand for about 5 minutes before cutting.
PER SERVING *198 cal., 11 g fat (5 g sat. fat), 153 mg chol., 648 mg sodium, 11 g carb., 1 g fiber, 13 g pro.* **Diabetic Exchanges:** *2 medium-fat meat, 1 starch.*

Good Morning Frittata

Small households can start the day right with this fast-fixing dish. Orange peppers add sunshiny sweetness and crunch.

—**MARY RELYEA** CANASTOTA, NY

START TO FINISH: 20 MIN.
MAKES: 2 SERVINGS

- 1 cup egg substitute
- ¼ cup fat-free milk
- ⅛ teaspoon pepper
  Dash salt
- ¼ cup chopped sweet orange pepper
- 2 green onions, thinly sliced
- ½ teaspoon canola oil
- ⅓ cup cubed fully cooked ham
- ¼ cup shredded reduced-fat cheddar cheese

1. In a small bowl, whisk the egg substitute, milk, pepper and salt; set aside. In an 8-in. ovenproof skillet, saute orange pepper and onions in oil until tender. Add ham; heat through. Reduce heat; top with egg mixture. Cover and cook for 4-6 minutes or until nearly set.

2. Uncover skillet; sprinkle with cheese. Broil 3-4 in. from the heat for 2-3 minutes or until eggs are completely set. Let stand for 5 minutes. Cut into wedges.

PER SERVING *169 cal., 6 g fat (3 g sat. fat), 23 mg chol., 727 mg sodium, 7 g carb., 1 g fiber, 21 g pro.* **Diabetic Exchanges:** *3 lean meat, ½ starch.*

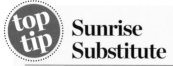 **Sunrise Substitute**

Egg substitute can replace whole eggs in many recipes with good results, especially in frittatas, omelets and quiches.

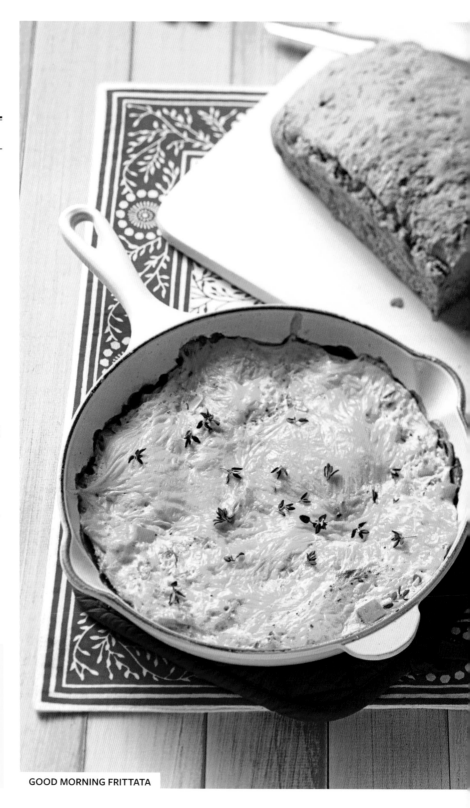

GOOD MORNING FRITTATA

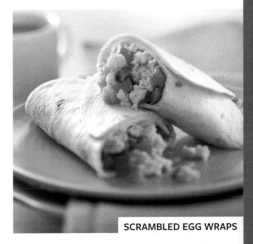

SCRAMBLED EGG WRAPS

Savory Apple-Chicken Sausage

Double or even triple this recipe when you're expecting a crowd. The sausage freezes well either cooked or raw.

—ANGELA BUCHANAN LONGMONT, CO

START TO FINISH: 25 MIN.
MAKES: 8 PATTIES

- 1 large tart apple, peeled and diced
- 2 teaspoons poultry seasoning
- 1 teaspoon salt
- ¼ teaspoon pepper
- 1 pound ground chicken

1. In a large bowl, combine the apple, poultry seasoning, salt and pepper. Crumble chicken over mixture and mix well. Shape into eight 3-in. patties.
2. In a large skillet coated with cooking spray, cook patties over medium heat for 5-6 minutes on each side or until no longer pink.
PER SERVING *1 patty equals 92 cal., 5 g fat (1 g sat. fat), 38 mg chol., 328 mg sodium, 4 g carb., 1 g fiber, 9 g pro.*
Diabetic Exchange: *1 medium-fat meat.*

SAVORY APPLE-CHICKEN SAUSAGE

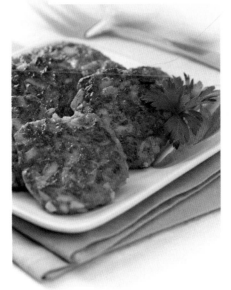

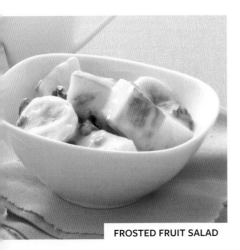

FROSTED FRUIT SALAD

Frosted Fruit Salad

I came up with this breakfast recipe that's easy, light and uses up the extra bananas and apples I always seem to have on hand.

—ANN FOX AUSTIN, TX

START TO FINISH: 10 MIN.
MAKES: 6 SERVINGS

- 2 large apples, cut into ¾-inch cubes
- 2 medium firm bananas, sliced
- 2 teaspoons lemon juice
- 1 carton (6 ounces) fat-free sugar-free raspberry yogurt
- ¼ cup raisins
- 1 tablespoon sunflower kernels

In a large bowl, combine apples and bananas. Sprinkle with lemon juice; toss to coat. Stir in the yogurt, raisins and sunflower kernels. Serve immediately.
PER SERVING *¾ cup equals 124 cal., 1 g fat (trace sat. fat), 1 mg chol., 31 mg sodium, 28 g carb., 3 g fiber, 3 g pro.*
Diabetic Exchange: *2 fruit.*

Scrambled Egg Wraps

Try this tasty morning meal, which also makes a fast lunch or light dinner, to fill your family up with protein and veggies.

—JANE SHAPTON IRVINE, CA

START TO FINISH: 20 MIN.
MAKES: 6 SERVINGS

- 1 medium sweet red pepper, chopped
- 1 medium green pepper, chopped
- 2 teaspoons canola oil
- 5 plum tomatoes, seeded and chopped
- 6 eggs
- ½ cup soy milk
- ¼ teaspoon salt
- 6 flour tortillas (8 inches), warmed

1. In a large nonstick skillet, saute peppers in oil until tender. Add tomatoes; saute 1-2 minutes longer.
2. Meanwhile, in a large bowl, whisk the eggs, soy milk and salt. Reduce heat to medium; add egg mixture to skillet. Cook and stir until eggs are completely set. Spoon ⅔ cup mixture down the center of each tortilla; roll up.
PER SERVING *258 cal., 10 g fat (2 g sat. fat), 212 mg chol., 427 mg sodium, 30 g carb., 1 g fiber, 12 g pro.* ***Diabetic Exchanges:*** *1½ starch, 1 lean meat, 1 vegetable, 1 fat.*

Makeover Noodle Kugel

You'll feel good about serving this fabulous, lightened-up brunch dish, especially now that it's lower in saturated fat by 8 g and in cholesterol by 115 mg.

—**CATHY TANG** REDMOND, WA

PREP: 15 MIN. • **BAKE:** 45 MIN. + STANDING
MAKES: 15 SERVINGS

- 1 package (12 ounces) yolk-free noodles
- 2 tablespoons butter, melted
- 2 cups (16 ounces) 1% cottage cheese
- 1½ cups sugar
- 4 eggs
- 1 cup egg substitute
- 1 cup (8 ounces) reduced-fat sour cream
- 1 cup reduced-fat ricotta cheese

TOPPING

- ½ cup cinnamon graham cracker crumbs (about 3 whole crackers)
- 1 tablespoon butter, melted

1. Cook noodles according to package directions; drain. Toss with butter; set aside.

2. In a large bowl, beat the cottage cheese, sugar, eggs, egg substitute, sour cream and ricotta cheese until well blended. Stir in noodles.

3. Transfer to a 13x9-in. baking dish coated with cooking spray. Combine cracker crumbs and butter; sprinkle over the top.

4. Bake, uncovered, at 350° for 45-50 minutes or until a thermometer reads 160°. Let stand for 10 minutes before cutting.

PER SERVING *271 cal., 6 g fat (3 g sat. fat), 73 mg chol., 235 mg sodium, 41 g carb., 1 g fiber, 13 g pro.* **Diabetic Exchanges:** *2½ starch, 1 lean meat, ½ fat.*

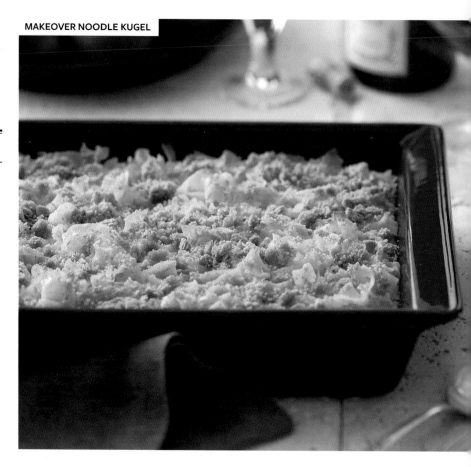

MAKEOVER NOODLE KUGEL

Makeover Toasted Granola

We pour milk over this homemade granola for a heart-smart breakfast, and we also sprinkle it over yogurt and ice cream for dessert. It's also wonderful to snack on right from the storage container!

—**SUSAN LAJEUNESSE** COLCHESTER, VT

PREP: 20 MIN. • **BAKE:** 1¼ HOURS + COOLING
MAKES: 10½ CUPS

- 1 cup packed brown sugar
- ⅓ cup water
- 4 cups old-fashioned oats
- 2 cups bran flakes
- 1 jar (12 ounces) toasted wheat germ
- 2 tablespoons all-purpose flour
- ¾ teaspoon salt
- ⅓ cup canola oil
- 2 teaspoons vanilla extract

1. In a large saucepan, bring brown sugar and water to a boil. Cook and stir until sugar is dissolved. Remove from the heat; set aside. In a large bowl, combine the oats, bran flakes, wheat germ, flour and salt. Stir oil and vanilla into sugar mixture; pour over oat mixture and toss to coat.

2. Transfer to two 15x10x1-in. baking pans coated with cooking spray. Bake at 250° for 1¼ to 1½ hours or until dry and lightly browned, stirring every 15 minutes. Cool completely on wire racks. Store in an airtight container.

PER SERVING *½ cup equals 202 cal., 6 g fat (1 g sat. fat), 0 chol., 118 mg sodium, 32 g carb., 4 g fiber, 8 g pro.* **Diabetic Exchanges:** *2 starch, 1 fat.*

Mediterranean Breakfast Pitas

Whether you turn to this pita recipe for breakfast or lunch, the healthy ingredients will keep you full throughout the day.

—JOSIE-LYNN BELMONT WOODBINE, GA

START TO FINISH: 25 MIN.
MAKES: 2 SERVINGS

- ¼ cup chopped sweet red pepper
- ¼ cup chopped onion
- 1 cup egg substitute
- ⅛ teaspoon salt
- ⅛ teaspoon pepper
- 1 small tomato, chopped
- ½ cup torn fresh baby spinach
- 1½ teaspoons minced fresh basil
- 2 whole pita breads
- 2 tablespoons crumbled feta cheese

1. In a small nonstick skillet coated with cooking spray, cook and stir red pepper and onion over medium heat for 3 minutes. Add the egg substitute, salt and pepper; cook and stir until set.
2. Combine the tomato, spinach and basil; spoon onto pitas. Top with egg mixture and sprinkle with feta cheese. Serve immediately.
PER SERVING *267 cal., 2 g fat (1 g sat. fat), 4 mg chol., 798 mg sodium, 41 g carb., 3 g fiber, 20 g pro.* **Diabetic Exchanges:** *2 starch, 2 lean meat, 1 vegetable.*

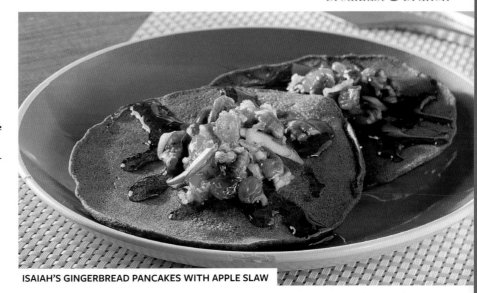

ISAIAH'S GINGERBREAD PANCAKES WITH APPLE SLAW

Isaiah's Gingerbread Pancakes with Apple Slaw

Perfect for weekend mornings, these gluten-free gingery pancakes are served with a sweet slaw. You can also swap in pears for the apples to change things up.

—SILVANA NARDONE BROOKLYN, NY

PREP: 25 MIN. • **COOK:** 5 MIN./BATCH
MAKES: 10 SERVINGS (3 CUPS SLAW)

- 2 cups gluten-free pancake mix
- 2 tablespoons brown sugar
- 1 tablespoon baking cocoa
- 1½ teaspoons ground ginger
- 1 teaspoon pumpkin pie spice
- ½ teaspoon baking soda
- 2 eggs, separated
- 1 cup rice milk
- ½ cup plus 1 tablespoon brewed coffee, room temperature
- 2 tablespoons canola oil
- 1 tablespoon molasses

SLAW
- 3 medium apples, grated
- ½ cup chopped pecans, toasted
- ¼ cup golden raisins
- 2 tablespoons lemon juice
- 1 tablespoon honey
  Maple syrup, warmed

1. In a large bowl, combine the first six ingredients. Combine the egg yolks, rice milk, coffee, oil and molasses; add to dry ingredients just until moistened. In a small bowl, beat egg whites on medium speed until stiff peaks form. Fold into the batter.
2. Pour batter by scant ¼ cupfuls onto a hot griddle coated with cooking spray; turn when bubbles form on top. Cook until the second side is golden brown.
3. Meanwhile, in a small bowl, combine the apples, pecans, raisins, lemon juice and honey. Serve with pancakes and the maple syrup.
NOTE *Read all ingredient labels for possible gluten content prior to use. Ingredient formulas can change, and production facilities vary among brands. If you're concerned that your brand may contain gluten, contact the company.*
PER SERVING *2 pancakes equals 225 cal., 8 g fat (1 g sat. fat), 42 mg chol., 231 mg sodium, 36 g carb., 2 g fiber, 3 g pro.* **Diabetic Exchanges:** *1½ starch, 1½ fat, ½ fruit.*

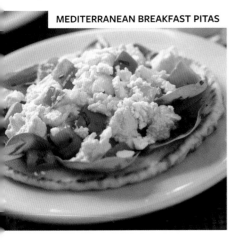

MEDITERRANEAN BREAKFAST PITAS

Delectable Granola

Be sure to remove this granola from the cookie sheets within 20 minutes of baking—otherwise the granola may stick to the sheets.

—**LORI STEVENS** RIVERTON, UT

PREP: 20 MIN. • **BAKE:** 30 MIN. + COOLING
MAKES: 11 CUPS

- 8 **cups old-fashioned oats**
- 1 **cup finely chopped almonds**
- 1 **cup finely chopped pecans**
- ½ **cup flaked coconut**
- ½ **cup packed brown sugar**
- ½ **cup canola oil**
- ½ **cup honey**
- ¼ **cup maple syrup**
- 2 **teaspoons ground cinnamon**
- 1½ **teaspoons salt**
- 2 **teaspoons vanilla extract**
  Plain yogurt, optional

1. In a large bowl, combine the oats, almonds, pecans and coconut. In a small saucepan, combine the brown sugar, oil, honey, maple syrup, cinnamon and salt. Heat for 3-4 minutes over medium heat until the sugar is dissolved. Remove from the heat; stir in vanilla. Pour over the oat mixture; stir to coat.

2. Transfer to two 15x10x1-in. baking pans coated with cooking spray. Bake at 350° for 25-30 minutes or until crisp, stirring every 10 minutes. Cool completely on wire racks. Store in an airtight container. Serve with yogurt if desired.

PER SERVING *½ cup equals 288 cal., 15 g fat (2 g sat. fat), 0 chol., 170 mg sodium, 36 g carb., 4 g fiber, 6 g pro. Diabetic Exchanges: 2½ starch, 2 fat.*

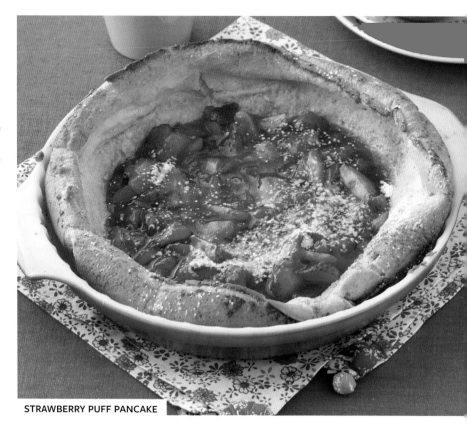

STRAWBERRY PUFF PANCAKE

Strawberry Puff Pancake

This recipe serves four, but if you just need it for two, use 2 eggs and ½ cup milk. It's yummy served with either strawberry or blueberry topping.

—**BRENDA MORTON** HALE CENTER, TX

START TO FINISH: 30 MIN.
MAKES: 4 SERVINGS

- 2 **tablespoons butter**
- 3 **eggs**
- ¾ **cup fat-free milk**
- 1 **teaspoon vanilla extract**
- ¾ **cup all-purpose flour**
- ⅛ **teaspoon salt**
- ⅛ **teaspoon ground cinnamon**
- ¼ **cup sugar**
- 1 **tablespoon cornstarch**
- ½ **cup water**
- 1 **cup sliced fresh strawberries**
  Confectioners' sugar

1. Place butter in a 9-in. pie plate; place in a 400° oven for 4-5 minutes or until melted. Meanwhile, in a small bowl, whisk the eggs, milk and vanilla. In another small bowl, combine the flour, salt and cinnamon; whisk into egg mixture until blended.

2. Pour into prepared pie plate. Bake for 15-20 minutes or until sides are crisp and golden brown.

3. In a small saucepan, combine the sugar and cornstarch. Stir in water until smooth; add strawberries. Cook and stir over medium heat until thickened. Coarsely mash strawberries. Serve with pancake. Dust with the confectioners' sugar.

PER SERVING *277 cal., 10 g fat (5 g sat. fat), 175 mg chol., 187 mg sodium, 38 g carb., 2 g fiber, 9 g pro. Diabetic Exchanges: 2½ starch, 1 medium-fat meat, 1 fat.*

Savory Omelet Cups

I replaced the pastry portion of this recipe with lighter crepe-like cups. Baked in tiny oven-proof dishes, they're filled with cheese, leeks, scallions, olives and some sun-dried tomatoes.

—**JOAN CHURCHILL** DOVER, NH

PREP: 40 MIN. • **BAKE:** 10 MIN.
MAKES: 4 SERVINGS

- ¼ **cup sun-dried tomatoes (not packed in oil)**
- ½ **cup water, divided**
- 3 **eggs**
- 6 **egg whites**
- 2 **tablespoons minced fresh cilantro**
- 4 **teaspoons butter, melted**
- ½ **teaspoon salt**
- ¼ **teaspoon pepper**
- ⅓ **cup shredded provolone cheese**
- 1 **cup chopped leeks (white portion only)**
- 2 **green onions, chopped**
- 1 **tablespoon olive oil**
- 2 **tablespoons chopped Greek olives**
- 2 **teaspoons minced fresh oregano or ½ teaspoon dried oregano**
- ¼ **cup grated Parmesan cheese**
- 1 **tablespoon honey**

1. Place tomatoes in a small bowl. Cover with ¼ cup water; let stand for 30 minutes. Meanwhile, in a large bowl, whisk the eggs, egg whites, cilantro, butter, salt, pepper and the remaining water.

2. Heat an 8-in. nonstick skillet coated with cooking spray; pour about ½ cup egg mixture into center of skillet. Lift and tilt pan to evenly coat bottom. Cook for 1½ to 2 minutes or until top appears dry; turn and cook for 30-45 seconds longer or until set.

3. Remove from pan and press into a 1-cup baking dish or ramekin coated with cooking spray. Repeat with remaining egg mixture, making three more omelet cups (coat skillet with cooking spray as needed). Sprinkle provolone cheese into cups.

4. Drain tomatoes; chop and set aside. In a large nonstick skillet, saute leeks and onions in oil until tender. Stir in the tomatoes, olives and oregano; cook over medium heat for 2-3 minutes. Spoon into omelet cups. Sprinkle with Parmesan cheese; drizzle with honey.

5. Bake at 350° for 10-12 minutes or until heated through.

PER SERVING *246 cal., 16 g fat (6 g sat. fat), 178 mg chol., 764 mg sodium, 12 g carb., 1 g fiber, 15 g pro.* **Diabetic Exchanges::** *2 lean meat, 2 fat, 1 vegetable.*

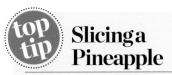

Slicing a Pineapple

Cut the crown and the rind from a pineapple. Slice off the base, and stand the pineapple upright. Follow the pattern of the eyes to cut diagonal wedge-shaped grooves in pineapple. Remove the wedges. Stand pineapple upright and cut off fruit next to, but not through, the core. Cut pieces into chunks or spears.

Warm Fruit Kabobs

We make these grilled kabobs for brunch, but they'd also be wonderful for dessert.

—**JANET SCHROEDER** STRAWBERRY POINT, IA

START TO FINISH: 30 MIN.
MAKES: 8 SERVINGS

- 1 **medium apple**
- 1 **medium banana**
- 1 **medium peach or nectarine**
- 1 **medium pear**
- 2 **slices fresh pineapple (1 inch thick)**
- 2 **tablespoons brown sugar**
- 2 **tablespoons lemon juice**
- 2 **tablespoons canola oil**
- 1 **teaspoon ground cinnamon**

1. Cut all of the fruit into 1-in. chunks. Alternately thread onto 16 soaked wooden skewers (using two skewers side by side for each kabob so fruit doesn't turn). In a small bowl, combine brown sugar, lemon juice, oil and the cinnamon.

2. Grill kabobs, uncovered, over medium heat 6 minutes or until heated through, turning often and basting frequently with brown sugar mixture.

PER SERVING *1 kabob equals 144 cal., 4 g fat (1 g sat. fat), 0 chol., 3 mg sodium, 29 g carb., 3 g fiber, 1 g pro.* **Diabetic Exchanges:** *2 fruit, ½ fat.*

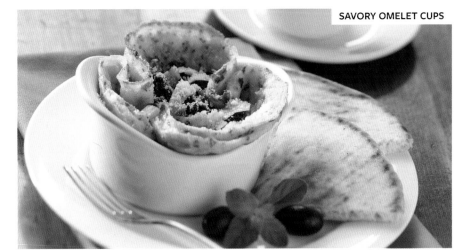

SAVORY OMELET CUPS

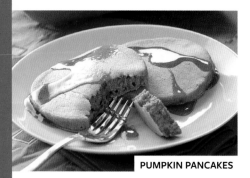

PUMPKIN PANCAKES

Pumpkin Pancakes

I created these pumpkin-flavored pancakes with two kinds of flour and a blend of spices. Serve them for brunch as a hearty eye-opener or for a change-of-pace dinner.

—VICKI FLODEN STORY CITY, IA

START TO FINISH: 20 MIN.
MAKES: 6 SERVINGS

- 1½ cups all-purpose flour
- ½ cup whole wheat flour
- 2 tablespoons brown sugar
- 2 teaspoons baking powder
- 1 teaspoon ground cinnamon
- ½ teaspoon salt
- ½ teaspoon ground ginger
- ½ teaspoon ground nutmeg
- 2 cups fat-free milk
- ½ cup canned pumpkin
- 1 egg white, lightly beaten
- 2 tablespoons canola oil

1. In a large bowl, combine the first eight ingredients. In a small bowl, combine the milk, pumpkin, egg white and oil; stir into dry ingredients just until moistened.

2. Pour batter by ¼ cupfuls onto a hot griddle coated with cooking spray; turn when bubbles form on top. Cook until second side is golden brown.

PER SERVING *2 pancakes equals 240 cal., 5 g fat (1 g sat. fat), 1 mg chol., 375 mg sodium, 41 g carb., 3 g fiber, 8 g pro.* **Diabetic Exchanges:** *2½ starch, 1 fat.*

Wholesome Whole-Grain Waffles

Here, I tweaked one of my waffle recipes. I added flax seed, substituted whole-wheat flour for some all-purpose, applesauce for some oil, and fat-free milk for whole. My family loved all the changes, and now it's a favorite breakfast treat we can all enjoy.

—JUDY PARKER MOORE, OK

PREP: 15 MIN. • **COOK:** 5 MIN./BATCH
MAKES: 12 WAFFLES

- 1 cup all-purpose flour
- 1 cup whole wheat flour
- 3 tablespoons ground flaxseed
- 3 teaspoons baking powder
- ½ teaspoon salt
- 2 eggs, separated
- 2 cups fat-free milk
- 3 tablespoons canola oil
- 3 tablespoons unsweetened applesauce
  Mixed fresh berries and confectioners' sugar, optional

1. In a large bowl, combine the flours, flax, baking powder and salt. Combine the egg yolks, milk, oil and applesauce; stir into dry ingredients until just moistened.

2. In a small bowl, beat egg whites until stiff peaks form; fold into batter.

3. Bake in a preheated waffle iron according to manufacturer's directions until golden brown. Serve with berries and confectioners' sugar if desired.

4. To freeze, arrange waffles in a single layer on sheet pans. Freeze overnight or until frozen. Transfer to a resealable plastic freezer bag. Waffles may be frozen for up to 2 months.

TO USE FROZEN WAFFLES *Reheat waffles in a toaster. Serve with berries and confectioners' sugar if desired.*

PER SERVING *2 waffles equals 278 cal., 11 g fat (1 g sat. fat), 70 mg chol., 456 mg sodium, 37 g carb., 4 g fiber, 11 g pro.* **Diabetic Exchanges:** *2½ starch, 1½ fat.*

WHOLESOME WHOLE-GRAIN WAFFLES

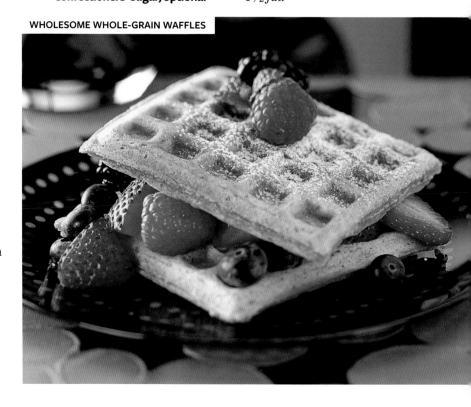

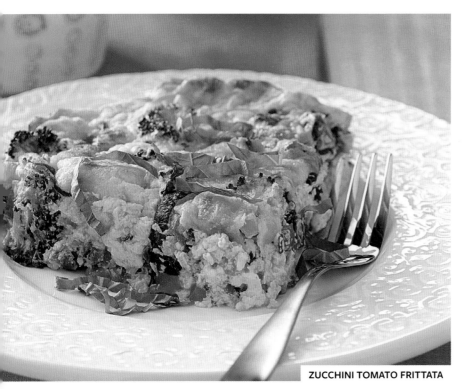

ZUCCHINI TOMATO FRITTATA

Black Forest Crepes

Cherries and chocolate are always great together, but the combination is even better when wrapped in warm crepes.

—**MARY RELYEA** CANASTOTA, NY

START TO FINISH: 20 MIN.
MAKES: 8 SERVINGS

- 1 **package (8 ounces) reduced-fat cream cheese, softened**
- ½ **cup reduced-fat sour cream**
- ½ **teaspoon vanilla extract**
- ⅔ **cup confectioners' sugar**
- 8 **prepared crepes (9 inches)**
- 1 **can (20 ounces) reduced-sugar cherry pie filling, warmed**
- ¼ **cup chocolate syrup**

1. In a small bowl, beat the cream cheese, sour cream and vanilla until smooth. Gradually beat in confectioners' sugar. Spread about 3 tablespoons over each crepe to within ½ in. of edges and roll up.

2. Arrange in an ungreased 13-in. x 9-in. baking dish. Bake, uncovered, at 350° for 5-7 minutes or until warm. To serve, top each crepe with ¼ cup pie filling and drizzle with 1½ teaspoons chocolate syrup.

PER SERVING *1 crepe equals 256 cal., 9 g fat (6 g sat. fat), 31 mg chol., 222 mg sodium, 39 g carb., 1 g fiber, 6 g pro.* **Diabetic Exchanges:** *2½ starch, 1½ fat.*

BLACK FOREST CREPES

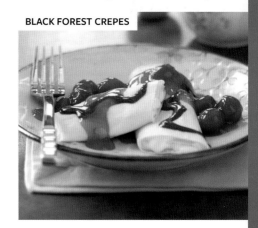

Zucchini Tomato Frittata

Frittata is Italian for omelet, and this one is packed full of veggies. Egg substitute and low-fat cheese lighten it up, making for a healthy morning meal.

—**KIM SOSEBEE** CLEVELAND, GA

PREP: 20 MIN. • **COOK:** 15 MIN.
MAKES: 4 SERVINGS

- ⅓ **cup sun-dried tomatoes (not packed in oil)**
- 1 **cup boiling water**
- 1½ **cups egg substitute**
- ½ **cup 2% cottage cheese**
- 2 **green onions, chopped**
- ¼ **cup minced fresh basil or 1 tablespoon dried basil**
- ⅛ **teaspoon crushed red pepper flakes**
- 1 **cup sliced zucchini**
- 1 **cup fresh broccoli florets**
- 1 **medium sweet red pepper, chopped**
- 2 **teaspoons canola oil**
- 2 **tablespoons grated Parmesan cheese**

1. Place tomatoes in a small bowl. Cover with boiling water; let stand for 5 minutes. Drain and set aside.

2. In a large bowl, whisk the egg substitute, cottage cheese, onions, basil, pepper flakes and reserved tomatoes; set aside.

3. In a 10-in. ovenproof skillet, saute the zucchini, broccoli and red pepper in oil until tender. Reduce heat; top with reserved egg mixture. Cover and cook for 4-6 minutes or until nearly set.

4. Uncover skillet. Sprinkle with Parmesan cheese. Broil 3-4 in. from the heat for 2-3 minutes or until eggs are completely set. Let stand for 5 minutes. Cut into wedges.

PER SERVING *138 cal., 4 g fat (1 g sat. fat), 6 mg chol., 484 mg sodium, 11 g carb., 3 g fiber, 15 g pro.* **Diabetic Exchanges:** *2 lean meat, 2 vegetable.*

Vanilla Fruit Salad

Peach pie filling is the secret ingredient in this crowd-pleasing salad. Make it throughout the year using whatever fruits are in season.

—**NANCY DODSON** SPRINGFIELD, IL

START TO FINISH: 20 MIN.
MAKES: 10 SERVINGS

- 1 **pound fresh strawberries, quartered**
- 1½ **cups seedless red and/or green grapes, halved**
- 2 **medium bananas, sliced**
- 2 **kiwifruit, peeled, sliced and quartered**
- 1 **cup cubed fresh pineapple**
- 1 **can (21 ounces) peach pie filling**
- 3 **teaspoons vanilla extract**

In a large bowl, combine the strawberries, grapes, bananas, kiwi and pineapple. Fold in pie filling and vanilla. Chill until serving.

PER SERVING *¾ cup equals 126 cal., trace fat (trace sat. fat), 0 chol., 12 mg sodium, 30 g carb., 3 g fiber, 2 g pro.* **Diabetic Exchange:** *2 fruit.*

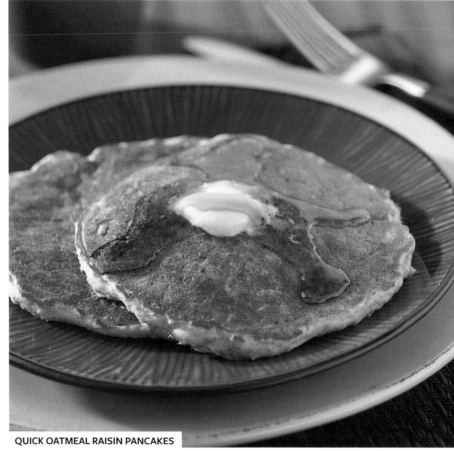
QUICK OATMEAL RAISIN PANCAKES

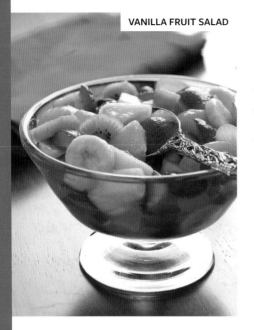
VANILLA FRUIT SALAD

Quick Oatmeal Raisin Pancakes

I found this recipe in a newspaper nearly 50 years ago and have used it ever since.

—**KAREL HURT** CORTEZ, CO

PREP: 15 MIN. • **COOK:** 10 MIN./BATCH
MAKES: 12 PANCAKES

- 2 **cups quick-cooking oats**
- 2 **cups buttermilk**
- ½ **cup egg substitute**
- 2 **tablespoons canola oil**
- ½ **cup all-purpose flour**
- 2 **tablespoons sugar**
- 1 **teaspoon baking powder**
- 1 **teaspoon baking soda**
- 1 **teaspoon ground cinnamon**
- ¼ **teaspoon salt**
- ½ **cup raisins**

1. In a small bowl, combine oats and buttermilk; let stand for 5 minutes. Stir in egg substitute and oil; set aside.
2. In a large bowl, combine the flour, sugar, baking powder, baking soda, cinnamon and salt. Stir in the wet ingredients just until moistened; add the raisins.
3. Pour batter by heaping ¼ cupfuls onto a hot griddle coated with cooking spray; turn when bubbles form on top. Cook until second side is golden brown.

PER SERVING *2 pancakes equals 274 cal., 7 g fat (1 g sat. fat), 3 mg chol., 505 mg sodium, 44 g carb., 3 g fiber, 10 g pro.* **Diabetic Exchanges:** *2 starch, 1 fruit, 1 fat.*

Sausage & Salsa Breakfast Burritos

The best of breakfast gets wrapped up snugly in a hand-held feast for this on-the-go meal and easy recipe.

—**MICHELLE BURNETT** EDEN, UT

START TO FINISH: 20 MIN.
MAKES: 6 SERVINGS

- **5 breakfast turkey sausage links**
- **2 cartons (8 ounces each) egg substitute**
- **½ cup salsa**
- **¼ teaspoon pepper**
- **6 whole wheat tortilla (8 inches), warmed**
- **½ cup shredded reduced-fat cheddar cheese**

1. Cook sausage links according to package directions. Meanwhile, in a large bowl, whisk the egg substitute, salsa and pepper. Pour into a large nonstick skillet coated with cooking spray. Cook and stir over medium heat until eggs are nearly set. Chop the sausage links. Add to egg mixture; cook and stir until completely set.

2. Spoon ⅓ cup egg mixture off center on each tortilla and sprinkle with 4 teaspoons cheese. Fold sides and ends over filling and roll up.

PER SERVING *265 cal., 10 g fat (3 g sat. fat), 25 mg chol., 602 mg sodium, 25 g carb., 2 g fiber, 18 g pro.* **Diabetic Exchanges:** *2 lean meat, 1½ starch, 1 fat.*

SAUSAGE & SALSA BREAKFAST BURRITOS

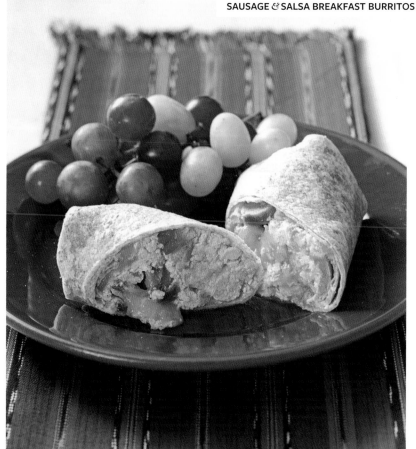

Breakfast Mushroom Cups

Enjoy these bite-sized stuffed mushrooms for a savory take on breakfast.

—**SARA MORRIS** LAGUNA BEACH, CA

START TO FINISH: 25 MIN.
MAKES: 2 SERVINGS

- **2 large portobello mushrooms, stems removed**
- **⅛ teaspoon garlic salt**
- **⅛ teaspoon pepper, divided**
- **1 small onion, chopped**
- **½ teaspoon olive oil**
- **1 cup fresh baby spinach**
- **½ cup egg substitute**
- **⅛ teaspoon salt**
- **¼ cup crumbled goat or feta cheese**
- **2 tablespoons minced fresh basil**

1. Place mushrooms on a 15x10x1-in. baking pan. Spray with cooking spray; sprinkle with garlic salt and a dash of pepper. Bake at 425° for 10 minutes or until tender.

2. In a large saucepan, saute onion in oil until tender. Stir in spinach and cook until wilted. In a small bowl, whisk egg substitute, salt and remaining pepper; add to pan. Cook and stir until set.

3. Spoon egg mixture into mushrooms; sprinkle with cheese and basil.

PER SERVING *126 cal., 5 g fat (2 g sat. fat), 18 mg chol., 472 mg sodium, 10 g carb., 3 g fiber, 11 g pro.* **Diabetic Exchanges:** *2 vegetable, 1 lean meat, ½ fat.*

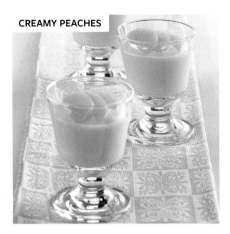
CREAMY PEACHES

Creamy Peaches

High in protein and virtually fat-free, this creamy breakfast treat can also double as a light dessert.

—DON PROKIDANSKY NEW PORT RICHEY, FL

START TO FINISH: 10 MIN.
MAKES: 4 SERVINGS

- 1 **can (15 ounces) sliced peaches in extra-light syrup, drained**
- 1½ **cups (12 ounces) fat-free cottage cheese**
- 4 **ounces fat-free cream cheese, cubed**
  Sugar substitute equivalent to 1 tablespoon sugar

1. Thinly slice four peach slices; set aside for garnish. Place remaining peaches in a food processor; add the cottage cheese. Cover and process until blended. Add cream cheese and sugar substitute; cover and process until blended.

2. Spoon into four serving dishes. Top with reserved peaches. Refrigerate until serving.

NOTE *This recipe was tested with Splenda no-calorie sweetener.*

PER SERVING *127 cal., trace fat (trace sat. fat), 6 mg chol., 443 mg sodium, 15 g carb., 1 g fiber, 15 g pro.* **Diabetic Exchanges:** *2 lean meat, ½ starch, ½ fruit.*

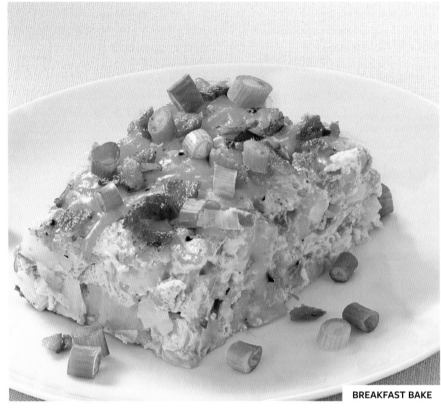
BREAKFAST BAKE

Breakfast Bake

I wanted to have scrambled eggs and hash browns one morning, so I created this dish. My wife loved it...and guess who's making breakfast more often now?

—HOWARD ROGERS EL PASO, TX

PREP: 15 MIN. • **BAKE:** 50 MIN.
MAKES: 6 SERVINGS

- 1½ **cups egg substitute**
- ½ **cup fat-free milk**
- 3½ **cups frozen O'Brien potatoes, thawed**
- 1⅓ **cups shredded reduced-fat cheddar cheese, divided**
- ½ **cup chopped sweet onion**
- 4 **tablespoons crumbled cooked bacon, divided**
- ½ **teaspoon salt**
- ½ **teaspoon salt-free seasoning blend**
- ¼ **teaspoon chili powder**
- 4 **green onions, chopped**

1. In a large bowl, whisk egg substitute and milk. Stir in the potatoes, 1 cup of cheese, onion, 2 tablespoons of bacon, salt, seasoning blend and chili powder. Pour into an 8-in. square baking dish coated with cooking spray.

2. Bake at 350° for 45-50 minutes or until a knife inserted near the center comes out clean. Sprinkle with remaining cheese and bacon. Bake 3-5 minutes longer or until cheese is melted. Sprinkle with green onions. Let stand for 5 minutes before cutting.

PER SERVING *219 cal., 6 g fat (4 g sat. fat), 22 mg chol., 682 mg sodium, 25 g carb., 3 g fiber, 17 g pro.* **Diabetic Exchanges:** *2 lean meat, 1½ starch.*

French Omelet

After first tasting a similar frittata at a restaurant, I went home and created my own low-fat version. I hope you like it!

—BERNICE MORRIS MARSHFIELD, MO

START TO FINISH: 20 MIN.
MAKES: 2 SERVINGS

- 2 eggs, lightly beaten
- ½ cup egg substitute
- ¼ cup fat-free milk
- ⅛ teaspoon salt
- ⅛ teaspoon pepper
- ¼ cup cubed fully cooked lean ham
- 1 tablespoon chopped onion
- 1 tablespoon chopped green pepper
- ¼ cup shredded reduced-fat cheddar cheese

1. In a small bowl, whisk the eggs, egg substitute, milk, salt and pepper. Coat a 10-in. nonstick skillet with cooking spray and place over medium heat. Add egg mixture to skillet (mixture should set immediately at edges).
2. As eggs set, push cooked edges toward the center, letting uncooked portion flow underneath. When the eggs are set, sprinkle the ham, onion and green pepper on one side and sprinkle with cheese; fold other side over filling. Slide omelet onto a plate.
PER SERVING *180 cal., 9 g fat (4 g sat. fat), 230 mg chol., 661 mg sodium, 4 g carb., trace fiber, 20 g pro.* **Diabetic Exchanges:** *3 lean meat, 1 fat.*

Gluten-Free Baked Oatmeal

Sometimes I treat myself to a few chocolate chips sprinkled on this fruity, delicious oatmeal. It's also good served with vanilla soy milk.

—JENNIFER BANYAY NORTHRIDGEVILLE, OH

PREP: 15 MIN. • **BAKE:** 30 MIN.
MAKES: 6 SERVINGS

- ½ cup raisins
- 1½ cups boiling water
- 2 cups gluten-free old-fashioned oats
- ⅓ cup packed brown sugar
- 1 teaspoon pumpkin pie spice
- ¼ teaspoon salt
- 1¼ cups fat-free milk
- 1 medium apple, peeled and finely chopped
- 2 tablespoons butter, melted
- ¼ cup chopped walnuts

1. Place raisins in a small bowl. Cover with boiling water; let stand 5 minutes.
2. Meanwhile, in a large bowl, combine the oats, brown sugar, pie spice and salt. Stir in the milk, apple and butter. Let stand for 5 minutes. Drain raisins; stir into oat mixture.
3. Transfer to an 8-in. square baking dish coated with cooking spray. Sprinkle with the walnuts. Bake, uncovered, at 350° for 30-35 minutes or until a knife inserted near the center comes out clean.
NOTE *Read all ingredient labels for possible gluten content prior to use. Ingredient formulas can change, and production facilities vary among brands. If you're concerned that your brand may contain gluten, contact the company.*
PER SERVING *⅔ cup equals 275 cal., 9 g fat (3 g sat. fat), 11 mg chol., 154 mg sodium, 45 g carb., 4 g fiber, 7 g pro.* **Diabetic Exchanges:** *2 starch, 1 fruit, 1 fat.*

FRENCH OMELET

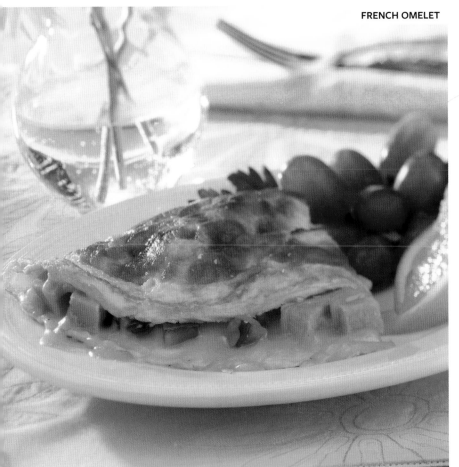

soups & sandwiches

You just can't beat the **classic combo** of a hot bowl of soup and a sandwich piled high with flavor. Serve as a satisfying lunch or speedy supper, but try these **stick-to-your-ribs** favorites soon!

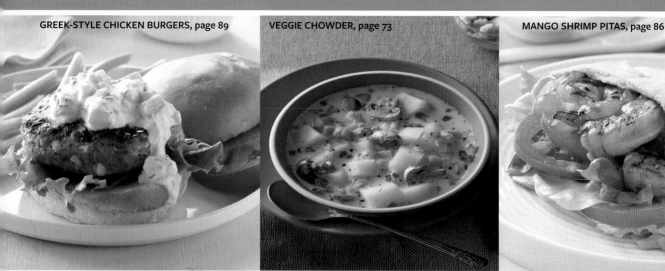

GREEK-STYLE CHICKEN BURGERS, page 89

VEGGIE CHOWDER, page 73

MANGO SHRIMP PITAS, page 86

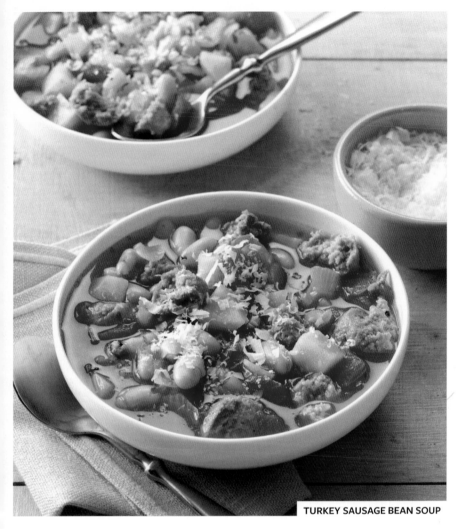

TURKEY SAUSAGE BEAN SOUP

1. In a Dutch oven, cook sausage, onion, fennel and celery root over medium heat 4-5 minutes or until sausage is no longer pink, breaking into crumbles; drain. Stir in tomatoes, water, bay leaves, beef base, Italian seasoning and pepper.
2. Bring to a boil. Reduce heat; simmer, covered, 20 minutes or until vegetables are tender. Stir in beans; heat through. Remove bay leaves. If desired, top servings with cheese.

PER SERVING *1 cup equals 168 cal., 4 g fat (1 g sat. fat), 20 mg chol., 585 mg sodium, 22 g carb., 6 g fiber, 11 g pro.* **Diabetic Exchanges:** *1½ starch, 1 medium-fat meat.*

Pulled Pork Sandwiches

You'll love the ease of this recipe—just throw everything in the slow cooker and get out of the kitchen. You hardly have to lift a finger for the delicious results!

—**TERRI MCKITRICK** DELAFIELD, WI

PREP: 15 MIN. • **COOK:** 7 HOURS
MAKES: 8 SERVINGS

- 1 can (8 ounces) tomato sauce
- 1 cup chopped onion
- 1 cup barbecue sauce
- 3 teaspoons chili powder
- 1 teaspoon ground cumin
- ½ teaspoon ground cinnamon
- 1 boneless pork sirloin roast (2 pounds), trimmed
- 8 seeded hamburger buns, split

1. In a 3-qt. slow cooker, combine the first six ingredients; add the pork. Spoon some of the sauce over pork. Cover and cook on low for 7 hours or until meat is tender.
2. Remove meat; shred with two forks. Return to slow cooker and heat through. Spoon ½ cup onto each bun.

PER SERVING *322 cal., 10 g fat (3 g sat. fat), 68 mg chol., 681 mg sodium, 29 g carb., 3 g fiber, 28 g pro.* **Diabetic Exchanges:** *3 lean meat, 2 starch.*

Turkey Sausage Bean Soup

This recipe is from my great-grandmother, though I've added a few ingredients to make it my own. Served with a side salad and some artisan bread, it's a wonderful, hearty family dinner.

—**TERREL PORTER-SMITH** LOS OSOS, CA

PREP: 15 MIN. • **COOK:** 25 MIN.
MAKES: 8 SERVINGS (2 QUARTS)

- 4 Italian turkey sausage links, casings removed
- 1 large onion, chopped
- 1 cup chopped fennel bulb
- 1 cup chopped celery root or peeled turnip
- 1 can (14½ ounces) no-salt-added diced tomatoes, undrained
- 3 cups water
- 4 bay leaves
- 1 tablespoon reduced-sodium beef base
- 2 teaspoons Italian seasoning
- ½ teaspoon pepper
- 2 cans (15 ounces each) white kidney or cannellini beans, rinsed and drained
  Shaved Parmesan cheese, optional

Turkey Florentine Sandwiches

I upgraded a lunchtime classic to this dinnertime feast with just a few basic ingredient tweaks. I hope you like it!

—KAREL REYNOLDS RUTHERFORDTON, NC

START TO FINISH: 20 MIN.
MAKES: 2 SERVINGS

- ½ cup sliced fresh mushrooms
- 2 teaspoons olive oil
- 1 cup fresh baby spinach
- 2 garlic cloves, minced
- 4 ounces sliced deli turkey breast
- 2 slices part-skim mozzarella cheese
- 4 slices whole wheat bread
  Cooking spray

1. In a small nonstick skillet, saute mushrooms in oil until tender. Add spinach and garlic; cook 1 minute longer.

2. Layer the spinach mixture, turkey and cheese on two bread slices; top with remaining bread. Spritz outsides of sandwiches with cooking spray. Cook on a panini maker or indoor grill for 4-5 minutes or until bread is browned and cheese is melted.

PER SERVING *346 cal., 14 g fat (5 g sat. fat), 35 mg chol., 937 mg sodium, 27 g carb., 4 g fiber, 27 g pro.* **Diabetic Exchanges:** *3 lean meat, 2 starch, 1 fat.*

TURKEY FLORENTINE SANDWICHES

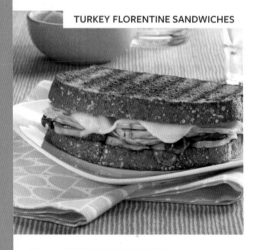

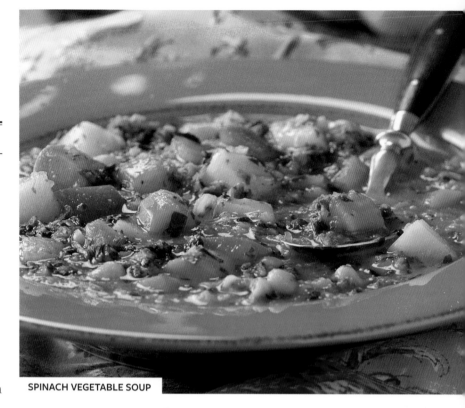

SPINACH VEGETABLE SOUP

Spinach Vegetable Soup

If you like your soup thick, you'll want to spoon up a bowl of this specialty! The unbeatable taste comes from fresh vegetables accented with fragrant herbs.

—JENNIFER NEILSEN WILLIAMSTON, NC

PREP: 15 MIN. • **COOK:** 25 MIN.
MAKES: 6 SERVINGS

- ½ cup chopped onion
- ½ cup chopped celery
- 1 tablespoon butter
- 2 cans (14½ ounces each) reduced-sodium chicken broth or vegetable broth
- 1½ cups diced peeled potatoes
- 1 small turnip, peeled and chopped
- 1 cup chopped carrot
- ½ cup chopped green pepper
- 1 teaspoon garlic powder
- 1 teaspoon each dried thyme, basil and rosemary, crushed
- 1 teaspoon rubbed sage
- ½ teaspoon salt
- ¼ teaspoon pepper
  Dash to ⅛ teaspoon cayenne pepper
- 2 packages (10 ounces each) frozen chopped spinach, thawed and well drained
- 1 can (14¾ ounces) cream-style corn

1. In a Dutch oven, saute onion and celery in butter until tender. Add the broth, potatoes, turnip, carrot, green pepper and seasonings. Bring to a boil. Reduce heat; cover and simmer for 15-20 minutes or until the vegetables are tender.

2. Stir in spinach and corn; cool slightly. Puree half of the soup in a blender; return to pan. Heat through.

PER SERVING *1⅓ cups equals 139 cal., 3 g fat (1 g sat. fat), 5 mg chol., 788 mg sodium, 26 g carb., 6 g fiber, 7 g pro.* **Diabetic Exchanges:** *2 vegetable, 1 starch, ½ fat.*

Thai Chicken Lettuce Wraps

This recipe is so flavorful and fresh tasting! The teachers and staff at my school love it because it's so much fun to put the wraps together yourself.

—LAUREEN PITTMAN RIVERSIDE, CA

PREP: 35 MIN.
MAKES: 6 SERVINGS

- ¼ cup rice vinegar
- 2 tablespoons lime juice
- 2 tablespoons reduced-fat mayonnaise
- 2 tablespoons reduced-fat creamy peanut butter
- 1 tablespoon brown sugar
- 1 tablespoon reduced-sodium soy sauce
- 2 teaspoons minced fresh gingerroot
- 1 teaspoon sesame oil
- 1 teaspoon Thai chili sauce
- 1 garlic clove, chopped
- 3 tablespoons canola oil
- ½ cup minced fresh cilantro

CHICKEN SALAD

- 2 cups cubed cooked chicken breast
- 1 small sweet red pepper, diced
- ½ cup chopped green onions
- ½ cup shredded carrot
- ½ cup unsalted dry roasted peanuts, chopped, divided
- 6 Bibb or Boston lettuce leaves

1. In a blender, combine the first 10 ingredients. While processing, gradually add oil in a steady stream; stir in cilantro. Set aside.

2. In a large bowl, combine the chicken, red pepper, onions, carrot and ¼ cup peanuts. Add dressing and toss to coat. Divide among lettuce leaves; sprinkle with remaining peanuts. Fold lettuce over filling.

PER SERVING *1½ cup chicken salad equals 284 cal., 19 g fat (2 g sat. fat), 38 mg chol., 222 mg sodium, 12 g carb., 2 g fiber, 19 g pro.* **Diabetic Exchanges:** *2 lean meat, 2 fat, 1 starch.*

Pea Soup with Quinoa

Low in fat and high in fiber, this soup is a definite keeper. Plus, it's so simple to make. You'll turn to it time and again!

—JANE HACKER MILWAUKEE, WI

PREP: 10 MIN. • **COOK:** 25 MIN.
MAKES: 4 SERVINGS

- 1 cup water
- ½ cup quinoa, rinsed
- 1 medium onion, chopped
- 2 teaspoons canola oil
- 2 cans (14½ ounces each) reduced-sodium chicken broth or vegetable broth
- 2 packages (10 ounces each) frozen peas
- ½ teaspoon salt
- ¼ teaspoon pepper
- 2 teaspoons reduced-fat plain yogurt

1. In a small saucepan, bring water to a boil. Add quinoa. Reduce heat; cover and simmer for 12-15 minutes or until water is absorbed.

2. Meanwhile, in a large saucepan, saute onion in oil until tender. Stir in broth and peas. Bring to a boil. Reduce heat; simmer, uncovered, for 5 minutes or until peas are tender. Cool slightly.

3. In a blender, process soup in batches until smooth. Return all to the pan. Stir in the salt, pepper and quinoa; heat through. Garnish each serving with ½ teaspoon yogurt.

NOTE *Look for quinoa in the cereal, rice or organic food aisle.*

PER SERVING *1½ cups equals 236 cal., 4 g fat (trace sat. fat), trace chol., 858 mg sodium, 38 g carb., 9 g fiber, 13 g pro.* **Diabetic Exchanges:** *2½ starch, ½ fat.*

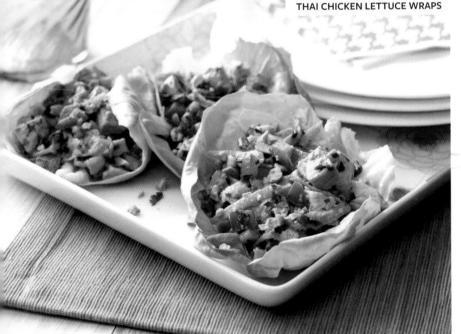

THAI CHICKEN LETTUCE WRAPS

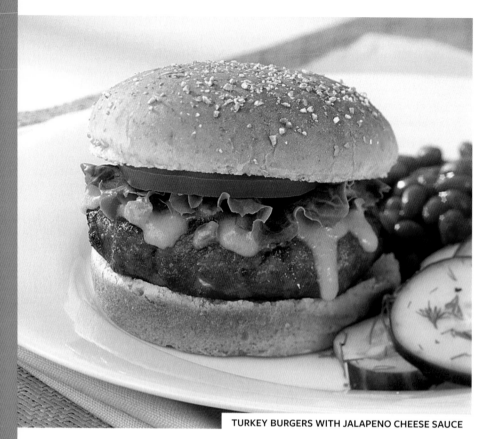

TURKEY BURGERS WITH JALAPENO CHEESE SAUCE

4. Serve on buns with lettuce, tomato and jalapeno cheese sauce.

NOTE *Wear disposable gloves when cutting hot peppers; the oils can burn skin. Avoid touching your face.*

PER SERVING *387 cal., 15 g fat (5 g sat. fat), 100 mg chol., 599 mg sodium, 33 g carb., 5 g fiber, 30 g pro.* **Diabetic Exchanges:** *3 lean meat, 2 starch, 1 fat.*

Zippy Burgers

Enhance lean ground beef with onion powder, chili powder and red pepper flakes. These satisfying burgers are sure to sizzle at any barbecue.

—TASTE OF HOME TEST KITCHEN

START TO FINISH: 20 MIN.
MAKES: 4 SERVINGS

- ¼ cup beer or beef broth
- 2 tablespoons Worcestershire sauce
- 2 teaspoons chili powder
- 1 teaspoon onion powder
- ½ teaspoon crushed red pepper flakes
- ¼ teaspoon salt
- ¼ teaspoon pepper
- 1 pound lean ground beef (90% lean)
- 4 hamburger buns, split

1. In a large bowl, combine the first seven ingredients. Crumble beef over mixture and mix well. Shape into four patties.
2. Using long-handled tongs, moisten a paper towel with cooking oil and lightly coat the grill rack. Grill hamburgers, covered, over medium heat or broil 4 in. from the heat for 6-8 minutes on each side or until a thermometer reads 160° and juices run clear. Serve on buns.

PER SERVING *314 cal., 12 g fat (4 g sat. fat), 70 mg chol., 557 mg sodium, 25 g carb., 2 g fiber, 25 g pro.* **Diabetic Exchanges:** *3 lean meat, 1½ starch.*

Turkey Burgers with Jalapeno Cheese Sauce

I took a burger recipe and replaced the beef with turkey and used low-fat cheese. To my delight, the result was even better than the original.

—VICKI SCHURK HAMDEN, CT

START TO FINISH: 25 MIN.
MAKES: 6 SERVINGS

- 3 slices whole wheat bread, torn
- 1 cup fat-free milk, divided
- 6 garlic cloves, minced
- 1½ teaspoons ground mustard
- ¼ teaspoon salt
- ¼ teaspoon pepper
- 1½ pounds lean ground turkey
- 1¼ teaspoons all-purpose flour
- ¾ cup shredded reduced-fat cheddar cheese
- 1 jalapeno pepper, seeded and chopped
- 6 whole wheat hamburger buns, split
- 6 lettuce leaves
- 6 slices tomato

1. In a large bowl, soak bread in ½ cup milk for 1 minute. Add the garlic, mustard, salt and pepper. Crumble turkey over mixture and mix well. Shape into six patties; set aside.
2. In a small saucepan, combine flour and remaining milk until smooth. Bring to a boil; cook and stir for 1-2 minutes or until thickened. Remove from the heat. Add cheese and jalapeno; stir until cheese is melted. Keep warm.
3. Using long-handled tongs, moisten a paper towel with cooking oil and lightly coat the grill rack. Grill patties, covered, over medium heat or broil 4 in. from the heat for 5-7 minutes on each side or until a meat thermometer reads 165° and juices run clear.

Vegetable Soup with Dumplings

Truly a complete meal in itself, this soup is loaded with vegetables. The fluffy carrot dumplings will have your family talking.
—**KAREN MAU** JACKSBORO, TN

PREP: 25 MIN. • **COOK:** 40 MIN.
MAKES: 10 SERVINGS

- 1½ **cups chopped onions**
- 4 **medium carrots, sliced**
- 3 **celery ribs, sliced**
- 2 **tablespoons canola oil**
- 3 **cups vegetable broth**
- 4 **medium potatoes, peeled and sliced**
- 4 **medium tomatoes, chopped**
- 2 **garlic cloves, minced**
- ½ **teaspoon salt**
- ½ **teaspoon pepper**
- ¼ **cup all-purpose flour**
- ½ **cup water**
- 1 **cup chopped cabbage**
- 1 **cup frozen peas**

CARROT DUMPLINGS

- 2¼ **cups reduced-fat biscuit/baking mix**
- 1 **cup shredded carrots**
- 1 **tablespoon minced fresh parsley**
- 1 **cup cold water**
- 10 **tablespoons shredded reduced-fat cheddar cheese**

1. In a Dutch oven, cook the onions, carrots and celery in oil for 6-8 minutes or until crisp-tender. Stir in the broth, potatoes, tomatoes, garlic, salt and pepper. Bring to a boil. Reduce heat; cover and simmer for 15-20 minutes or until vegetables are tender.

2. In a small bowl, combine flour and water until smooth; stir into vegetable mixture. Bring to a boil; cook and stir for 2 minutes or until thickened. Stir in the cabbage and peas.

3. For dumplings, in a small bowl, combine baking mix, carrots and parsley. Stir in the water until moistened. Drop in 10 mounds onto simmering soup. Cover and simmer for 15 minutes or until a toothpick inserted in a dumpling comes out clean (do not lift cover while simmering). Garnish with cheese.

PER SERVING *258 cal., 7 g fat (2 g sat. fat), 5 mg chol., 826 mg sodium, 44 g carb., 5 g fiber, 8 g pro.* **Diabetic Exchanges:** *2 starch, 2 vegetable, 1 fat.*

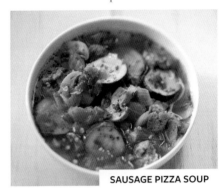

SAUSAGE PIZZA SOUP

Sausage Pizza Soup

If you love pizza but know you shouldn't have it, try this healthy alternative. You won't believe how delicious this soup is. It curbs any pizza cravings you might have.
—**BETH SHERER** MILWAUKEE, WI

PREP: 10 MIN. • **COOK:** 25 MIN.
MAKES: 4 SERVINGS

- ½ **pound Italian turkey sausage links, casings removed**
- 1 **medium zucchini, sliced**
- 1 **cup sliced fresh mushrooms**
- 1 **small onion, chopped**
- 1 **can (14½ ounces) no-salt-added diced tomatoes**
- 1 **cup water**
- 1 **cup reduced-sodium chicken broth**
- 1 **teaspoon dried basil**
- ¼ **teaspoon pepper**
  Minced fresh basil and crushed red pepper flakes, optional

In a large saucepan, cook the sausage, zucchini, mushrooms and onion over medium heat until meat is no longer pink; drain. Add the tomatoes, water, broth, dried basil and pepper. Bring to a boil. Reduce heat; simmer, uncovered, for 15 minutes. Sprinkle with fresh basil and pepper flakes if desired.

PER SERVING *1 cup equals 128 cal., 5 g fat (1 g sat. fat), 34 mg chol., 528 mg sodium, 9 g carb., 3 g fiber, 12 g pro.* **Diabetic Exchanges:** *2 vegetable, 1 medium-fat meat.*

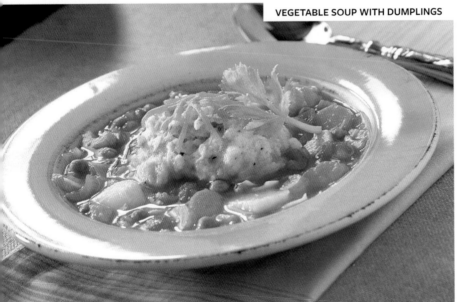

VEGETABLE SOUP WITH DUMPLINGS

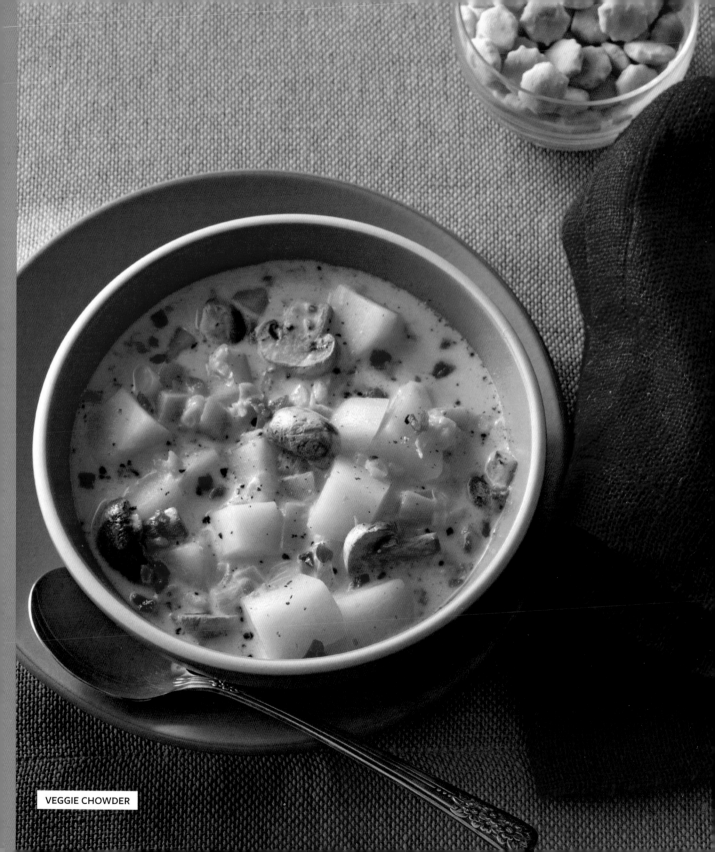

VEGGIE CHOWDER

Veggie Chowder

This brothy soup isn't too heavy, so it's perfect with a hearty sandwich. The great flavor is a wonderful way to get kids to eat their vegetables.

—VICKI KERR PORTLAND, ME

START TO FINISH: 30 MIN.
MAKES: 6 SERVINGS (1¾ QUARTS)

- 2 **cups cubed peeled potatoes**
- 2 **cups reduced-sodium chicken broth**
- 1 **cup chopped carrots**
- ½ **cup chopped onion**
- 1 **can (14¾ ounces) cream-style corn**
- 1 **can (12 ounces) fat-free evaporated milk**
- ¾ **cup shredded reduced-fat cheddar cheese**
- ½ **cup sliced fresh mushrooms**
- ¼ **teaspoon pepper**
- 2 **tablespoons bacon bits**

1. In a large saucepan, combine potatoes, broth, carrots and onion; bring to a boil. Reduce heat; simmer, uncovered, 10-15 minutes or until vegetables are tender.

2. Add corn, milk, cheese, mushrooms and pepper; cook and stir 4-6 minutes longer or until heated through. Sprinkle with bacon bits.

PER SERVING *1 cup equals 178 cal., 3 g fat (2 g sat. fat), 12 mg chol., 554 mg sodium, 29 g carb., 2 g fiber, 11 g pro. Diabetic Exchanges: 2 starch, ½ fat.*

top tip

Soup-er Secret

To chop carrots for soup, peel, remove the ends and cut the carrots into quarters. Then let the food processor do the chopping!
—MARION K. WATERLOO, IA

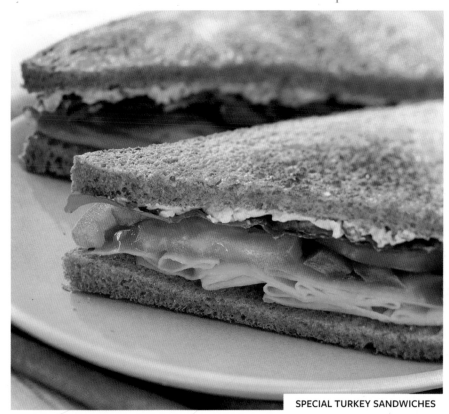

SPECIAL TURKEY SANDWICHES

Special Turkey Sandwiches

Every Saturday night, my family's tradition is to have lunch for dinner. With a rich cream cheese spread, these turkey sandwiches have become a favorite.

—MARIA L. C. BERTRAM WALTHAM, MA

START TO FINISH: 25 MIN.
MAKES: 4 SERVINGS

- 4 **ounces reduced-fat cream cheese**
- ½ **cup finely chopped fresh spinach**
- ½ **cup minced fresh basil**
- ⅓ **cup shredded Parmesan cheese**
- 1 **garlic clove, minced**
- ½ **large red onion, sliced**
- 2 **tablespoons dry red wine or reduced-sodium beef broth**
- 8 **slices whole wheat bread, toasted**
- ¾ **pound sliced deli turkey**
- 8 **slices tomato**
- 8 **lettuce leaves**

1. In a small bowl, beat the cream cheese, spinach, basil, cheese and garlic until blended; set aside. In a small skillet, cook onion in wine until tender; set aside.

2. Place four slices of toast on a broiler pan; top with turkey. Place remaining toast on broiler pan; spread with cream cheese mixture.

3. Broil 3-4 in. from the heat for 2-3 minutes or until heated through. Layer the onion, tomato and lettuce over turkey. Top with remaining toast.

PER SERVING *348 cal., 11 g fat (6 g sat. fat), 63 mg chol., 1,426 mg sodium, 36 g carb., 5 g fiber, 29 g pro. Diabetic Exchanges: 3 lean meat, 2 starch, 1½ fat.*

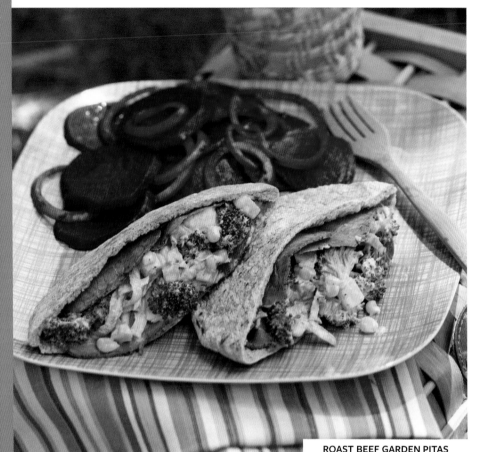

ROAST BEEF GARDEN PITAS

Prosciutto Egg Panini

Change up the usual bacon and egg sandwich by piling on prosciutto instead. It's a great for breakfast, lunch and dinner!

—ERIN RENOUF MYLROIE SANTA CLARA, UT

START TO FINISH: 30 MIN.
MAKES: 8 SERVINGS

- 3 **eggs**
- 2 **egg whites**
- 6 **tablespoons fat-free milk**
- 1 **green onion, thinly sliced**
- 1 **tablespoon Dijon mustard**
- 1 **tablespoon maple syrup**
- 8 **slices sourdough bread**
- 8 **thin slices prosciutto or deli ham**
- ½ **cup shredded sharp cheddar cheese**
- 8 **teaspoons butter**

1. In a small bowl, whisk the eggs, egg whites, milk and onion. Coat a large skillet with cooking spray and place over medium heat. Add egg mixture; cook and stir over medium heat until completely set.

2. Combine mustard and syrup; spread over four bread slices. Layer with scrambled eggs, prosciutto and cheese; top with remaining bread. Butter outsides of sandwiches.

3. Cook on a panini maker or indoor grill for 3-4 minutes or until bread is browned and cheese is melted. Cut each panini in half to serve.

PER SERVING *228 cal., 10 g fat (5 g sat. fat), 111 mg chol., 640 mg sodium, 21 g carb., 1 g fiber, 13 g pro.* **Diabetic Exchanges:** *1½ starch, 1½ fat, 1 lean meat.*

Roast Beef Garden Pitas

Featuring fresh veggies coated with a special horseradish dressing and topped with roast beef, these pitas appeal to all.

—NICOLE FILIZETTI JACKSONVILLE, FL

START TO FINISH: 20 MIN.
MAKES: 3 SERVINGS

- 3 **whole wheat pita pocket halves**
- ⅓ **pound thinly sliced deli roast beef**
- ¼ **cup chopped fresh broccoli**
- ¼ **cup frozen corn, thawed**
- ¼ **cup chopped seeded peeled cucumber**
- 2 **tablespoons shredded carrot**
- 2 **tablespoons finely chopped celery**
- 2 **tablespoons thinly sliced green onion**

DRESSING

- 1½ **teaspoons prepared horseradish**
- 1½ **teaspoons mayonnaise**
- 1½ **teaspoons reduced-fat sour cream**
- ½ **teaspoon Dijon mustard**
- ⅛ **teaspoon salt**
- ⅛ **teaspoon pepper**

1. Line pita halves with roast beef. In a small bowl, combine the broccoli, corn, cucumber, carrot, celery and onion.

2. In another bowl, combine the dressing ingredients. Pour over vegetable mixture; toss to coat. Fill pita halves.

PER SERVING *172 cal., 5 g fat (1 g sat. fat), 30 mg chol., 579 mg sodium, 20 g carb., 3 g fiber, 14 g pro.* **Diabetic Exchanges:** *2 lean meat, 1 starch, ½ fat.*

Southwestern Bean Chowder

My young children love this soup as much as my husband does. I like using white kidney beans—they have a terrific texture.

—JULI MEYERS HINESVILLE, GA

PREP: 20 MIN. • **COOK:** 35 MIN.
MAKES: 8 SERVINGS (2 QUARTS)

- 2 cans (15 ounces each) white kidney or cannellini beans, rinsed and drained, divided
- 1 medium onion, chopped
- ¼ cup chopped celery
- ¼ cup chopped green pepper
- 1 tablespoon olive oil
- 2 garlic cloves, minced
- 3 cups vegetable broth
- 1½ cups frozen corn, thawed
- 1 medium carrot, shredded
- 1 can (4 ounces) chopped green chilies
- 1 tablespoon ground cumin
- ½ teaspoon chili powder
- 4½ teaspoons cornstarch
- 2 cups 2% milk
- 1 cup (4 ounces) shredded cheddar cheese
    Minced fresh cilantro and additional shredded cheddar cheese, optional

1. In a small bowl, mash one can beans with a fork; set aside.

2. In a Dutch oven, saute the onion, celery and pepper in oil until tender. Add garlic; cook 1 minute longer. Stir in the mashed beans, broth, corn, carrot, chilies, cumin, chili powder and remaining beans. Bring to a boil. Reduce heat; simmer, uncovered, for 20 minutes.

3. Combine cornstarch and milk until smooth. Stir into bean mixture. Bring to a boil; cook and stir for 2 minutes or until thickened. Stir in cheese until melted. Serve with cilantro and additional cheese if desired.

PER SERVING *1 cup equals 236 cal., 8 g fat (4 g sat. fat), 20 mg chol., 670 mg sodium, 31 g carb., 6 g fiber, 11 g pro.* **Diabetic Exchanges:** *2 starch, 1 lean meat, ½ fat.*

Smoked Turkey & Slaw Wraps

Crunchy, colorful coleslaw adds a tangy twist to these wholesome wraps. Serve them for lunch or dinner—they're wonderful either way.

—DEBORAH WILLIAMS PEORIA, AZ

START TO FINISH: 15 MIN.
MAKES: 4 SERVINGS

- 1 cup shredded green cabbage
- ½ cup shredded red cabbage
- 1 small carrot, grated
- 1 green onion, thinly sliced
- 3 tablespoons reduced-fat mayonnaise
- 1 tablespoon lemon juice
- 2 teaspoons Dijon mustard
- ¼ teaspoon sugar
- 4 whole wheat tortillas (8 inches), room temperature
- ½ pound sliced deli smoked turkey
- 1 small tomato, sliced

1. In a small bowl, combine the first four ingredients. Combine the mayonnaise, lemon juice, mustard and sugar; pour over cabbage mixture and toss to coat.

2. Spoon cabbage mixture down the center of each tortilla. Top with turkey and tomato; roll up.

PER SERVING *260 cal., 8 g fat (1 g sat. fat), 24 mg chol., 761 mg sodium, 28 g carb., 3 g fiber, 17 g pro.* **Diabetic Exchanges:** *2 lean meat, 1½ starch, 1 vegetable, 1 fat.*

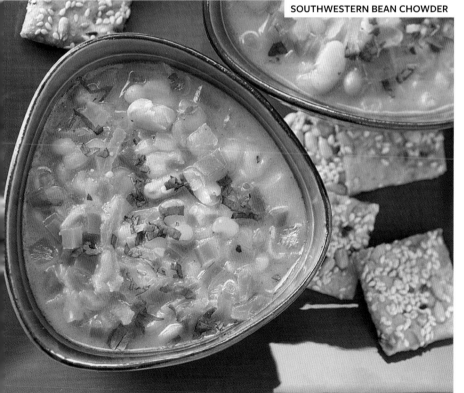

SOUTHWESTERN BEAN CHOWDER

Italian Beef Sandwiches

It takes very little effort to make these delicious sandwiches—the slow cooker does all the hard work for you.

—CHER SCHWARTZ ELLISVILLE, MO

PREP: 20 MIN. • **COOK:** 8 HOURS
MAKES: 12 SERVINGS

- 1 beef rump roast or bottom round roast (3 pounds)
- 3 cups reduced-sodium beef broth
- 1 envelope Italian salad dressing mix
- 1 teaspoon garlic powder
- 1 teaspoon onion powder
- 1 teaspoon dried parsley flakes
- 1 teaspoon dried basil
- 1 teaspoon dried oregano
- 1 teaspoon pepper
- 1 large onion, julienned
- 1 large green pepper, julienned
- 4½ teaspoons olive oil
- 12 hamburger buns, split
- 12 slices reduced-fat provolone cheese

1. Cut roast in half; place in a 4-qt. slow cooker. Combine the broth, dressing mix and seasonings; pour over meat. Cover and cook on low for 8 hours or until tender.

2. Remove roast; cool slightly. Skim fat from cooking juices; reserve 1 cup juices. Shred beef and return to slow cooker. Stir in reserved cooking juices; heat through.

3. Meanwhile, in a large skillet, saute the onion and green pepper in oil until tender.

4. Using a slotted spoon, place beef on bun bottoms; layer with cheese and vegetables. Replace bun tops.

PER SERVING *346 cal., 12 g fat (5 g sat. fat), 79 mg chol., 707 mg sodium, 25 g carb., 2 g fiber, 32 g pro.* **Diabetic Exchanges:** *4 lean meat, 1½ starch, 1 fat.*

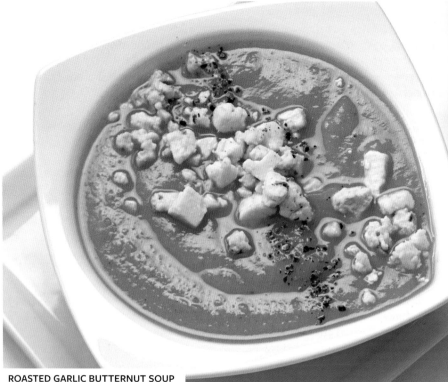

ROASTED GARLIC BUTTERNUT SOUP

Roasted Garlic Butternut Soup

This lower-fat soup is creamy, packs a lot of flavor and offers 545 mg of potassium.

—ROBIN HAAS CRANSTON, RI

PREP: 35 MIN. • **COOK:** 20 MIN.
MAKES: 9 SERVINGS (2¼ QUARTS)

- 1 whole garlic bulb
- 1 teaspoon olive oil
- 1 medium butternut squash (3 pounds), peeled and cubed
- 1 medium sweet potato, peeled and cubed
- 1 large onion, chopped
- 2 tablespoons butter
- 3¼ cups water
- 1 can (14½ ounces) reduced-sodium chicken broth
- 1 teaspoon paprika
- ½ teaspoon pepper
- ¼ teaspoon salt
- 9 tablespoons crumbled blue cheese

1. Remove papery outer skin from garlic (do not peel or separate cloves). Cut top off of garlic bulb. Brush with oil; wrap in heavy-duty foil. Bake at 425° for 30-35 minutes or until softened. Cool for 10-15 minutes.

2. Meanwhile, in a Dutch oven, saute the squash, sweet potato and onion in butter until crisp-tender. Add the water, broth, paprika, pepper and salt; squeeze softened garlic into pan. Bring to a boil. Reduce heat; cover and simmer for 20-25 minutes or until vegetables are tender. Cool slightly.

3. In a food processor, process soup in batches until smooth. Return all to pan and heat through. Ladle into bowls; top with blue cheese.

PER SERVING *1 cup soup with 1 tablespoon blue cheese equals 144 cal., 6 g fat (3 g sat. fat), 13 mg chol., 340 mg sodium, 21 g carb., 5 g fiber, 4 g pro.* **Diabetic Exchanges:** *1 starch, 1 fat.*

Jamaican Jerk Turkey Wraps

After tasting these wraps at a neighborhood party, I had to get the recipe! The grilled turkey tenderloin and light jalapeno dressing make them oh-so-good.

—MARY ANN DELL PHOENIXVILLE, PA

PREP: 20 MIN. • **GRILL:** 20 MIN.
MAKES: 4 SERVINGS

- 2 **cups broccoli coleslaw mix**
- 1 **medium tomato, seeded and chopped**
- 3 **tablespoons reduced-fat coleslaw dressing**
- 1 **jalapeno pepper, seeded and chopped**
- 1 **tablespoon prepared mustard**
- 1½ **teaspoons Caribbean jerk seasoning**
- 2 **turkey breast tenderloins (8 ounces each)**
- 4 **fat-free flour tortillas (8 inches)**

1. In a large bowl, toss the coleslaw mix, tomato, coleslaw dressing, chopped jalapeno and prepared mustard; set aside.

2. Rub seasoning over turkey tenderloins. Moisten a paper towel with cooking oil; using long-handled tongs, rub on grill rack to coat lightly. Grill turkey, covered, over medium heat or broil 4 in. from heat 8-10 minutes on each side or until a thermometer reads 165°. Let stand 5 minutes.

3. Grill tortillas, uncovered, over medium heat for 45-55 seconds on each side or until warmed. Thinly slice turkey; place down the center of tortillas. Top with coleslaw mixture and roll up.

NOTE *Wear disposable gloves when cutting hot peppers; the oils can burn skin. Avoid touching your face.*

PER SERVING *295 cal., 4 g fat (1 g sat. fat), 59 mg chol., 658 mg sodium, 34 g carb., 3 g fiber, 31 g pro.* **Diabetic Exchanges:** *3 lean meat, 2 starch, 1 vegetable, ½ fat.*

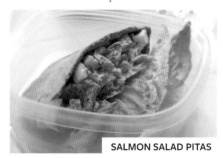

SALMON SALAD PITAS

Salmon Salad Pitas

I know these pitas are good because my husband and sons don't even mind having them the next day as leftovers.

—CHERYL BAINBRIDGE BLOOMINGTON, IN

PREP: 25 MIN. + CHILLING
MAKES: 4 SERVINGS

- 1 **salmon fillet (1 pound)**
- ¼ **cup chopped celery**
- ¼ **cup chopped seeded peeled cucumber**
- ¼ **cup reduced-fat sour cream**
- ¼ **cup fat-free mayonnaise**
- 1 **tablespoon minced chives**
- 1 **tablespoon minced fresh dill**
- 1 **teaspoon Italian seasoning**
- ¼ **teaspoon salt**
- ⅛ **teaspoon white pepper**
- 4 **romaine leaves**
- 4 **whole wheat pita pocket halves**

1. Place 2 in. of water in a large skillet; bring to a boil. Reduce heat; carefully add salmon. Poach, uncovered, for 6-12 minutes or until fish is firm and flakes easily with a fork. Remove salmon with a slotted spatula. Cool.

2. In a large bowl, combine the celery, cucumber, sour cream, mayonnaise and seasonings. Flake the salmon; stir into salad mixture. Cover and refrigerate for at least 1 hour. Serve in lettuce-lined pita breads.

PER SERVING *331 cal., 15 g fat (4 g sat. fat), 74 mg chol., 522 mg sodium, 22 g carb., 3 g fiber, 27 g pro.* **Diabetic Exchanges:** *3 lean meat, 1½ starch, 1 fat.*

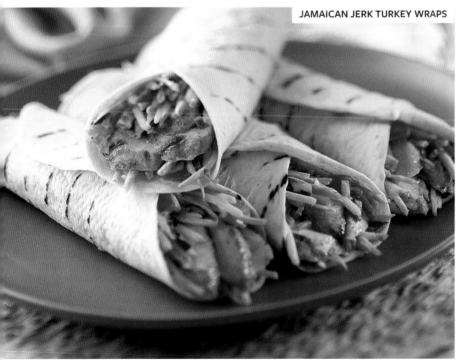

JAMAICAN JERK TURKEY WRAPS

Couscous Meatball Soup

Dip some fresh crusty bread into a bowl of this soup and you've got yourself the perfect pick-me-up on a chilly day.

—**JONATHAN PACE** SAN FRANCISCO, CA

PREP: 25 MIN. • **COOK:** 40 MIN.
MAKES: 10 SERVINGS (2½ QUARTS)

- 1 **pound lean ground beef (90% lean)**
- 2 **teaspoons dried basil**
- 2 **teaspoons dried oregano**
- ½ **teaspoon salt**
- 1 **large onion, finely chopped**
- 2 **teaspoons canola oil**
- 8 **cups chopped collard greens**
- 8 **cups chopped fresh kale**
- 2 **cartons (32 ounces each) vegetable stock**
- 1 **tablespoon white wine vinegar**
- ½ **teaspoon crushed red pepper flakes**
- ¼ **teaspoon pepper**
- 1 **package (8.8 ounces) Israeli couscous**

1. In a small bowl, combine the beef, basil, oregano and salt. Shape into ½-in. balls. In a large nonstick skillet coated with cooking spray, brown meatballs; drain. Remove meatballs and set aside.

2. In the same skillet, brown onion in oil. Add greens and kale; cook for 6-7 minutes longer or until wilted.

3. In a Dutch oven, combine the greens mixture, meatballs, stock, vinegar, pepper flakes and pepper. Bring to a boil. Reduce heat; cover and simmer for 10 minutes. Return to a boil. Stir in couscous. Reduce heat; cover and simmer for 10-15 minutes or until couscous is tender, stirring once.

PER SERVING *1 cup equals 202 cal., 5 g fat (2 g sat. fat), 28 mg chol., 583 mg sodium, 26 g carb., 2 g fiber, 13 g pro.* ***Diabetic Exchanges:*** *1½ starch, 1 lean meat, 1 vegetable.*

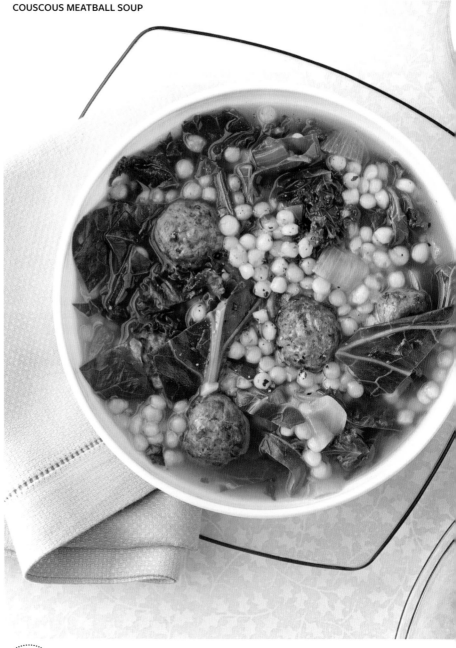

top tip

Simple Substitutions

Don't have any kale on hand for this recipe? Chop up some fresh spinach instead. Don't like things too spicy? Simply leave out the red pepper flakes.

Garden Tuna Pita Sandwiches

A well-balanced meal packed into a pita makes it a breeze to carry a healthy lunch. If you're not big on tuna, you can go with canned chicken instead.

—**BECKY CLARK** WARRIOR, AL

START TO FINISH: 20 MIN.
MAKES: 3 SERVINGS

- 2 pouches (one 5 ounces, one 2½ ounces) light water-packed tuna
- ¾ cup 2% cottage cheese
- ½ cup chopped cucumber
- ¼ cup reduced-fat mayonnaise
- ¼ cup shredded carrot
- 2 tablespoons minced fresh chives
- 2 tablespoons minced fresh parsley
- ½ teaspoon dill weed
- ¼ teaspoon salt
  Dash pepper
- 6 whole wheat pita pocket halves
- 1 cup fresh baby spinach
- 6 slices tomato

In a small bowl, combine the first 10 ingredients. Line pita halves with spinach and tomato; fill each with ⅓ cup tuna mixture.

PER SERVING *362 cal., 10 g fat (2 g sat. fat), 36 mg chol., 1,114 mg sodium, 39 g carb., 5 g fiber, 31 g pro.* **Diabetic Exchanges:** *3 lean meat, 2 starch, 1 vegetable, 1 fat.*

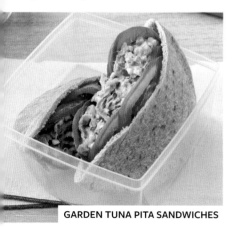

GARDEN TUNA PITA SANDWICHES

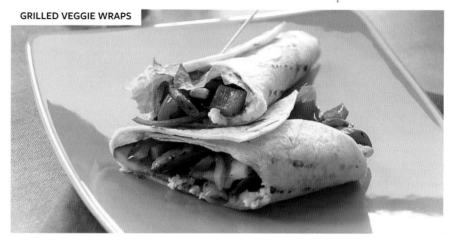

GRILLED VEGGIE WRAPS

Grilled Veggie Wraps

The key to this recipe's success is the three-cheese spread. My father is strictly a meat-and-potatoes man, but he definitely liked these wraps!

—**BRITANI SEPANSKI** INDIANAPOLIS, IN

PREP: 15 MIN. + MARINATING • **GRILL:** 15 MIN.
MAKES: 4 SERVINGS

- 2 tablespoons balsamic vinegar
- 1½ teaspoons minced fresh basil
- 1½ teaspoons olive oil
- 1½ teaspoons molasses
- ¾ teaspoon minced fresh thyme
- ⅛ teaspoon salt
- ⅛ teaspoon pepper
- 1 medium zucchini, cut lengthwise into ¼-inch slices
- 1 medium sweet red pepper, cut into 1-inch pieces
- 1 medium red onion, cut into ½-inch slices
- 4 ounces whole fresh mushrooms, cut into ½-inch pieces
- 4 ounces fresh sugar snap peas
- ½ cup crumbled feta cheese
- 3 tablespoons reduced-fat cream cheese
- 2 tablespoons grated Parmesan cheese
- 1 tablespoon reduced-fat mayonnaise
- 4 flour tortillas (8 inches)
- 4 romaine leaves

1. In a resealable plastic bag, combine the first seven ingredients; add vegetables. Seal bag and turn to coat; refrigerate for 2 hours, turning once.

2. Drain and reserve marinade. Transfer vegetables to a grill wok or basket. Grill, uncovered, over medium-high heat for 5 minutes, stirring frequently.

3. Set aside 1 teaspoon marinade. Turn vegetables; baste with remaining marinade. Grill 5-8 minutes longer or until tender, stirring frequently. Meanwhile, in a small bowl, combine cheeses and mayonnaise; set aside.

4. Brush one side of each tortilla with reserved marinade. Place tortillas, marinade side down, on grill for 1-3 minutes or until lightly toasted.

5. Spread 3 tablespoons of cheese mixture over ungrilled side of each tortilla. Top with romaine and 1 cup grilled vegetables; roll up.

NOTE *If you do not have a grill wok or basket, use a disposable foil pan. Poke holes in the bottom of the pan with a meat fork to allow liquid to drain.*

PER SERVING *332 cal., 14 g fat (6 g sat. fat), 26 mg chol., 632 mg sodium, 39 g carb., 4 g fiber, 13 g pro.* **Diabetic Exchanges:** *2 starch, 2 vegetable, 2 fat.*

Corn Soup with Pico de Gallo

Once my family gets a whiff of this Southwestern soup, it doesn't take them long to reach the dinner table. The blend of seasonings and succulent pico de gallo add to its fabulous flavor.

—**ELAINE SWEET** DALLAS, TX

PREP: 50 MIN. • **COOK:** 20 MIN.
MAKES: 6 SERVINGS

- **3** corn tortillas (6 inches), cut into 1-inch strips
- **4** medium ears sweet corn, husks removed
- **½** teaspoon canola oil
- **½** teaspoon each salt, pepper and paprika
- **1** medium red onion, chopped
- **1** bacon strip, chopped
- **6** garlic cloves, minced
- **¼** cup all-purpose flour
- **3** cups reduced-sodium chicken broth
- **1** cup fat-free milk
- **1** can (4 ounces) chopped green chilies
- **1** teaspoon ground cumin
- **1** teaspoon dried oregano
- **½** cup minced fresh cilantro
- **¼** cup lime juice

PICO DE GALLO

- **2** plum tomatoes, chopped
- **1** medium ripe avocado, peeled and chopped
- **1** small serrano pepper, seeded and chopped
- **1** garlic clove, minced
- **¼** teaspoon salt
- **¼** teaspoon pepper

1. Place tortilla strips on a baking sheet coated with cooking spray; bake at 350° for 8-10 minutes or until crisp.
2. Rub corn with canola oil; sprinkle with seasonings. Moisten a paper towel with cooking oil; using long-handled tongs, lightly coat the grill rack.
3. Grill corn, covered, over medium heat for 10-12 minutes or until tender, turning frequently. Cool slightly; cut corn from cobs and set aside.
4. In a large saucepan, saute onion and bacon for 5 minutes; add garlic, cook 1 minute longer. Stir in flour until blended; gradually add broth. Bring to a boil; cook and stir for 2 minutes or until thickened. Add corn, milk, chilies, cumin and oregano; heat through. Remove from heat; stir in the cilantro and lime juice.

5. Combine pico de gallo ingredients. Serve with soup and tortilla strips.
NOTE *Wear disposable gloves when cutting hot peppers; the oils can burn skin. Avoid touching your face.*
PER SERVING *217 cal., 8 g fat (1 g sat. fat), 3 mg chol., 740 mg sodium, 33 g carb., 6 g fiber, 8 g pro. Diabetic Exchanges: 2 starch, 1½ fat.*

Cranberry BBQ Turkey Sandwiches

Put leftover turkey to good use in this slightly sweet sandwich. Keep the meat warm in a slow cooker at your next potluck, and you're sure to impress guests.

—**SUSAN MATTHEWS** ROCKFORD, IL

PREP: 10 MIN. • **COOK:** 30 MIN.
MAKES: 12 SERVINGS

- **1** can (14 ounces) jellied cranberry sauce
- **1** cup reduced-sodium beef broth
- **¼** cup sugar
- **¼** cup ketchup
- **2** tablespoons cider vinegar
- **1** tablespoon Worcestershire sauce
- **1** teaspoon yellow mustard
- **¼** teaspoon garlic powder
- **⅛** teaspoon seasoned salt
- **⅛** teaspoon paprika
- **6** cups shredded cooked turkey breast
- **12** sandwich buns, split

1. In a large saucepan, combine the first 10 ingredients. Bring to a boil. Reduce heat; simmer, uncovered, for 20 minutes or until sauce is thickened.
2. Stir in turkey; simmer 4-5 minutes longer or until heated through. Spoon ½ cup onto each bun.
PER SERVING *296 cal., 3 g fat (1 g sat. fat), 61 mg chol., 388 mg sodium, 41 g carb., 1 g fiber, 25 g pro. Diabetic Exchanges: 3 lean meat, 2½ starch.*

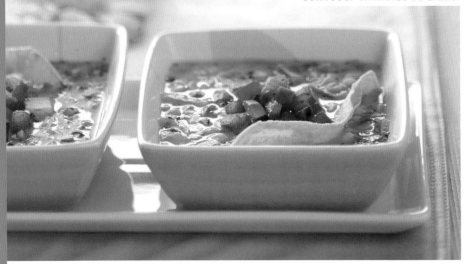

CORN SOUP WITH PICO DE GALLO

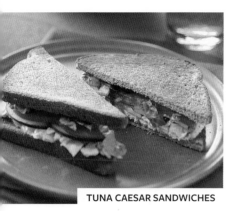

TUNA CAESAR SANDWICHES

Tuna Caesar Sandwiches

Tuna sandwiches are wonderfully versatile. Feel free to add whichever ingredients you'd like to make this sandwich your own.

—**GLORIA BRADLEY** NAPERVILLE, IL

START TO FINISH: 20 MIN.
MAKES: 4 SERVINGS

- 2 **cans (5 ounces each) white water-packed tuna, drained and flaked**
- ¼ **cup marinated quartered artichoke hearts, drained and chopped**
- ¼ **cup finely chopped onion**
- ¼ **cup reduced-fat mayonnaise**
- 3 **tablespoons grated Parmesan cheese**
- 2 **teaspoons lemon juice**
- 1 **teaspoon Dijon mustard**
- 8 **slices whole wheat bread, toasted**
- 16 **cucumber slices**
- 8 **slices tomato**
- 2 **cups shredded lettuce**

In a small bowl, combine the first seven ingredients. Spread over four slices of toast. Top with cucumber, tomato, lettuce and remaining toast.

PER SERVING *338 cal., 12 g fat (3 g sat. fat), 38 mg chol., 797 mg sodium, 30 g carb., 5 g fiber, 27 g pro.* ***Diabetic Exchanges:*** *3 lean meat, 2 starch, 1 fat.*

Makeover Cauliflower Soup

Creamy soups are soul-warming and satisfying, and this healthy recipe is certainly no exception.

—**DORIS WATT DAVIS** HELLERTOWN, PA

PREP: 30 MIN. • **COOK:** 30 MIN.
MAKES: 11 SERVINGS (2¾ QUARTS)

- 2 **celery ribs, chopped**
- 1 **small onion, chopped**
- 1 **medium carrot, chopped**
- 2 **tablespoons butter**
- 1 **large head cauliflower (2 pounds), broken into florets**
- 6 **cups reduced-sodium chicken broth**
- ½ **cup all-purpose flour**
- 2 **cups 2% milk**
- ¾ **cup fat-free half-and-half**
- 1 **tablespoon minced fresh parsley**
- 1 **teaspoon salt**
- 1 **teaspoon dill weed**
- ¼ **teaspoon white pepper**

1. In a Dutch oven, saute the celery, onion and carrot in butter for 3-5 minutes or until crisp-tender. Stir in the cauliflower and broth; bring to a boil. Reduce heat; cover and simmer for 15-20 minutes or until tender. Cool slightly.

2. In a blender, process vegetable mixture in batches until smooth. Return all to the pan. Heat over medium heat.

3. In a small bowl, whisk flour and milk until smooth; stir into puree. Bring to a boil; cook and stir for 2 minutes or until thickened. Reduce heat; stir in the half-and-half, parsley, salt, dill and pepper. Heat through.

PER SERVING *1 cup equals 106 cal., 3 g fat (2 g sat. fat), 9 mg chol., 641 mg sodium, 14 g carb., 3 g fiber, 6 g pro.* ***Diabetic Exchanges:*** *1 vegetable, ½ starch, ½ fat.*

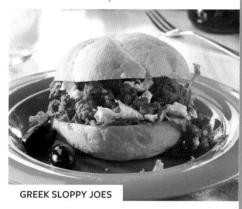

GREEK SLOPPY JOES

Greek Sloppy Joes

It's amazing how a little feta cheese adds a whole new depth of flavor to a simple sloppy joe recipe. I enjoy filling a pita with any leftovers the next day.

—**SONYA LABBE** WEST HOLLYWOOD, CA

START TO FINISH: 25 MIN.
MAKES: 6 SERVINGS

- 1 **pound lean ground beef (90% lean)**
- 1 **small red onion, chopped**
- 2 **garlic cloves, minced**
- 1 **can (15 ounces) tomato sauce**
- 1 **teaspoon dried oregano**
- 2 **cups chopped romaine**
- 6 **kaiser rolls, split and toasted**
- ½ **cup crumbled feta cheese**

1. In a large skillet, cook beef, onion and garlic over medium heat for 6-8 minutes or until beef is no longer pink, breaking up beef into crumbles; drain. Stir in tomato sauce and oregano. Bring to a boil. Reduce heat; simmer, uncovered, 8-10 minutes or until the sauce is slightly thickened, stirring occasionally.

2. Place romaine on roll bottoms; top with meat mixture. Sprinkle with feta cheese; replace tops.

PER SERVING *335 cal., 10 g fat (4 g sat. fat), 52 mg chol., 767 mg sodium, 36 g carb., 3 g fiber, 23 g pro.* ***Diabetic Exchanges:*** *3 lean meat, 2 starch, 1 vegetable.*

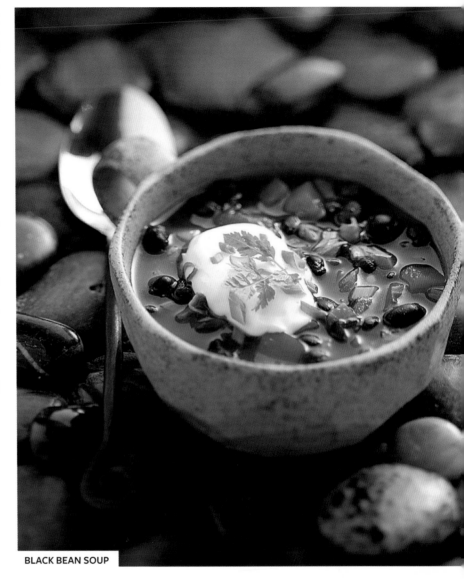

top tip

Full of Beans

It's easy to thicken Southwestern soups without adding flour. Simply stir pureed cooked beans into the soup and heat through.

Black Bean Soup

Fill your tummy without expanding your waistline when you dig into a bowl of this soup. If you want to add meat, use lean beef or chicken to pack in extra protein.

—ANGEE OWENS LUFKIN, TX

PREP: 20 MIN. • **COOK:** 25 MIN.
MAKES: 8 SERVINGS (2 QUARTS)

- 3 **cans (15 ounces each) black beans, rinsed and drained, divided**
- 3 **celery ribs with leaves, chopped**
- 1 **large onion, chopped**
- 1 **medium sweet red pepper, chopped**
- 1 **jalapeno pepper, seeded and chopped**
- 2 **tablespoons olive oil**
- 4 **garlic cloves, minced**
- 2 **cans (14½ ounces each) reduced-sodium chicken broth or vegetable broth**
- 1 **can (14½ ounces) diced tomatoes with green peppers and onions, undrained**
- 3 **teaspoons ground cumin**
- 1½ **teaspoons ground coriander**
- 1 **teaspoon Louisiana-style hot sauce**
- ¼ **teaspoon pepper**
- 1 **bay leaf**
- 1 **teaspoon lime juice**
- ½ **cup reduced-fat sour cream**
- ¼ **cup chopped green onions**

1. In a small bowl, mash one can black beans; set aside. In a large saucepan, saute the celery, onion, red pepper and jalapeno in oil until tender. Add garlic; cook 1 minute longer.

BLACK BEAN SOUP

2. Stir in the broth, tomatoes, cumin, coriander, hot sauce, pepper, bay leaf, remaining beans and reserved mashed beans. Bring to a boil. Reduce heat; cover and simmer for 15 minutes.

3. Discard bay leaf. Stir in lime juice. Garnish each serving with 1 tablespoon of sour cream and 1½ teaspoons of green onion.

CHICKEN BLACK BEAN SOUP *Add 2 cups cubed cooked chicken with the broth.*

NOTE *Wear disposable gloves when cutting hot peppers; the oils can burn skin. Avoid touching your face.*
PER SERVING *1 cup equals 222 cal., 5 g fat (1 g sat. fat), 5 mg chol., 779 mg sodium, 32 g carb., 9 g fiber, 11 g pro.*
***Diabetic Exchanges:** 2 starch, 1 lean meat, 1 vegetable, 1 fat.*

Broiled Vegetable Sandwiches

I like to serve veggies on a toasted bun with fresh basil, mayo and a dash of jalapeno pepper. You don't even miss the meat!

—**JANE JACKSON** RANDOLPH, IA

START TO FINISH: 30 MIN.
MAKES: 2 SERVINGS

- 6 slices peeled eggplant (¼ inch thick)
- ½ cup sliced yellow summer squash (¼ inch thick)
- ⅓ cup sliced zucchini (¼ inch thick)
- 2 slices red onion (¼ inch thick)
  Cooking spray
- 1 teaspoon Italian seasoning
  Dash cayenne pepper
- 2 hard rolls, split and toasted
- 5 teaspoons reduced-fat mayonnaise
- 2 fresh basil leaves
- 2 fresh spinach leaves
- 1 cup julienned roasted sweet red peppers
- 2 slices tomato
- 2 teaspoons minced seeded jalapeno pepper
- ⅛ teaspoon pepper

1. In a large bowl, combine the eggplant, yellow squash, zucchini and onion. Spray lightly with cooking spray. Add Italian seasoning and cayenne; toss to coat.

2. If broiling the vegetables, arrange on a 15x10x1-in. baking pan coated with cooking spray. If grilling the vegetables, transfer to a grill wok or basket. Broil 4-6 in. from the heat or grill, covered, over medium heat for 5-7 minutes on each side or until tender and lightly browned.

3. Spread roll bottoms with mayonnaise; layer with the basil, spinach, red peppers, tomato and jalapeno. Sprinkle with pepper. Top with vegetables; replace roll tops.

NOTE *Wear disposable gloves when cutting hot peppers; the oils can burn skin. Avoid touching your face.*

PER SERVING *290 cal., 7 g fat (1 g sat. fat), 4 mg chol., 869 mg sodium, 44 g carb., 5 g fiber, 8 g pro. Diabetic Exchanges: 2 starch, 2 vegetable, 1 fat.*

Low-Fat Potato Soup

My husband usually doesn't care for low-fat dishes. So he was quite surprised to find, after polishing off a bowl of this rich-tasting soup, that it has only 2 grams of fat per serving. Yum!

—**NATALIE WARF** SPRING LAKE, NC

START TO FINISH: 30 MIN.
MAKES: 5 SERVINGS

- 1¾ cups diced peeled potatoes
- 1 medium onion, chopped
- ¼ cup chopped celery
- 1 can (14½ ounces) reduced-sodium chicken broth
- ⅛ teaspoon pepper
- 3 tablespoons cornstarch
- 1 can (12 ounces) fat-free evaporated milk, divided
- 1 cup (4 ounces) shredded reduced-fat cheddar cheese

1. In a large saucepan, combine the potatoes, onion, celery, broth and pepper. Bring to a boil. Reduce heat; cover and simmer for 15-18 minutes or until vegetables are tender.

2. Combine cornstarch and ¼ cup milk until smooth; stir into potato mixture. Add the remaining milk. Bring to a boil; cook and stir for 2 minutes or until thickened. Remove from the heat. Stir in cheese until melted.

PER SERVING *1 cup equals 178 cal., 2 g fat (0 sat. fat), 9 mg chol., 274 mg sodium, 26 g carb., 0 fiber, 14 g pro. Diabetic Exchanges: 2 starch, 1 medium-fat meat.*

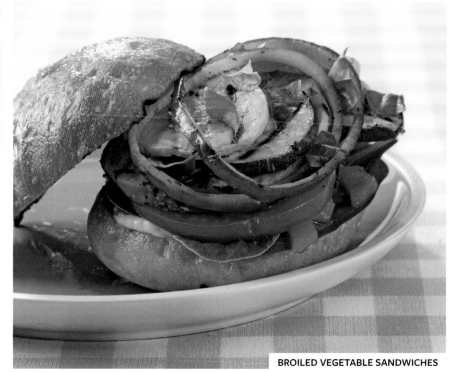

BROILED VEGETABLE SANDWICHES

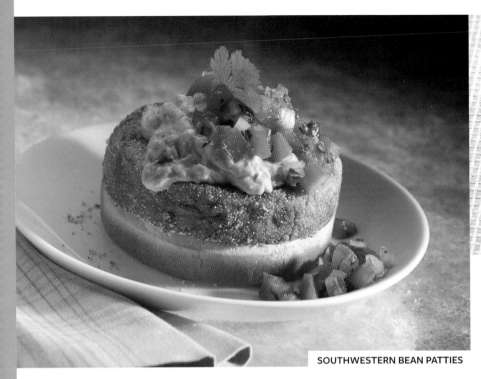

SOUTHWESTERN BEAN PATTIES

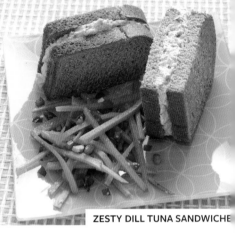

ZESTY DILL TUNA SANDWICHE

Southwestern Bean Patties

When I first served this recipe, the Southwest flavor and guacamole topping received especially high marks. It was a real hit with everyone!

—**DEBBY CHIORINO** PT. HUENEME, CA

START TO FINISH: 30 MIN.
MAKES: 6 SERVINGS

- 1 **small onion, chopped**
- ¼ **cup finely chopped sweet red pepper**
- 5 **teaspoons canola oil, divided**
- 1 **garlic clove, minced**
- 1 **can (16 ounces) fat-free refried beans**
- ¾ **cup dry bread crumbs**
- 1 **can (4 ounces) chopped green chilies, drained**
- 2 **tablespoons minced fresh cilantro**
- ¼ **teaspoon ground cumin**
- ⅛ **teaspoon pepper**
- ⅓ **cup cornmeal**
- 6 **hamburger buns, split**
- ½ **cup guacamole**
- ½ **cup salsa**

1. In a large nonstick skillet, saute onion and red pepper in 1½ teaspoons of oil until tender. Add the garlic; cook 1 minute longer.

2. In a large bowl, combine the refried beans, bread crumbs, chilies, cilantro, cumin, pepper and onion mixture; mix well. Shape into six patties; coat in cornmeal.

3. In the same skillet, cook patties in batches in remaining oil over medium-high heat for 2-3 minutes on each side or until lightly browned.

4. Place patties on bun bottoms (save bun tops for another use). Top each with 4 teaspoons of guacamole and 4 teaspoons of salsa.

PER SERVING *312 cal., 9 g fat (1 g sat. fat), 0 chol., 801 mg sodium, 46 g carb., 8 g fiber, 11 g pro.* **Diabetic Exchanges:** *3 starch, 1 lean meat, 1 fat.*

Zesty Dill Tuna Sandwiches

I absolutely love tuna salad, so I brought together all of my favorite things to make what I think is the best tuna salad sandwich ever. What a treat for lunch!

—**JENNY DUBINSKY** INWOOD, WV

START TO FINISH: 15 MIN.
MAKES: 2 SERVINGS

- 1 **can (5 ounces) light water-packed tuna, drained**
- ¼ **cup reduced-fat mayonnaise**
- 1 **tablespoon grated Parmesan cheese**
- 1 **tablespoon sweet pickle relish**
- 1 **tablespoon minced fresh parsley**
- 1 **teaspoon spicy brown mustard**
- ¼ **teaspoon dill weed**
- ⅛ **teaspoon onion powder**
- ⅛ **teaspoon curry powder**
- ⅛ **teaspoon garlic powder**
- 4 **slices whole wheat bread**

In a small bowl, combine the first 10 ingredients. Spread over two slices of bread. Top with remaining bread.

PER SERVING *346 cal., 13 g fat (3 g sat. fat), 34 mg chol., 877 mg sodium, 29 g carb., 4 g fiber, 27 g pro.* **Diabetic Exchanges:** *3 lean meat, 2 starch, 1½ fat.*

Hearty Pita Tacos

Just because you're eating healthy doesn't mean you have to skimp on flavor. Our 9-year-old daughter enjoys helping us make these tasty sandwiches, so it's all the more satisfying when we sit down to eat.

—**JAMIE VALOCCHI** MESA, AZ

START TO FINISH: 30 MIN.
MAKES: 6 SERVINGS

- 1 **pound lean ground beef (90% lean)**
- 1 **small sweet red pepper, chopped**
- 2 **green onions, chopped**
- 1 **can (16 ounces) kidney beans, rinsed and drained**
- ¾ **cup frozen corn**
- ⅔ **cup taco sauce**
- 1 **can (2¼ ounces) sliced ripe olives, drained**
- ½ **teaspoon garlic salt**
- ¼ **teaspoon onion powder**
- ¼ **teaspoon dried oregano**
- ¼ **teaspoon paprika**
- ¼ **teaspoon pepper**
- 6 **whole wheat pita pocket halves**
- 6 **tablespoons shredded reduced-fat cheddar cheese**
  Sliced avocado and additional taco sauce, optional

1. In a large skillet, cook the beef, red pepper and onions over medium heat until meat is no longer pink; drain. Stir in the beans, corn, taco sauce, olives and seasonings; heat through.

2. Spoon ¾ cup beef mixture into each pita half. Sprinkle with cheese. Serve with avocado and additional taco sauce if desired.

PER SERVING *339 cal., 10 g fat (4 g sat. fat), 52 mg chol., 787 mg sodium, 38 g carb., 8 g fiber, 26 g pro.* **Diabetic Exchanges:** *3 lean meat, 2½ starch.*

Chicken Tortilla Soup

The fresh lime and cilantro in this zesty soup remind me of warmer climates, a nice bonus on blustery days in northern Michigan. I lightened up the original recipe by simply baking the tortilla strips instead of frying them.

—**MARIANNE MORGAN** TRAVERSE CITY, MI

START TO FINISH: 30 MIN.
MAKES: 6 SERVINGS

- 3 **corn tortillas (6 inches), cut into ¼-inch strips**
- 4 **teaspoons olive oil, divided**
- ¼ **teaspoon salt**
- ¾ **pound boneless skinless chicken breasts, cut into ½-inch chunks**
- 1 **large onion, chopped**
- 5 **cups reduced-sodium chicken broth**
- 1 **pound red potatoes, cut into ½-inch cubes**
- 1 **cup frozen corn**
- 1 **can (4 ounces) chopped green chilies**
- ¼ **cup minced fresh cilantro**
- ¼ **teaspoon pepper**
- 3 **tablespoons lime juice**

1. In a large resealable plastic bag, combine tortilla strips, 1 teaspoon oil and salt. Seal bag and shake to coat. Arrange tortilla strips on an ungreased baking sheet. Bake at 400° for 8-10 minutes or until crisp, stirring once. Remove to paper towels to cool.

2. In a large saucepan, saute chicken in remaining oil until no longer pink and lightly browned. Add onion; cook and stir until onion is tender. Add the broth and potatoes.

3. Bring to a boil. Reduce heat; cover and simmer for 10 minutes. Add the corn, chilies, cilantro and pepper. Cook until heated through. Stir in lime juice. Garnish with tortilla strips.

PER SERVING *1½ cups equals 221 cal., 4 g fat (1 g sat. fat), 33 mg chol., 757 mg sodium, 27 g carb., 4 g fiber, 19 g pro.* **Diabetic Exchanges:** *2 starch, 2 lean meat, ½ fat.*

CHICKEN TORTILLA SOUP

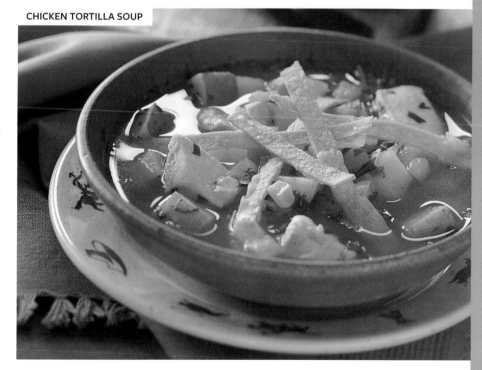

Mango Shrimp Pitas

Mango, ginger and curry combine with a splash of lime to coat juicy, grilled shrimp in this recipe. Stuffed in pitas, shrimp becomes a handheld lunch! You could also serve the shrimp on a bed of rice.

—**BEVERLY OFERRALL** LINKWOOD, MD

PREP: 15 MIN. + MARINATING • **GRILL:** 10 MIN.
MAKES: 4 SERVINGS

- ½ cup mango chutney
- 3 tablespoons lime juice
- 1 teaspoon grated fresh gingerroot
- ½ teaspoon curry powder
- 1 pound uncooked large shrimp, peeled and deveined
- 2 pita breads (6 inches), halved
- 8 Bibb or Boston lettuce leaves
- 1 large tomato, thinly sliced

1. In a small bowl, combine the chutney, lime juice, ginger and curry. Pour ½ cup marinade into a large resealable plastic bag; add the shrimp. Seal bag and turn to coat; refrigerate for at least 15 minutes. Cover and refrigerate remaining marinade.

2. Drain and discard marinade. Thread shrimp onto four metal or soaked wooden skewers. Moisten a paper towel with cooking oil; using long-handled tongs, lightly coat the grill rack.

3. Grill shrimp, covered, over medium heat or broil 4 in. from the heat for 6-8 minutes or until shrimp turn pink, turning frequently.

4. Fill pita halves with lettuce, tomato and shrimp; spoon reserved chutney mixture over filling.

PER SERVING *230 cal., 2 g fat (trace sat. fat), 138 mg chol., 410 mg sodium, 29 g carb., 1 g fiber, 22 g pro.* **Diabetic Exchanges:** *3 lean meat, 2 starch.*

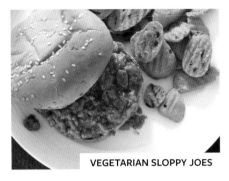

VEGETARIAN SLOPPY JOES

Vegetarian Sloppy Joes

Sloppy joes without the meat? It can be done! This recipe still tastes like the old favorite, while staying vegetarian-friendly.

—**LINDA WINTER** OAK HARBOR, WA

START TO FINISH: 25 MIN.
MAKES: 6 SERVINGS

- 2 teaspoons butter
- 1 small onion, finely chopped
- 1 package (12 ounces) frozen vegetarian meat crumbles
- ½ teaspoon pepper
- 2 tablespoons all-purpose flour
- ⅔ cup ketchup
- 1 can (8 ounces) no-salt-added tomato sauce
- 6 hamburger buns, split and toasted

1. In a large nonstick skillet coated with cooking spray, melt butter over medium-high heat. Add onion; cook and stir until tender. Stir in meat crumbles and pepper; heat through.

2. Sprinkle flour over mixture and stir until blended. Stir in ketchup and tomato sauce. Bring to a boil; cook and stir 1-2 minutes or until thickened. Serve on buns.

NOTE *Vegetarian meat crumbles are a nutritious protein source made from soy. Look for them in the natural foods freezer section.*

PER SERVING *273 cal., 6 g fat (2 g sat. fat), 4 mg chol., 815 mg sodium, 39 g carb., 5 g fiber, 15 g pro.* **Diabetic Exchanges:** *2½ starch, 2 lean meat.*

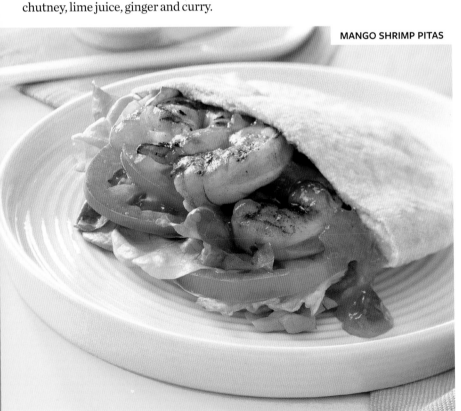

MANGO SHRIMP PITAS

Tomato Mushroom Soup

My husband and I were never too fond of tomato soup, but we were hooked once we gave this recipe a chance. I make a batch every week now!

—CHRIS NELSON ALLIANCE, OH

START TO FINISH: 30 MIN.
MAKES: 4 SERVINGS

- 1 **cup sliced fresh mushrooms**
- 2 **tablespoons chopped onion**
- 2 **tablespoons butter**
- 1 **garlic clove, minced**
- 3 **tablespoons all-purpose flour**
- 1 **can (14½ ounces) reduced-sodium chicken broth**
- 2 **cups chopped seeded peeled plum tomatoes**
- 2 **tablespoons minced fresh basil or 2 teaspoons dried basil**
- 1 **tablespoon sugar**
- ½ **teaspoon salt**
- ⅛ **teaspoon pepper**

1. In a large saucepan, saute mushrooms and onion in butter until tender. Add garlic; cook 1 minute longer. Remove vegetables with a slotted spoon and set aside. In the same pan, combine flour and broth until smooth. Bring to a boil; cook and stir for 1-2 minutes or until thickened.

2. Return mushroom mixture to saucepan. Add the tomatoes, basil, sugar, salt and pepper. Cook over medium heat for 5 minutes or until heated through.

PER SERVING *95 cal., 5 g fat (3 g sat. fat), 12 mg chol., 506 mg sodium, 11 g carb., 1 g fiber, 3 g pro.* **Diabetic Exchanges:** *2 vegetable, 1½ fat.*

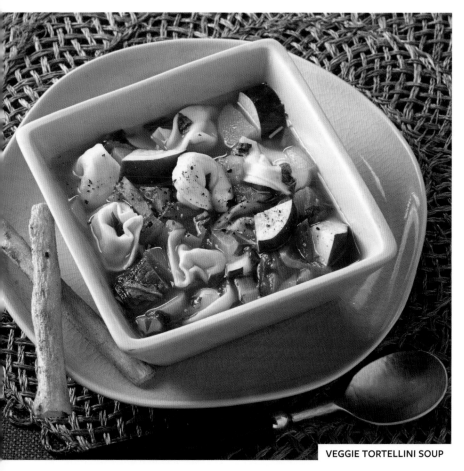

VEGGIE TORTELLINI SOUP

Veggie Tortellini Soup

Italian cuisine has more to offer than pizza and spaghetti. Just check out this healthy, mouthwatering soup! I've served it to company for years; most ask for the recipe.

—PRISCILLA GILBERT
INDIAN HARBOUR BEACH, FL

PREP: 15 MIN. • **COOK:** 20 MIN.
MAKES: 7 SERVINGS

- 3 **medium carrots, chopped**
- 1 **large onion, chopped**
- 1 **tablespoon olive oil**
- 4 **garlic cloves, minced**
- 2 **cans (14½ ounces each) vegetable broth**
- 2 **medium zucchini, chopped**
- 4 **plum tomatoes, chopped**
- 2 **cups refrigerated cheese tortellini**
- ⅓ **cup chopped fresh spinach**
- 1 **teaspoon minced fresh rosemary or ¼ teaspoon dried rosemary, crushed**
- ¼ **teaspoon pepper**
- 1 **tablespoon red wine vinegar**

1. In a Dutch oven, saute carrots and onion in oil until onion is tender. Add garlic; cook 1 minute longer.

2. Stir in the broth, zucchini, tomatoes, tortellini, spinach, rosemary and pepper. Bring to a boil. Reduce heat; cover and simmer for 8-10 minutes or until tortellini are tender. Just before serving, stir in vinegar.

PER SERVING *155 cal., 5 g fat (2 g sat. fat), 13 mg chol., 693 mg sodium, 24 g carb., 3 g fiber, 6 g pro.* **Diabetic Exchanges:** *1 starch, 1 vegetable, ½ fat.*

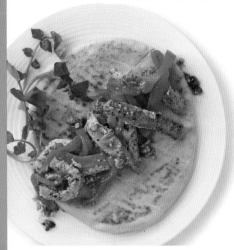

PEPPERED PORK PITAS

Peppered Pork Pitas

Tender pork and sweet red peppers create family-friendly sandwiches. These are especially good with garlic mayo, but you can have fun experimenting with your own variations.

—KATHERINE WHITE CLEMMONS, NC

START TO FINISH: 20 MIN.
MAKES: 4 SERVINGS

- 1 **pound boneless pork loin chops, cut into thin strips**
- 1 **tablespoon olive oil**
- 2 **teaspoons coarsely ground pepper**
- 2 **garlic cloves, minced**
- 1 **jar (12 ounces) roasted sweet red peppers, drained and julienned**
- 4 **whole pita breads, warmed**

In a small bowl, combine the pork, oil, pepper and garlic; toss to coat. In a large skillet, saute pork mixture until no longer pink. Add red peppers; heat through. Serve with pita breads.
PER SERVING *380 cal., 11 g fat (3 g sat. fat), 55 mg chol., 665 mg sodium, 37 g carb., 2 g fiber, 27 g pro.* **Diabetic Exchanges:** *3 lean meat, 2 starch, 1 fat.*

Carrot Broccoli Soup

This soup is a staple at our house. It's fast, easy and filled to the brim with carrots and broccoli. Even picky eaters will like it.

—SANDY SMITH LONDON, ON

PREP: 15 MIN. • **COOK:** 20 MIN.
MAKES: 4 SERVINGS

- 1 **medium onion, chopped**
- 2 **medium carrots, chopped**
- 2 **celery ribs, chopped**
- 1 **tablespoon butter**
- 3 **cups fresh broccoli florets**
- 3 **cups fat-free milk, divided**
- ¾ **teaspoon salt**
- ½ **teaspoon dried thyme**
- ⅛ **teaspoon pepper**
- 3 **tablespoons all-purpose flour**

1. In a large saucepan coated with cooking spray, cook the onion, carrots and celery in butter for 3 minutes. Add broccoli; cook 3 minutes longer. Stir in 2¾ cups milk, salt, thyme and pepper.
2. Bring to a boil. Reduce heat; cover and simmer for 5-10 minutes or until vegetables are tender. Combine the flour and the remaining milk until smooth; gradually stir into soup. Bring to a boil; cook for 2 minutes longer or until thickened.
PER SERVING *168 cal., 4 g fat (3 g sat. fat), 14 mg chol., 633 mg sodium, 24 g carb., 4 g fiber, 10 g pro.* **Diabetic Exchanges:** *2 vegetable, 1 fat-free milk, ½ fat.*

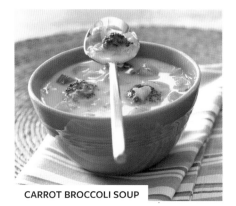

CARROT BROCCOLI SOUP

Marinated Chicken Sandwiches

Sweet brown sugar, zesty mustard and ginger perks up ordinary chicken in these sandwiches. Top each with the type of cheese you like best.

—RUTH LEE TROY, ON

PREP: 20 MIN. + MARINATING • **GRILL:** 10 MIN.
MAKES: 6 SERVINGS

- ½ **cup reduced-sodium soy sauce**
- ¼ **cup packed brown sugar**
- ¼ **cup ketchup**
- 1 **tablespoon canola oil**
- 1 **tablespoon molasses**
- 1 **teaspoon garlic powder**
- 1 **teaspoon minced fresh gingerroot**
- 1 **teaspoon prepared mustard**
- 6 **boneless skinless chicken breast halves (6 ounces each)**
- 3 **tablespoons reduced-fat mayonnaise**
- 6 **kaiser rolls, split and toasted**
- 6 **lettuce leaves**
- 6 **slices (½ ounce each) reduced-fat Swiss cheese**

1. In a large resealable plastic bag, combine the first eight ingredients; add chicken. Seal bag and turn to coat; refrigerate for at least 1 hour.
2. Drain and discard marinade. Using long-handled tongs, moisten a paper towel with cooking oil and lightly coat the grill rack. Grill chicken, covered, over medium heat or broil 4 in. from the heat for 4-6 minutes on each side or until a thermometer reads 170°.
3. Spread mayonnaise over bottom of rolls; top with chicken, lettuce and cheese. Replace roll tops.
PER SERVING *430 cal., 12 g fat (3 g sat. fat), 103 mg chol., 595 mg sodium, 34 g carb., 2 g fiber, 45 g pro.* **Diabetic Exchanges:** *5 lean meat, 2 starch.*

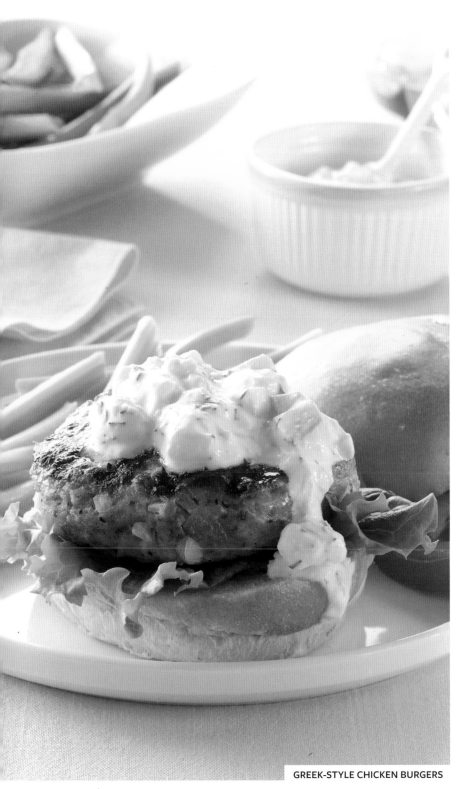

Greek-Style Chicken Burgers

The original recipe for these burgers called for lamb or beef, but I decided to substitute ground chicken to decrease the fat.

—**JUDY PUSKAS** WALLACEBURG, ON

PREP: 25 MIN. + CHILLING • **GRILL:** 10 MIN.
MAKES: 4 SERVINGS

SAUCE
- ⅓ **cup fat-free plain Greek yogurt**
- ¼ **cup chopped peeled cucumber**
- ¼ **cup crumbled reduced-fat feta cheese**
- 1½ **teaspoons snipped fresh dill**
- 1½ **teaspoons lemon juice**
- 1 **small garlic clove, minced**

BURGERS
- 1 **medium onion, finely chopped**
- ¼ **cup dry bread crumbs**
- 1 **tablespoon dried oregano**
- 1 **tablespoon lemon juice**
- 2 **garlic cloves, minced**
- ½ **teaspoon salt**
- ¼ **teaspoon pepper**
- 1 **pound ground chicken**
- 4 **hamburger buns, split**
- 4 **lettuce leaves**
- 4 **tomato slices**

1. In a small bowl, mix the sauce ingredients; refrigerate until serving.
2. In a large bowl, combine the first seven burger ingredients. Add chicken; mix lightly but thoroughly. Shape into four ½-in.-thick patties.
3. Moisten a paper towel with cooking oil; using long-handled tongs, rub on grill rack to coat lightly. Grill burgers, covered, over medium heat or broil 4 in. from heat 5-7 minutes on each side or until a thermometer reads 165°. Serve on buns with lettuce, tomato and sauce.
PER SERVING *350 cal., 12 g fat (4 g sat. fat), 78 mg chol., 732 mg sodium, 35 g carb., 3 g fiber, 27 g pro.* **Diabetic Exchanges:** *3 lean meat, 2 starch, 1 vegetable.*

GREEK-STYLE CHICKEN BURGERS

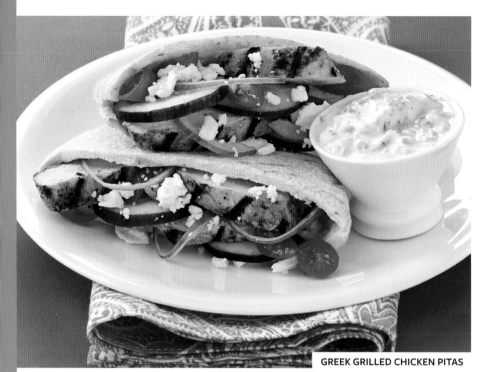

Chipotle Beef Sandwiches

A jar of chipotle salsa makes it a cinch to spice up beef sirloin for mouthwatering sandwiches. This slow cooker recipe is definitely good when you're hosting a party.

—**JESSICA RING** MADISON, WI

PREP: 25 MIN. • **COOK:** 7 HOURS
MAKES: 10 SERVINGS

- 1 large sweet onion, halved and thinly sliced
- 1 beef sirloin tip roast (3 pounds)
- 1 jar (16 ounces) chipotle salsa
- ½ cup beer or nonalcoholic beer
- 1 envelope Lipton beefy onion soup mix
- 10 kaiser rolls, split

1. Place onion in a 5-qt. slow cooker. Cut roast in half; place over onion. Combine the salsa, beer and soup mix. Pour over top. Cover and cook on low for 7-8 hours or until meat is tender.
2. Remove roast. Shred meat with two forks and return to the slow cooker; heat through. Using a slotted spoon, spoon shredded meat onto rolls.
PER SERVING *362 cal., 9 g fat (3 g sat. fat), 72 mg chol., 524 mg sodium, 37 g carb., 2 g fiber, 31 g pro.* **Diabetic Exchanges:** *3 lean meat, 2½ starch.*

GREEK GRILLED CHICKEN PITAS

Greek Grilled Chicken Pitas

I took one of my mother's recipes, then switched a few things to make it healthier and take advantage of fresh veggies.

—**BLAIR LONERGAN** ROCHELLE, VA

PREP: 20 MIN. + MARINATING • **GRILL:** 10 MIN.
MAKES: 4 SERVINGS

- ½ cup balsamic vinaigrette
- 1 pound boneless skinless chicken breast halves

CUCUMBER SAUCE
- 1 cup plain Greek yogurt
- ½ cup finely chopped cucumber
- ¼ cup finely chopped red onion
- 1 tablespoon minced fresh parsley
- 1 tablespoon lime juice
- 1 garlic clove, minced
- ¼ teaspoon salt
- ⅛ teaspoon pepper

PITAS
- 8 pita pocket halves
- ½ cup sliced cucumber
- ½ cup grape tomatoes, chopped
- ½ cup sliced red onion
- ½ cup crumbled feta cheese

1. Pour vinaigrette into a large resealable plastic bag. Add the chicken; seal bag and turn to coat. Refrigerate for at least 4 hours or overnight. In a small bowl, combine the sauce ingredients; chill until serving.
2. Drain and discard marinade. If grilling the chicken, moisten a paper towel with cooking oil; using long-handled tongs, lightly coat the grill rack. Grill chicken, covered, over medium heat or broil 4 in. from the heat for 4-7 minutes on each side or until a thermometer reads 170°.
3. Cut chicken into strips. Fill each pita half with chicken, cucumber, tomatoes, onion and cheese; drizzle with sauce.
PER SERVING *428 cal., 14 g fat (6 g sat. fat), 85 mg chol., 801 mg sodium, 41 g carb., 3 g fiber, 33 g pro.* **Diabetic Exchanges:** *3 starch, 3 lean meat, 1 fat.*

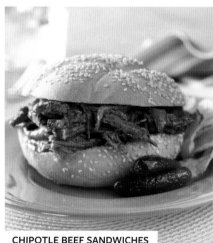

CHIPOTLE BEEF SANDWICHES

Sweet Potato Minestrone

My daughters love how comforting this soup is, and I love that it's high in beta-carotene and other nutrients. It's a win-win!

—**HELEN VAIL** GLENSIDE, PA

PREP: 15 MIN. • **COOK:** 20 MIN.
MAKES: 14 SERVINGS (ABOUT 3½ QUARTS)

- **4 cans (14½ ounces each) reduced-sodium beef or vegetable broth**
- **3 cups water**
- **2 medium sweet potatoes, peeled and cubed**
- **1 medium onion, chopped**
- **4 garlic cloves, minced**
- **2 teaspoons Italian seasoning**
- **6 cups shredded cabbage**
- **1 package (7 ounces) small pasta shells**
- **2 cups frozen peas**

1. In a soup kettle, combine the broth, water, sweet potatoes, onion, garlic and Italian seasoning; bring to a boil. Reduce heat; cover and simmer for 10 minutes.

2. Return to a boil. Add the cabbage, pasta and peas; cook for 8-10 minutes or until the pasta and vegetables are tender.

PER SERVING *1 cup equals 127 cal., 1 g fat (0 sat. fat), 0 chol., 67 mg sodium, 23 g carb., 0 fiber, 6 g pro.* **Diabetic Exchange:** *1½ starch.*

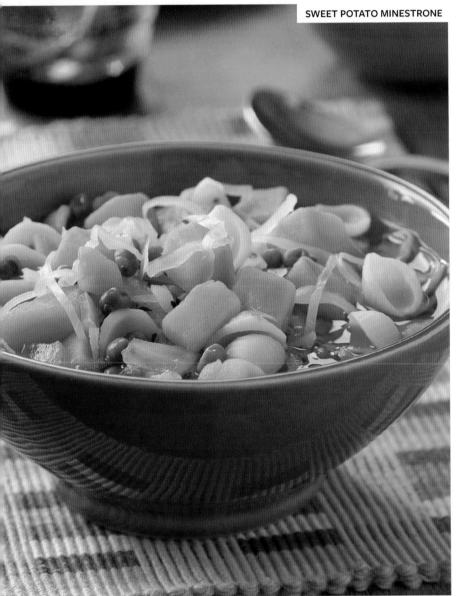

SWEET POTATO MINESTRONE

Turkey Reubens

Even those who are diehard fans of the classic Reuben will enjoy this lighter take on the popular sandwich.

—**ELIZABETH MYERS** WILLIAMSPORT, PA

START TO FINISH: 25 MIN.
MAKES: 4 SERVINGS

- **8 slices rye bread**
- **½ pound thinly sliced deli turkey**
- **½ cup sauerkraut, rinsed and well drained**
- **4 slices reduced-fat Swiss cheese**
- **¼ cup fat-free Thousand Island salad dressing**

1. On four slices of bread, layer the turkey, sauerkraut, cheese and salad dressing. Top with remaining bread. Spritz both sides of sandwiches with butter-flavored cooking spray.

2. In a large nonstick skillet over medium heat, toast sandwiches on both sides until cheese is melted.

PER SERVING *310 cal., 8 g fat (3 g sat. fat), 35 mg chol., 1,398 mg sodium, 39 g carb., 5 g fiber, 22 g pro.* **Diabetic Exchanges:** *2½ starch, 2 lean meat, ½ fat.*

Chunky Sausage Lentil Soup

Lentils are an inexpensive and nutritious power food. My husband just loves this soup, and I like that it freezes well.

—**D. LEE SCAR** EAST HANOVER, NJ

PREP: 30 MIN. • **COOK:** 40 MIN.
MAKES: 10 SERVINGS (3½ QUARTS)

- 8 cups water
- 1 package (16 ounces) dried lentils, rinsed
- 1 package (19½ ounces) Italian turkey sausage links, casings removed and crumbled
- 2 medium onions, chopped
- 2 celery ribs, chopped
- 2 medium carrots, cut into ¼-inch slices
- 6 garlic cloves, minced
- 3 cans (14½ ounces each) reduced-sodium beef broth
- 1 can (28 ounces) crushed tomatoes
- 1 medium red potato, diced
- 1½ teaspoons dried thyme
- 1½ teaspoons coarsely ground pepper
   Salad croutons, optional

1. In a large saucepan, bring water and lentils to a boil. Reduce heat; cover and simmer for 18-22 minutes or until lentils are tender. Drain. In a Dutch oven, cook the sausage, onions, celery and carrots over medium heat until meat is no longer pink and vegetables are tender; drain. Add garlic; cook 2 minutes longer.

2. Stir in the broth, tomatoes, potato, thyme and pepper. Bring to a boil. Reduce heat; simmer, uncovered, for 15-20 minutes or until potato is tender. Stir in lentils; heat through. Serve with croutons if desired.

FREEZE OPTION *Reserving croutons for later, freeze cooled soup in freezer containers. To use, partially thaw in refrigerator overnight. Heat through in a saucepan, stirring occasionally and adding a little broth or water if necessary. Top each serving with croutons if desired.*

PER SERVING *1⅓ cups equals 314 cal., 6 g fat (1 g sat. fat), 36 mg chol., 681 mg sodium, 43 g carb., 17 g fiber, 24 g pro.* **Diabetic Exchanges:** *3 lean meat, 2 starch, 2 vegetable.*

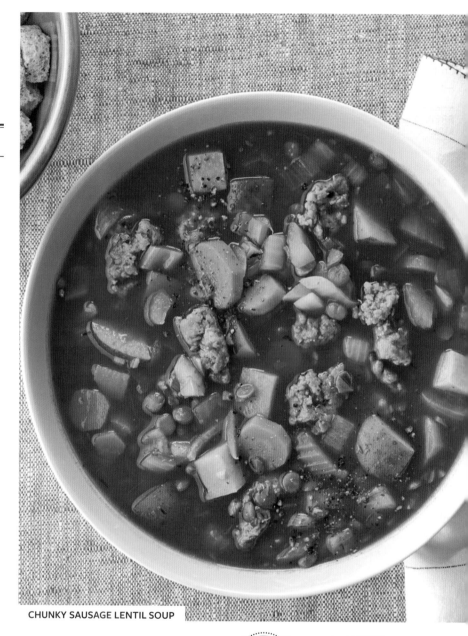

CHUNKY SAUSAGE LENTIL SOUP

top tip

Preparing Potatoes

When preparing lots of potatoes, peel, dice and place them in cold water to prevent any discoloration.

Roasted Tomato & Garlic Soup

Serve this tomato soup as a meal starter or on its own with fresh-baked bread.

—LIZZIE MUNRO BROOKLYN, NY

PREP: 55 MIN. • **COOK:** 30 MIN.
MAKES: 4 SERVINGS

- 3 **whole garlic bulbs**
- 3 **tablespoons olive oil, divided**
- 2½ **pounds large tomatoes, quartered and seeded**
- ¼ **teaspoon salt, divided**
- ¼ **teaspoon pepper, divided**
- 1 **medium onion, chopped**
- 5 **garlic cloves, minced**
- 1 **tablespoon minced fresh or 1 teaspoon dried thyme**
- 2 **cups chicken stock**
- ½ **cup half-and-half cream**

1. Preheat oven to 350°. Remove papery outer skin from garlic bulbs, but do not peel or separate the cloves. Cut off top of garlic bulbs, exposing individual cloves; drizzle with 2 tablespoons oil. Wrap in foil.
2. Place tomatoes in a 15x10x1-in. foil-lined baking pan; sprinkle with ⅛ teaspoon each salt and pepper. Bake garlic bulbs and tomatoes for 40-45 minutes or until cloves are soft and tomatoes are tender. Unwrap and cool 10 minutes.
3. In a large saucepan, heat remaining oil over medium heat. Add onion; cook and stir until tender. Add minced garlic, thyme and tomatoes. Squeeze garlic from skin; add to pan. Add stock. bring to a boil. Reduce heat; simmer, uncovered, 20-25 minutes or until flavors are blended, breaking up tomatoes with a spoon.
4. Remove soup from heat; cool slightly. Process in batches in a blender until smooth. Return soup to the pan; add cream and remaining salt and pepper. Heat through.

PER SERVING *252 cal., 14 g fat (4 g sat. fat), 15 mg chol., 438 mg sodium, 27 g carb., 5 g fiber, 8 g pro.* **Diabetic Exchanges:** *2½ fat, 1½ starch.*

Grilled Turkey Sandwiches

Switch it up on the grill tonight—give these sandwiches a try. The herbed marinade makes the meat extra juicy and tender.

—MARY DETWEILER MIDDLEFIELD, OH

PREP: 20 MIN. + MARINATING • **GRILL:** 10 MIN.
MAKES: 6 SERVINGS

- ½ **cup chicken broth**
- ¼ **cup olive oil**
- 4½ **teaspoons finely chopped onion**
- 1 **tablespoon white wine vinegar**
- 2 **teaspoons dried parsley flakes**
- ½ **teaspoon salt**
- ½ **teaspoon rubbed sage**
- ⅛ **teaspoon pepper**
- 6 **turkey breast cutlets (about 1 pound)**
- 6 **whole wheat hamburger buns, split**
- 6 **lettuce leaves**
- 6 **tomato slices**

1. In a large resealable plastic bag, combine the first eight ingredients; add turkey. Seal bag and turn to coat; refrigerate for 12 hours or overnight, turning occasionally.
2. Drain and discard marinade. Using long-handled tongs, moisten a paper towel with cooking oil and lightly coat the grill rack.
3. Prepare grill for indirect heat, using a drip pan. Place turkey over drip pan and grill, covered, over indirect medium heat or broil 4 in. from the heat for 3-4 minutes on each side or until no longer pink. Serve on buns with lettuce and tomato.

PER SERVING *232 cal., 6 g fat (1 g sat. fat), 47 mg chol., 373 mg sodium, 24 g carb., 4 g fiber, 23 g pro.* **Diabetic Exchanges:** *2 lean meat, 1½ starch, ½ fat.*

GRILLED TURKEY SANDWICHES

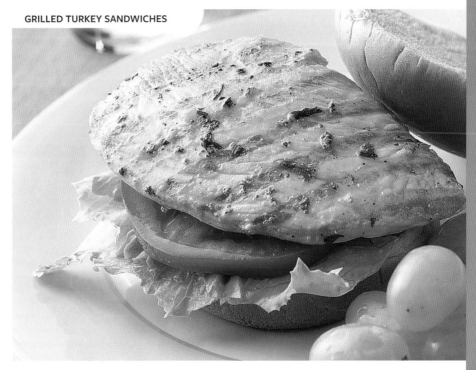

beef, pork & lamb

Dig into a **hearty dinner** tonight! Whether you're following a special diet or not, these **mouthwatering entrees** are sure to rise to the top of your list of most-requested suppers.

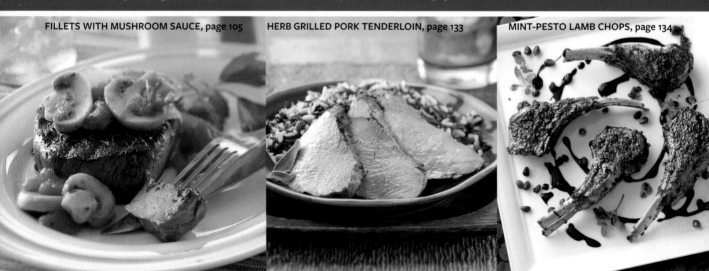

FILLETS WITH MUSHROOM SAUCE, page 105   HERB GRILLED PORK TENDERLOIN, page 133   MINT-PESTO LAMB CHOPS, page 134

until meat is tender. Let stand for 10 minutes before slicing.

PER SERVING *202 cal., 7 g fat (2 g sat. fat), 66 mg chol., 306 mg sodium, 8 g carb., 1 g fiber, 26 g pro.* **Diabetic Exchanges:** *3 lean meat, ½ starch.*

Veggie-Topped Swiss Steak

Round steak turns so tender when you put it in a slow cooker. I like to serve this dish with mashed potatoes.

—LORSKYNY, TASTE OF HOME ONLINE COMMUNITY

PREP: 35 MIN. • **COOK:** 6 HOURS
MAKES: 6 SERVINGS

- 1½ **pounds beef top round steak**
- ¼ **cup all-purpose flour**
- 2 **teaspoons ground mustard**
- ¾ **teaspoon salt**
- ¼ **teaspoon pepper**
- 2 **tablespoons canola oil**
- 2 **tablespoons butter**
- 1 **can (14½ ounces) diced tomatoes**
- 2 **celery ribs, finely chopped**
- 2 **medium carrots, grated**
- 1 **medium onion, finely chopped**
- 2 **tablespoons Worcestershire sauce**
- 1 **tablespoon brown sugar**

1. Cut steak into serving-size pieces. In a large resealable plastic bag, combine the flour, mustard, salt and pepper. Add beef, a few pieces at a time, and shake to coat.
2. In a large skillet, brown meat in oil and butter on both sides. Transfer meat to a 3-qt. slow cooker. Combine the tomatoes, celery, carrots, onion, Worcestershire sauce and brown sugar; pour over meat.
3. Cover and cook on low for 6-8 hours or until meat is tender.

PER SERVING *287 cal., 12 g fat (4 g sat. fat), 74 mg chol., 524 mg sodium, 16 g carb., 3 g fiber, 28 g pro.* **Diabetic Exchanges:** *4 lean meat, 1 vegetable, 1 fat, ½ starch.*

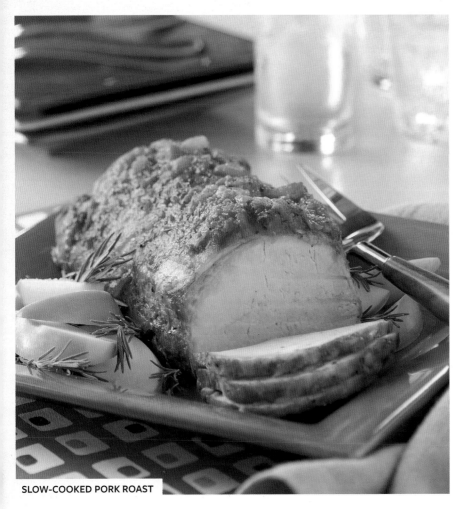

SLOW-COOKED PORK ROAST

Slow-Cooked Pork Roast

When you've got a jam-packed day ahead, turn to this slow cooker recipe. It'll be a favorite in your home in no time.

—MARION LOWERY MEDFORD, OR

PREP: 20 MIN. • **COOK:** 6 HOURS + STANDING
MAKES: 12 SERVINGS

- 2 **cans (8 ounces each) unsweetened crushed pineapple, undrained**
- 1 **cup barbecue sauce**
- 2 **tablespoons unsweetened apple juice**
- 1 **tablespoon minced fresh rosemary or 1 teaspoon dried rosemary, crushed**
- 1 **teaspoon minced garlic**
- 2 **teaspoons grated lemon peel**
- 1 **teaspoon liquid smoke, optional**
- ½ **teaspoon salt**
- ¼ **teaspoon pepper**
- 1 **boneless pork loin roast (3 to 4 pounds)**

1. In a large saucepan, combine the first nine ingredients. Bring to a boil. Reduce heat; simmer, uncovered, for 3 minutes.
2. Meanwhile, cut roast in half. In a nonstick skillet coated with cooking spray, brown pork roast on all sides.
3. Place roast in a 5-qt. slow cooker. Pour sauce over roast and turn to coat. Cover and cook on low for 6-7 hours or

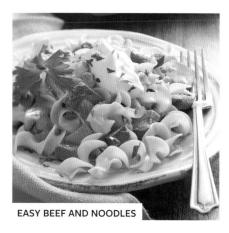

EASY BEEF AND NOODLES

Easy Beef and Noodles

My family loves this lighter version of beef
Stroganoff. Using roast beef from the deli
saves the hours spent cooking a whole
roast. I serve this entree with a green salad.

—PAMELA SHANK PARKERSBURG, WV

START TO FINISH: 25 MIN.
MAKES: 2 SERVINGS

- 2½ cups uncooked yolk-free noodles
- ⅓ cup sliced fresh mushrooms
- ⅓ cup chopped onion
- 1 tablespoon olive oil
- 1¼ cups reduced-sodium beef broth
- 6 ounces deli roast beef, cubed
- ⅛ teaspoon pepper
- 2 tablespoons fat-free sour cream, optional
- 2 teaspoons minced fresh parsley

1. Cook noodles according to package
directions. In a large skillet, saute
mushrooms and onion in oil until
tender. Add the broth, roast beef and
pepper. Bring to a boil. Reduce heat;
simmer, uncovered, for 10 minutes.
2. Drain noodles; stir into skillet. Top
with sour cream if desired. Garnish
with parsley.
PER SERVING *375 cal., 10 g fat (2 g sat.
fat), 50 mg chol., 778 mg sodium, 42 g
carb., 3 g fiber, 26 g pro. **Diabetic
Exchanges:** 3 starch, 3 lean meat,
1½ fat.*

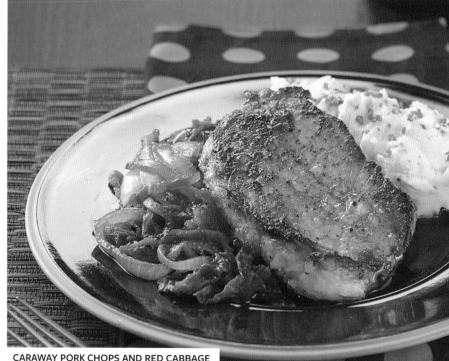

CARAWAY PORK CHOPS AND RED CABBAGE

Caraway Pork Chops and Red Cabbage

My husband loves cooked red cabbage, so I
created a savory one-skillet supper that my
18-year-old son also enjoys. Try it with
mashed potatoes.

—JUDY REBMAN FREDERICK, IL

PREP: 20 MIN. • **COOK:** 20 MIN.
MAKES: 4 SERVINGS

- 4 boneless pork loin chops (5 ounces each)
- 1¼ teaspoons caraway seeds, divided
- 1 teaspoon rotisserie chicken seasoning
- 1 teaspoon brown sugar
- 1 tablespoon canola oil
- 4 cups shredded red cabbage
- 1 medium apple, peeled and thinly sliced
- ½ small onion, sliced
- 1 tablespoon water
- 1 tablespoon red wine vinegar
- ½ teaspoon salt
- ½ teaspoon reduced-sodium chicken bouillon granules
- 4 tablespoons apple jelly

1. Season pork chops with 1 teaspoon
caraway seeds, chicken seasoning and
brown sugar. In a large nonstick skillet
coated with cooking spray, brown chops
in oil. Remove and keep warm.
2. Add the cabbage, apple, onion, water,
vinegar, salt, bouillon granules and
remaining caraway seeds to the skillet.
Cover and cook over medium heat for
10 minutes, stirring occasionally.
3. Place chops over cabbage mixture;
top each with 1 tablespoon apple jelly.
Cover and cook 10-12 minutes longer or
until meat is tender.
PER SERVING *319 cal., 12 g fat (3 g sat.
fat), 68 mg chol., 523 mg sodium, 25 g
carb., 2 g fiber, 29 g pro. **Diabetic
Exchanges:** 4 lean meat, 1 starch,
1 vegetable, 1 fat.*

Biscuit-Topped Shepherd's Pies

This comforting and cozy meal is sure to warm up cool nights. If you don't have ramekins, just spoon the mixture into an 8-in. square baking dish.

—JOSEPHINE PIRO EASTON, PA

PREP: 30 MIN. • **BAKE:** 10 MIN.
MAKES: 6 SERVINGS

- 1 **pound lean ground beef (90% lean)**
- 1 **medium onion, chopped**
- 1 **celery rib, finely chopped**
- 1 **package (16 ounces) frozen peas and carrots, thawed and drained**
- 1 **can (15 ounces) Italian tomato sauce**
- ¼ **teaspoon pepper**
- 1 **cup reduced-fat biscuit/baking mix**
- 2 **tablespoons grated Parmesan cheese**
- ¼ **teaspoon dried rosemary, crushed**
- ½ **cup fat-free milk**
- 2 **tablespoons butter, melted**

1. In a large nonstick skillet, cook the beef, onion and celery over medium heat until meat is no longer pink; drain. Add the vegetables, tomato sauce and pepper; cook and stir for 5-6 minutes or until heated through. Spoon into six 8-oz. ramekins coated with cooking spray; set aside.

2. In a small bowl, combine the biscuit mix, cheese and rosemary. Stir in milk and butter just until moistened. Spoon dough over meat mixture; place ramekins on a baking sheet.

3. Bake at 425° for 10-12 minutes or until golden brown.

PER SERVING *311 cal., 12 g fat (5 g sat. fat), 59 mg chol., 771 mg sodium, 31 g carb., 5 g fiber, 22 g pro.* **Diabetic Exchanges:** *2 lean meat, 1½ starch, 1 vegetable, 1 fat.*

Fiesta Grilled Flank Steak

Whether you broil your steak or grill it, this marinade's lime and pineapple juice will help tenderize it.

—ROXANNE CHAN ALBANY, CA

PREP: 20 MIN. + MARINATING • **GRILL:** 15 MIN.
MAKES: 4 SERVINGS

- ½ **cup unsweetened pineapple juice**
- 1 **tablespoon lime juice**
- ½ **teaspoon garlic salt**
- ½ **teaspoon ground cumin**
- 1 **beef flank steak (1 pound)**
- 1 **cup cubed fresh pineapple**
- ½ **cup salsa verde**
- 1 **medium ripe avocado, peeled and cubed**
- 1 **green onion, finely chopped**
- 1 **tablespoon minced fresh cilantro**

1. In a large resealable plastic bag, combine the pineapple juice, lime juice, garlic salt and cumin. Score the surface of the beef, making diamond shapes ¼ in. deep; place in bag. Seal bag and turn to coat; refrigerate for 8 hours or overnight.

2. In a small bowl, combine the pineapple, salsa, avocado, green onion and cilantro. Cover and chill until serving.

3. Drain beef and discard marinade. Using long-handled tongs, moisten a paper towel with cooking oil and lightly coat the grill rack. Grill steak, covered, over medium heat or broil 4 in. from the heat for 6-8 minutes on each side or until meat reaches desired doneness (for medium-rare, a meat thermometer should read 145°; medium, 160°; well-done, 170°).

4. Let stand for 5 minutes; thinly slice across the grain. Serve with salsa.

PER SERVING *274 cal., 15 g fat (4 g sat. fat), 54 mg chol., 322 mg sodium, 12 g carb., 4 g fiber, 24 g pro.* **Diabetic Exchanges:** *3 lean meat, 1 fat, ½ fruit.*

FIESTA GRILLED FLANK STEAK

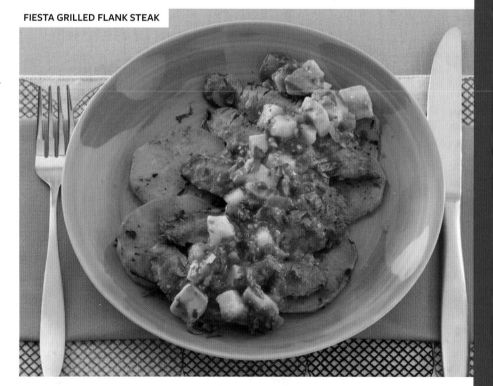

Tangy Pork Chops

I've used this recipe for many years and always get compliments when I serve it. The saucy onion-and-pepper topping is a match for the juicy chops.

—MRS. THOMAS MAUST BERLIN, PA

PREP: 30 MIN. • **BAKE:** 20 MIN.
MAKES: 6 SERVINGS

- 6 **bone-in pork loin chops (7 ounces each)**
- 2 **teaspoons canola oil**
- 2 **celery ribs, finely chopped**
- 1 **small onion, finely chopped**
- 1 **tablespoon butter**
- ½ **cup ketchup**
- ¼ **cup water**
- 2 **tablespoons cider vinegar**
- 1 **tablespoon brown sugar**
- 1 **tablespoon lemon juice**
- 1 **tablespoon Worcestershire sauce**
- ¼ **teaspoon salt**
- ⅛ **teaspoon pepper**
- 1 **small onion, thinly sliced**
- 1 **large green pepper, cut into rings**

1. In a large nonstick skillet coated with cooking spray, brown chops in oil in batches. Transfer to a 13x9-in. baking dish coated with cooking spray.
2. In the same pan, saute celery and chopped onion in butter until tender. Stir in the ketchup, water, vinegar, brown sugar, lemon juice, Worcestershire sauce, salt and pepper. Bring to a boil. Reduce heat; cover and simmer for 15-20 minutes or until slightly reduced.
3. Pour sauce over chops. Top with sliced onion and pepper rings. Cover and bake at 350° for 20-25 minutes or until a thermometer reads 160°.
PER SERVING *284 cal., 12 g fat (4 g sat. fat), 91 mg chol., 469 mg sodium, 12 g carb., 1 g fiber, 31 g pro.* **Diabetic Exchanges:** *4 lean meat, 1 starch, ½ fat.*

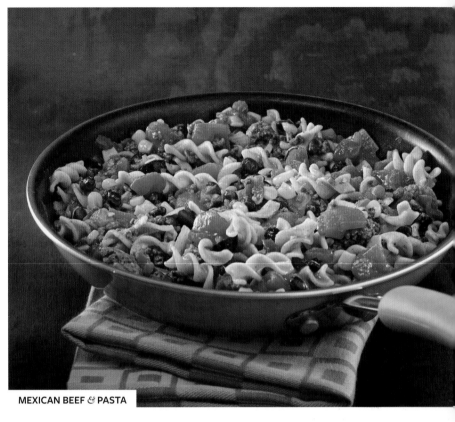

MEXICAN BEEF & PASTA

Mexican Beef & Pasta

Your family will love my hearty skillet supper that uses healthier ingredients.

—CHRISTINE RICHARDSON

MAPLE GROVE, MN

START TO FINISH: 30 MIN.
MAKES: 8 SERVINGS

- 3 **cups uncooked whole wheat spiral pasta**
- 1 **pound lean ground beef (90% lean)**
- 1 **small onion, chopped**
- 2 **cans (14½ ounces each) no-salt-added diced tomatoes, undrained**
- 1 **can (15 ounces) black beans, rinsed and drained**
- 1 **cup frozen corn, thawed**
- 1 **cup chunky salsa**
- 1 **can (4 ounces) chopped green chilies**
- 1 **can (2¼ ounces) sliced ripe olives, drained**
- 3 **tablespoons taco seasoning**
- ½ **cup reduced-fat sour cream**
  Crushed tortilla chips, optional

1. Cook pasta according to package directions; drain. Meanwhile, in a large skillet, cook beef and onion over medium heat until meat is no longer pink; drain.
2. Stir in the pasta, tomatoes, beans, corn, salsa, green chilies, olives and taco seasoning. Bring to a boil. Reduce heat; simmer, uncovered, for 8-10 minutes or until heated through. Serve with sour cream and chips if desired.
PER SERVING *1¼ cups of beef mixture with 1 tablespoon reduced-fat sour cream equals 305 cal., 7 g fat (3 g sat. fat), 40 mg chol., 737 mg sodium, 40 g carb., 7 g fiber, 20 g pro.* **Diabetic Exchanges:** *2 starch, 2 lean meat, 2 vegetable.*

Marinated Pork Loin

Beautifully glazed with a mouthwatering marinade, this entree is relatively low in fat but still moist and tender.

—PAULA YOUNG TIFFIN, OH

PREP: 20 MIN. • **BAKE:** 1 HOUR + STANDING
MAKES: 12 SERVINGS

- 1 **cup orange juice**
- ¾ **cup apricot preserves**
- 2 **tablespoons plus ¼ cup sherry or vegetable broth, divided**
- 3 **tablespoons lemon juice**
- 2 **tablespoons olive oil**
- 1 **tablespoon curry powder**
- 1 **tablespoon Worcestershire sauce**
- 1 **teaspoon dried thyme**
- ½ **teaspoon pepper**
- 1 **boneless whole pork loin roast (3 pounds)**
- 1 **tablespoon cornstarch**

1. In a small bowl, combine the orange juice, preserves, 2 tablespoons sherry, lemon juice, oil, curry, Worcestershire sauce, thyme and pepper. Pour ¾ cup marinade into a large resealable plastic bag; add the pork. Seal bag and turn to coat; refrigerate overnight, turning occasionally. Set aside 1 cup remaining marinade for sauce; cover and refrigerate. Cover and refrigerate the rest of the marinade for basting.

2. Drain and discard marinade; place pork on a rack in a shallow roasting pan. Bake, uncovered, at 350° for 1 to 1¼ hours or until a thermometer reads 145°, basting occasionally with the reserved marinade. Transfer to a serving platter. Let stand for 10 minutes before slicing.

3. Meanwhile, in a small saucepan, combine cornstarch with the remaining sherry and 1 cup marinade. Bring to a boil; cook and stir for 2 minutes or until thickened. Serve with roast.

PER SERVING *229 cal., 8 g fat (3 g sat. fat), 55 mg chol., 51 mg sodium, 15 g carb., trace fiber, 22 g pro.* **Diabetic Exchanges:** *3 lean meat, 1 starch, ½ fat.*

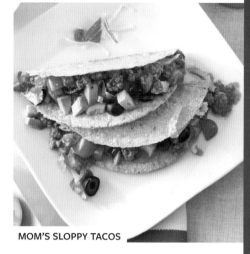

MOM'S SLOPPY TACOS

Mom's Sloppy Tacos

No matter how hectic weeknights become, there's always time to serve a great meal with recipes like this!

—KAMI JONES AVONDALE, AZ

START TO FINISH: 30 MIN.
MAKES: 6 SERVINGS

- 1½ **pounds extra-lean ground beef (95% lean)**
- 1 **can (15 ounces) tomato sauce**
- ¾ **teaspoon garlic powder**
- ½ **teaspoon salt**
- ¼ **teaspoon pepper**
- ¼ **teaspoon cayenne pepper**
- 12 **taco shells, warmed**
  Optional toppings: shredded lettuce and cheese, chopped tomatoes, avocado and olives

1. In a large skillet, cook beef over medium heat until no longer pink. Stir in the tomato sauce, garlic powder, salt, pepper and cayenne. Bring to a boil. Reduce heat; simmer, uncovered, for 10 minutes.

2. Fill each taco shell with ¼ cup beef mixture and toppings of your choice.

PER SERVING *264 cal., 10 g fat (4 g sat. fat), 65 mg chol., 669 mg sodium, 17 g carb., 1 g fiber, 25 g pro.* **Diabetic Exchanges:** *3 lean meat, 1 starch, 1 fat.*

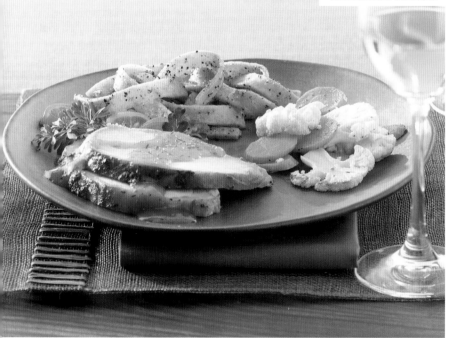

MARINATED PORK LOIN

Chili Beef Pasta

Right after I got married, my aunt gave me her recipe for skillet spaghetti and told me it was a perfect weeknight meal. Over the years I've changed up the ingredients and played with the seasonings to make it a healthier dish, but my family still loves it.

—**KRISTEN KILLIAN** DEPEW, NY

START TO FINISH: 30 MIN.
MAKES: 6 SERVINGS

- 1 **pound lean ground beef (90% lean)**
- 2 **tablespoons dried minced onion**
- 2 **teaspoons dried oregano**
- 2 **teaspoons chili powder**
- ½ **teaspoon garlic powder**
- ⅛ **teaspoon salt**
- 3 **cups tomato juice**
- 2 **cups water**
- 1 **can (6 ounces) tomato paste**
- 1 **teaspoon sugar**
- 8 **ounces uncooked whole wheat spiral pasta**
  Chopped tomatoes and minced fresh oregano, optional

1. In a Dutch oven, cook beef over medium heat 6-8 minutes or until no longer pink, breaking into crumbles; drain. Stir in seasonings.
2. Add tomato juice, water, tomato paste and sugar to pan; bring to a boil. Stir in pasta. Reduce heat; simmer, covered, 20-22 minutes or until pasta is tender, stirring occasionally. If desired, top with tomatoes and oregano.
PER SERVING *1⅓ cups equals 319 cal., 7 g fat (2 g sat. fat), 47 mg chol., 442 mg sodium, 41 g carb., 6 g fiber, 24 g pro. Diabetic Exchanges: 3 lean meat, 2 starch, 1 vegetable.*

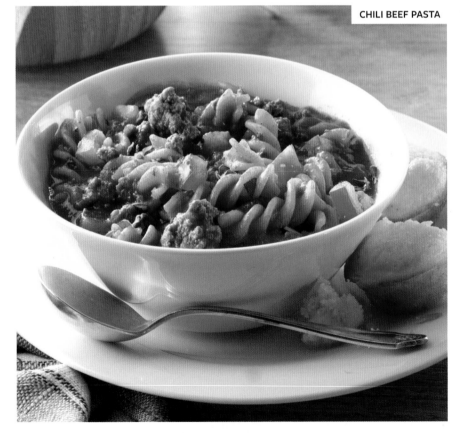

CHILI BEEF PASTA

Crumb-Crusted Pork Roast with Vegetables

Combine pork and roasted veggies with a savory crumb coating for a hearty meal.
—**TASTE OF HOME TEST KITCHEN**

PREP: 25 MIN. • **BAKE:** 1 HOUR + STANDING
MAKES: 8 SERVINGS

- 1 **boneless pork loin roast (2 pounds)**
- 4 **teaspoons honey**
- 1 **tablespoon molasses**
- 1½ **teaspoons spicy brown mustard**
- 2 **teaspoons rubbed sage**
- 1 **teaspoon dried thyme**
- 1 **teaspoon dried rosemary, crushed**
- ½ **cup soft whole wheat bread crumbs**
- 2 **tablespoons grated Parmesan cheese**
- 1 **large rutabaga, peeled and cubed**
- 1 **large sweet potato, peeled and cubed**
- 1 **large celery root, peeled and cubed**
- 1 **large onion, cut into wedges**
- 2 **tablespoons canola oil**
- ½ **teaspoon salt**
- ¼ **teaspoon pepper**

1. Preheat oven to 350°. Place roast on a rack in a shallow roasting pan coated with cooking spray. In a small bowl, mix honey, molasses and mustard; brush over roast.
2. In a large bowl, mix sage, thyme and rosemary. In another small bowl, toss bread crumbs with Parmesan cheese and 2 teaspoons of the herb mixture; press onto roast.
3. Add vegetables, oil, salt and pepper to remaining herb mixture; toss to coat. Arrange vegetables around roast.
4. Roast 1 to 1½ hours or until a thermometer reads 145°. Remove from pan; let stand 10 minutes before slicing. Serve with vegetables.
PER SERVING *302 cal., 10 g fat (2 g sat. fat), 57 mg chol., 313 mg sodium, 29 g carb., 5 g fiber, 25 g pro. Diabetic Exchanges: 3 lean meat, 2 starch, ½ fat.*

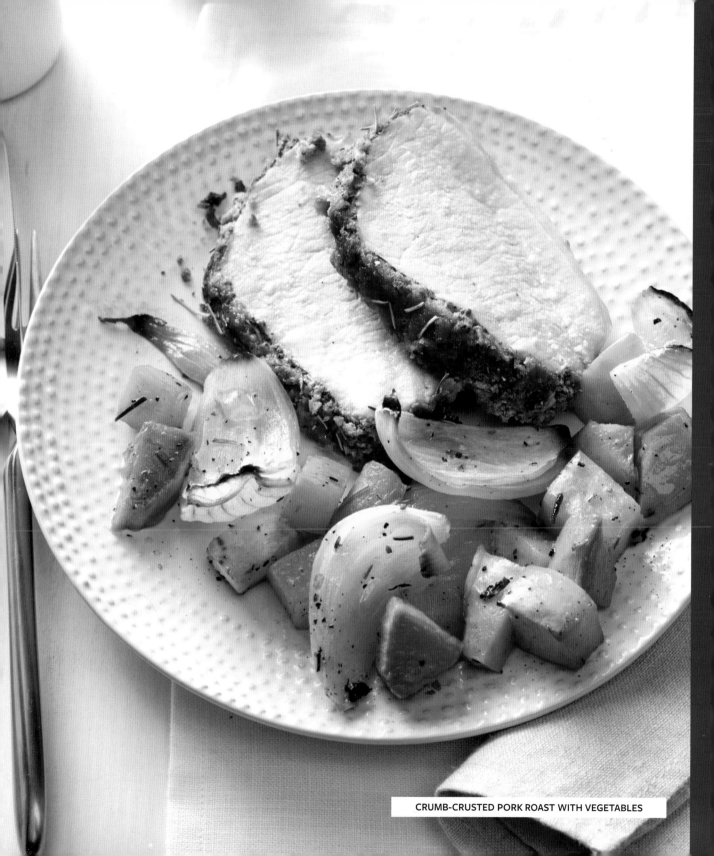

CRUMB-CRUSTED PORK ROAST WITH VEGETABLES

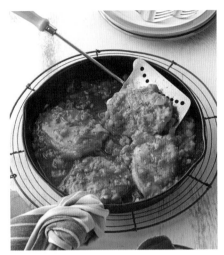

SOUTHWESTERN PINEAPPLE PORK CHOPS

Southwestern Pineapple Pork Chops

My husband and I love visiting the Southwest. After a recent trip, I decided to add a Southwestern flair to a few of our favorite healthy dishes like this one!

—LISA VARNER EL PASO, TX

START TO FINISH: 30 MIN.
MAKES: 4 SERVINGS

- 4 boneless pork loin chops (5 ounces each)
- ½ teaspoon garlic pepper blend
- 1 tablespoon canola oil
- 1 can (8 ounces) unsweetened crushed pineapple, undrained
- 1 cup medium salsa
  Minced fresh cilantro

Sprinkle pork chops with pepper blend. In a large skillet, brown chops in oil. Remove and keep warm. In the same skillet, combine pineapple and salsa. Bring to a boil. Return chops to the pan. Reduce heat; cover and simmer for 15-20 minutes or until tender. Sprinkle with cilantro.

PER SERVING *274 cal., 12 g fat (3 g sat. fat), 68 mg chol., 315 mg sodium, 13 g carb., trace fiber, 27 g pro.* **Diabetic Exchanges:** *4 lean meat, 1 fat, ½ fruit.*

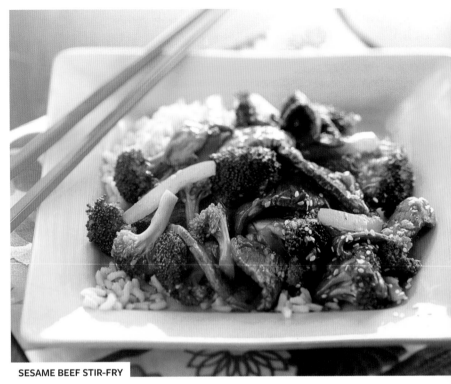

SESAME BEEF STIR-FRY

Sesame Beef Stir-Fry

Soy sauce and gingerroot add robust flavor to this quick stir-fry. Perfect for two, it couldn't be simpler to prepare.

—CHARLENE CHAMBERS ORMOND BEACH, FL

START TO FINISH: 30 MIN.
MAKES: 2 SERVINGS

- 2 teaspoons cornstarch
- ½ cup reduced-sodium beef broth
- 4 teaspoons reduced-sodium soy sauce
- 1 tablespoon minced fresh gingerroot
- 1 garlic clove, minced
- ½ pound beef top sirloin steak, thinly sliced
- 2 teaspoons sesame seeds, toasted, divided
- 2 teaspoons peanut or canola oil, divided
- 2 cups fresh broccoli florets
- 1 small sweet yellow pepper, julienned
- 1 cup hot cooked brown rice

1. In a small bowl, combine the first five ingredients until blended; set aside.

2. In a large nonstick skillet or wok, stir-fry beef and 1 teaspoon sesame seeds in 1 teaspoon oil until no longer pink. Remove and keep warm.

3. Stir-fry broccoli in remaining oil for 2 minutes. Add pepper; stir-fry for 4-6 minutes longer or until vegetables are crisp-tender.

4. Stir cornstarch mixture and add to the pan. Bring to a boil; cook and stir for 2 minutes or until thickened.

5. Add beef; heat through. Serve with rice. Sprinkle with the remaining sesame seeds.

PER SERVING *2 cups stir-fry with ½ cup rice equals 363 cal., 12 g fat (3 g sat. fat), 47 mg chol., 606 mg sodium, 33 g carb., 5 g fiber, 31 g pro.* **Diabetic Exchanges:** *3 lean meat, 2 starch, 1 vegetable, 1 fat.*

Tangy Barbecued Pork Chops

Not only are these pork chops tasty, they're also lower in carbs! Serve them with mashed potatoes for a homey touch.

—NELLA PARKER HERSEY, MI

PREP: 35 MIN. • **BAKE:** 25 MIN.
MAKES: 6 SERVINGS

- 1 **medium onion, sliced**
- ½ **cup water**
- 3 **tablespoons cider vinegar**
- 2 **tablespoons sugar**
- 1 **tablespoon prepared mustard**
- 1 **lemon slice**
- ¼ **teaspoon salt**
- ¼ **teaspoon pepper**
- ⅛ **teaspoon crushed red pepper flakes**
- ½ **cup ketchup**
- 2 **tablespoons Worcestershire sauce**
- 1 **teaspoon liquid smoke, optional**
- 6 **bone-in pork loin chops (7 ounces each)**
- 1 **tablespoon canola oil**

1. In a small saucepan, combine the first nine ingredients. Bring to a boil. Reduce heat; simmer, uncovered, for 20 minutes. Stir in the ketchup, Worcestershire sauce and liquid smoke if desired; heat through. Discard lemon.

2. Meanwhile, in a large skillet, brown pork chops in oil in batches. Transfer to a 13x9-in baking dish coated with cooking spray; pour sauce over chops.

3. Cover and bake at 350° for 25-30 minutes or until a thermometer reads 160°.

PER SERVING *279 cal., 11 g fat (3 g sat. fat), 86 mg chol., 500 mg sodium, 13 g carb., 1 g fiber, 31 g pro.* **Diabetic Exchanges:** *4 lean meat, 1 starch.*

Slow Cooker Fajitas

I love fajitas from Mexican restaurants, but when I tried preparing them at home, the meat was always too chewy. Then I tried this recipe in my slow cooker, and my husband and I enjoyed every bite.

—KATIE URSO SENECA, IL

PREP: 25 MIN. • **COOK:** 8 HOURS
MAKES: 8 SERVINGS

- 1 **each medium green, sweet red and yellow peppers, cut into ½-inch strips**
- 1 **sweet onion, cut into ½-inch strips**
- 2 **pounds beef top sirloin steaks, cut into thin strips**
- ¾ **cup water**
- 2 **tablespoons red wine vinegar**
- 1 **tablespoon lime juice**
- 1 **teaspoon ground cumin**
- 1 **teaspoon chili powder**
- ½ **teaspoon salt**
- ½ **teaspoon garlic powder**
- ½ **teaspoon pepper**
- ½ **teaspoon cayenne pepper**
- 8 **flour tortillas (8 inches), warmed**
- ½ **cup salsa**
- ½ **cup shredded reduced-fat cheddar cheese**
- 8 **teaspoons minced fresh cilantro**

1. Place peppers and onion in a 5-qt. slow cooker. Top with beef. Combine the water, vinegar, lime juice and seasonings; pour over meat. Cover and cook on low for 8-10 hours or until the meat is tender.

2. Using a slotted spoon, place about ¾ cup meat mixture down the center of each tortilla. Top with salsa, cheese and cilantro; roll up.

PER SERVING *335 cal., 10 g fat (3 g sat. fat), 69 mg chol., 564 mg sodium, 32 g carb., 2 g fiber, 29 g pro.* **Diabetic Exchanges:** *3 lean meat, 2 starch, 1 vegetable.*

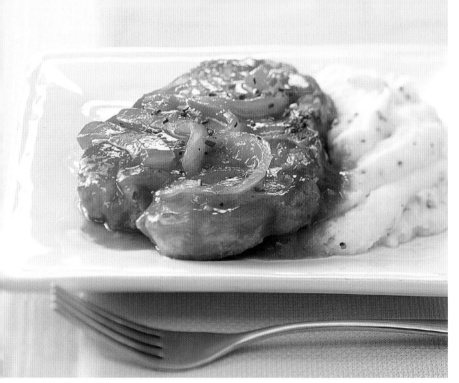

TANGY BARBECUED PORK CHOPS

Sesame-Pepper Flank Steak

Peppery yet sweet, this tender flank steak is a perfect excuse to heat up the grill.

—**VERA REID** LARAMIE, WY

PREP: 10 MIN. + MARINATING • **GRILL:** 15 MIN.
MAKES: 8 SERVINGS

- ¼ **cup sugar**
- ¼ **cup reduced-sodium soy sauce**
- 4 **green onions, sliced**
- 4 **garlic cloves, minced**
- 1 **tablespoon sesame seeds**
- 1 **tablespoon minced fresh gingerroot**
- 1 **tablespoon sesame oil**
- 2 **teaspoons pepper**
- 1 **beef flank steak (2 pounds)**

1. In a large resealable plastic bag, combine first eight ingredients. Score surface of beef with shallow diagonal cuts, making diamond shapes; place in bag. Seal bag and turn to coat; refrigerate for 8 hours or overnight.
2. Drain and discard marinade. Using long-handled tongs, moisten a paper towel with cooking oil and lightly coat the grill rack. Grill beef, covered, over medium heat or broil 4 in. from heat for 6-8 minutes on each side or until meat reaches desired doneness (for medium-rare, a thermometer should read 145°; medium, 160°; well-done, 170°).
3. Let stand for 5 minutes; thinly slice across the grain.
PER SERVING *3 ounces equals 197 cal., 9 g fat (4 g sat. fat), 54 mg chol., 220 mg sodium, 5 g carb., trace fiber, 23 g pro.* **Diabetic Exchanges:** *3 lean meat, 1½ fat.*

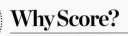

Why Score?

Scoring the surface of a flank steak prevents the edges from curling up when grilling.

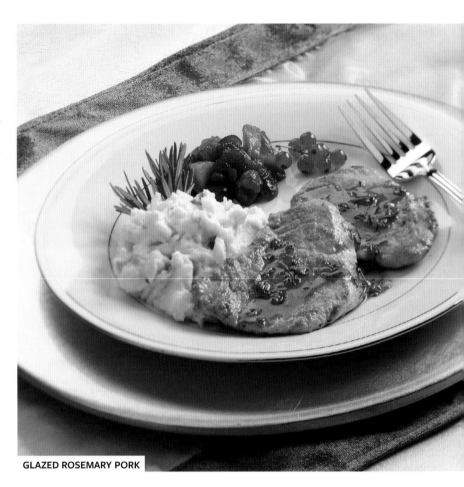

GLAZED ROSEMARY PORK

Glazed Rosemary Pork

This delicately seasoned pork is both fancy enough for a dinner party, but easy enough to make anytime.

—**BARBARA SISTRUNK** FULTONDALE, AL

START TO FINISH: 20 MIN.
MAKES: 6 SERVINGS

- 3 **tablespoons honey**
- 2 **teaspoons plus 1 tablespoon olive oil, divided**
- 1 **tablespoon Dijon mustard**
- 1 **tablespoon minced fresh rosemary or 1 teaspoon dried rosemary, crushed**
- 1 **teaspoon balsamic vinegar**
- 4 **garlic cloves, minced**
- ⅛ **teaspoon salt**
- ⅛ **teaspoon pepper**
- 2 **pork tenderloins (1 pound each), cut into 1-inch slices**

1. In a small bowl, combine the honey, 2 teaspoons oil, mustard, rosemary, vinegar, garlic, salt and pepper; set aside. Flatten pork slices to ½-in. thickness. In a large nonstick skillet, saute pork in remaining oil for 1 minute on each side or until browned.
2. Transfer to a 13x9-in. baking dish coated with cooking spray. Spoon honey mixture over the meat. Bake, uncovered, at 350° for 10-12 minutes or until a thermometer reads 160°.
PER SERVING *259 cal., 9 g fat (2 g sat. fat), 91 mg chol., 174 mg sodium, 10 g carb., trace fiber, 32 g pro.* **Diabetic Exchanges:** *4 lean meat, ½ starch.*

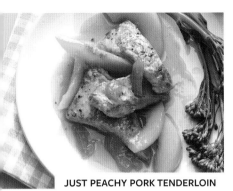

JUST PEACHY PORK TENDERLOIN

Just Peachy Pork Tenderloin

I decided to pair pork and ripe peaches together one night. We have a no-plate-licking rule in my home, but I licked my plate clean this time!

—JULIA GOSLIGA ADDISON, VERMONT

START TO FINISH: 20 MIN.
MAKES: 4 SERVINGS

- 1 pork tenderloin (1 pound), cut into 12 slices
- ½ teaspoon salt
- ¼ teaspoon pepper
- 2 teaspoons olive oil
- 4 medium peaches, peeled and sliced
- 1 tablespoon lemon juice
- ¼ cup peach preserves

1. Flatten each tenderloin slice to ¼-in. thickness. Sprinkle with salt and pepper. In a large nonstick skillet over medium heat, cook pork in oil until the juices run clear. Remove and keep warm.
2. Add peaches and lemon juice, stirring to loosen browned bits. Cook and stir over medium heat 3-4 minutes or until the peaches are tender. Stir in the pork and preserves; heat through.
PER SERVING 241 cal., 6 g fat (2 g sat. fat), 63 mg chol., 340 mg sodium, 23 g carb., 2 g fiber, 23 g pro. **Diabetic Exchanges:** 3 lean meat, 1 fruit, ½ starch, ½ fat.

Fillets with Mushroom Sauce

Dress up grilled tenderloin steaks with a delicious onion, mushroom and tomato sauce. The sauce can be whipped up while the meat is on the grill, which saves you lots of time!

—CAROLYN BRINKMEYER AURORA, CO

START TO FINISH: 25 MIN.
MAKES: 4 SERVINGS

- 4 beef tenderloin steaks (4 ounces each)
- 1 large onion, cut into ½-inch slices
- ½ pound fresh mushrooms, thickly sliced
- 2 tablespoons butter
- 1 can (14½ ounces) diced tomatoes, undrained
- ¼ cup water
- ½ teaspoon dried basil
- ½ teaspoon beef bouillon granules
- ⅛ teaspoon pepper

1. Grill, covered, over medium heat or broil 4 in. from the heat for 6-9 minutes on each side or until meat reaches desired doneness (for medium-rare, a thermometer should read 145°; medium, 160°; well-done, 170°).
2. Meanwhile, in a large skillet, saute onion and mushrooms in butter until tender. Stir in the tomatoes, water, basil, bouillon and pepper. Bring to a boil; cook and stir over medium heat for 5 minutes or until thickened. Serve with beef.
PER SERVING 278 cal., 14 g fat (0 sat. fat), 70 mg chol., 299 mg sodium, 10 g carb., 0 fiber, 26 g pro. **Diabetic Exchanges:** 3 lean meat, 2 vegetable, 1½ fat.

FILLETS WITH MUSHROOM SAUCE

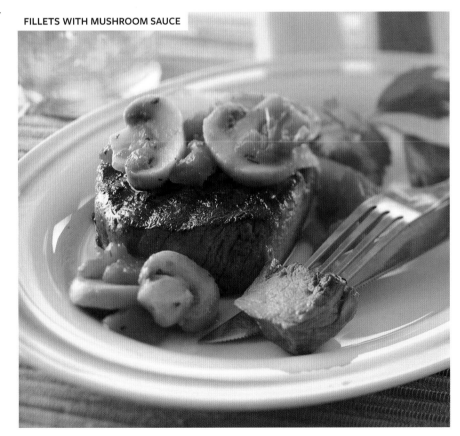

Ginger Steak Fried Rice

Perfect for a weeknight meal, all the ingredients for this recipe come together in one pan. Just serve with rice for a complete dinner. The steak will cut more easily if you partially freeze it ahead of time.

—**SIMONE GARZA** EVANSVILLE, IN

START TO FINISH: 30 MIN.
MAKES: 4 SERVINGS

- 2 **eggs, lightly beaten**
- 2 **teaspoons olive oil**
- 1 **beef top sirloin steak (¾ pound), cut into thin strips**
- 4 **tablespoons reduced-sodium soy sauce, divided**
- 1 **package (12 ounces) broccoli coleslaw mix**
- 1 **cup frozen peas**
- 2 **tablespoons grated fresh gingerroot**
- 3 **garlic cloves, minced**
- 2 **cups cold cooked brown rice**
- 4 **green onions, sliced**

1. In a large nonstick skillet coated with cooking spray, cook and stir eggs over medium heat until no liquid egg remains, breaking up eggs into small pieces. Remove from pan; wipe skillet clean if necessary.

2. In same pan, heat oil over medium-high heat. Add beef; stir-fry for 1-2 minutes or until no longer pink. Stir in 1 tablespoon soy sauce; remove from the pan.

3. Add coleslaw mix, peas, ginger and garlic to same pan; cook and stir until coleslaw mix is crisp-tender. Add rice and remaining soy sauce, tossing to combine rice with vegetable mixture and heat through. Stir in cooked eggs, beef and green onions; heat through.

PER SERVING *1½ cups equals 346 cal., 9 g fat (3 g sat. fat), 140 mg chol., 732 mg sodium, 36 g carb., 6 g fiber, 29 g pro.* **Diabetic Exchanges:** *3 lean meat, 2 starch, 1 vegetable, ½ fat.*

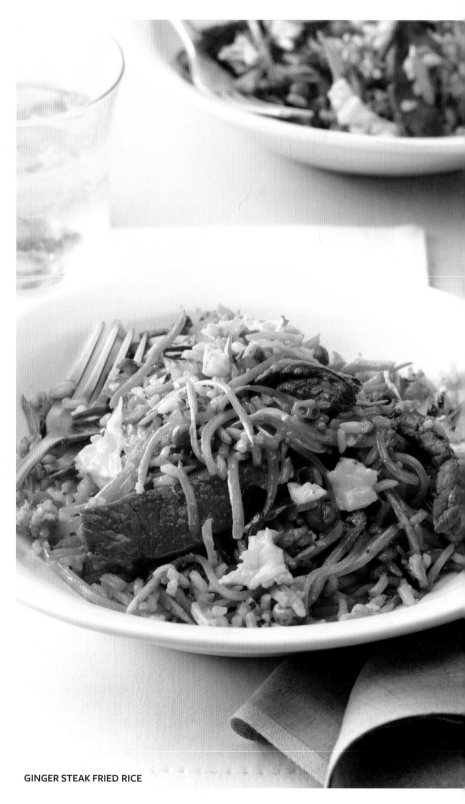

GINGER STEAK FRIED RICE

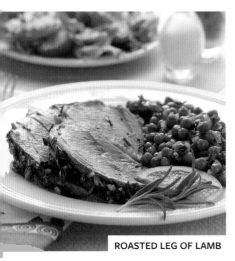

ROASTED LEG OF LAMB

Roasted Leg of Lamb

Rubbing rosemary, garlic and onion into this delectable roasted lamb takes the flavor to a whole new level.

—**SUZY HORVATH** MILWAUKIE, OR

PREP: 10 MIN. • **BAKE:** 2 HOURS + STANDING
MAKES: 10-12 SERVINGS

- ⅓ **cup olive oil**
- ¼ **cup minced fresh rosemary**
- ¼ **cup finely chopped onion**
- 4 **garlic cloves, minced**
- ½ **teaspoon salt**
- ¼ **teaspoon pepper**
- 1 **bone-in leg of lamb (5 to 6 pounds), trimmed**

1. Preheat oven to 325°. Combine the oil, rosemary, onion, garlic, salt and pepper; rub over lamb. Place fat side up on a rack in a shallow roasting pan.
2. Bake, uncovered, 2 to 2½ hours or until meat reaches desired doneness (for medium-rare, a thermometer should read 145°; medium, 160°; well-done, 170°), basting occasionally with pan juices. Let stand 15 minutes before slicing.
PER SERVING *212 cal., 12 g fat (3 g sat. fat), 85 mg chol., 137 mg sodium, 1 g carb., trace fiber, 24 g pro.* **Diabetic Exchanges:** *3 lean meat, 2 fat.*

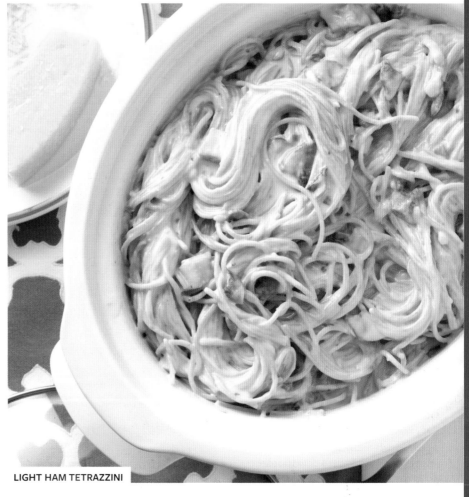

LIGHT HAM TETRAZZINI

Light Ham Tetrazzini

Feed a hungry crowd in a flash! If you're bringing this tetrazzini to a potluck, cook and add the spaghetti to the slow cooker just before heading out. No one will suspect this recipe is light.

—**SUSAN BLAIR** STERLING, MI

PREP: 15 MIN. • **COOK:** 4 HOURS
MAKES: 10 SERVINGS

- 2 **cans (10¾ ounces each) reduced-fat reduced-sodium condensed cream of mushroom soup, undiluted**
- 2 **cups sliced fresh mushrooms**
- 2 **cups cubed fully cooked ham**
- 1 **cup fat-free evaporated milk**
- ¼ **cup white wine or water**
- 2 **teaspoons prepared horseradish**
- 1 **package (14½ ounces) uncooked multigrain spaghetti**
- 1 **cup shredded Parmesan cheese**

1. In a 5-qt. slow cooker, combine the soup, mushrooms, ham, milk, wine and horseradish. Cover and cook on low for 4 hours.
2. Cook spaghetti according to package directions; drain. Add spaghetti and cheese to slow cooker; toss to coat.
PER SERVING *1 cup equals 279 cal., 5 g fat (2 g sat. fat), 26 mg chol., 734 mg sodium, 37 g carb., 4 g fiber, 20 g pro.* **Diabetic Exchanges:** *2½ starch, 1 lean meat, ½ fat.*

Mexican Meat Loaf

Welcome your family to the table with this Southwest-inspired meat loaf. It's comfort food at its healthy best!

—**MARY RELYEA** CANASTOTA, NY

PREP: 25 MIN. • **BAKE:** 55 MIN. + STANDING
MAKES: 8 SERVINGS

- 1 large onion, chopped
- 1 large sweet red pepper, chopped
- 3 garlic cloves, minced
- 1 tablespoon olive oil
- 1 cup dry bread crumbs
- 2 teaspoons chili powder
- 1 teaspoon salt
- 1 teaspoon dried oregano
- ½ teaspoon ground cumin
- ½ teaspoon pepper
- 1 can (14½ ounces) diced tomatoes with mild green chilies, divided
- ⅓ cup plain yogurt
- 1 egg, lightly beaten
- 2 pounds lean ground beef (90% lean)

1. In a large nonstick skillet, saute the onion, red pepper and garlic in oil until tender. Transfer to a large bowl. Stir in the bread crumbs, chili powder, salt, oregano, cumin, pepper, ⅔ cup diced tomatoes with green chilies, yogurt and egg. Crumble beef over mixture and mix well.

2. Shape into a loaf and place in an 11x7-in. baking dish coated with cooking spray. Spoon the remaining diced tomatoes over top. Bake, uncovered, at 350° for 55-60 minutes or until no pink remains and a meat thermometer reads 160°. Drain if necessary; let stand for 15 minutes before slicing.

PER SERVING *1 slice equals 296 cal., 13 g fat (5 g sat. fat), 98 mg chol., 672 mg sodium, 18 g carb., 3 g fiber, 26 g pro. Diabetic Exchanges: 3 lean meat, 1 starch, ½ fat.*

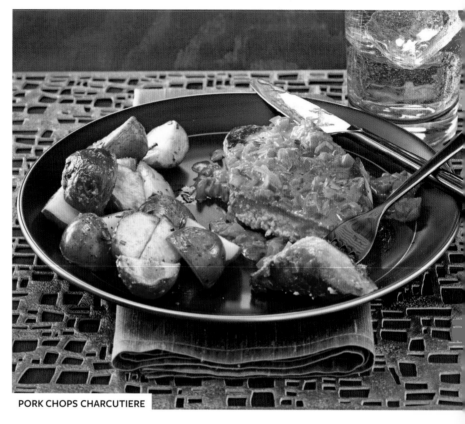

PORK CHOPS CHARCUTIERE

Pork Chops Charcutiere

The peppery mustard sauce spooned over these tender chops makes for a savory meal any night of the week.

—**MONIQUE HOOKER** DESOTO, WI

PREP: 25 MIN. • **COOK:** 25 MIN.
MAKES: 4 SERVINGS

- 4 boneless pork loin chops (5 ounces each)
- 1 to 3 teaspoons pepper
- 4½ teaspoons olive oil
- 1 small onion, finely chopped
- 4 shallots, finely chopped
- 1 cup reduced-sodium beef broth
- ½ cup white wine or additional reduced-sodium beef broth
- 2 tablespoons Dijon mustard
- 2 tablespoons chopped celery leaves or minced fresh parsley

1. Sprinkle pork chops with pepper. In a large nonstick skillet coated with cooking spray, brown chops in oil. Remove and keep warm. In the same skillet, saute onion and shallots until tender. Add broth and wine, stirring to loosen browned bits from skillet. Bring to a boil. Reduce heat; simmer, uncovered, for 3 minutes.

2. Return chops to skillet. Cover and cook 8-10 minutes longer or until meat is tender. Place chops on a serving platter and keep warm. Stir mustard into skillet. Return to a boil. Reduce heat; simmer, uncovered, for 12-15 minutes or until sauce is thickened. Spoon sauce over chops; sprinkle with celery leaves.

PER SERVING *292 cal., 13 g fat (4 g sat. fat), 70 mg chol., 339 mg sodium, 11 g carb., 1 g fiber, 29 g pro. Diabetic Exchanges: 4 lean meat, 1 starch, 1 fat.*

Slow-Cooked Stew

You can't beat this combination of melt-in-your-mouth beef and colorful vegetables in a thick sauce over noodles.

—DIANE DELANEY HARRISBURG, PA

PREP: 20 MIN. • **COOK:** 9 HOURS
MAKES: 10 SERVINGS

- 4 cups reduced-sodium V8 juice
- 3 tablespoons quick-cooking tapioca
- 1 tablespoon sugar
- ¼ teaspoon pepper
- 2 cups frozen cut green beans
- 2 cups fresh baby carrots, halved lengthwise
- 2 celery ribs, thinly sliced
- 1 small onion, chopped
- 1½ pounds beef stew meat, cut into 1-inch cubes
  Hot cooked noodles

In a large bowl, combine the V8 juice, tapioca, sugar and pepper; let stand for 15 minutes. In a 5-qt. slow cooker, combine the beans, carrots, celery and onion. Top with beef. Add V8 mixture. Cover and cook on low for 9-10 hours or until beef is tender. Serve over noodles.

PER SERVING *1 cup equals 156 cal., 5 g fat (2 g sat. fat), 42 mg chol., 141 mg sodium, 13 g carb., 2 g fiber, 14 g pro.* **Diabetic Exchanges:** *2 lean meat, 1 vegetable.*

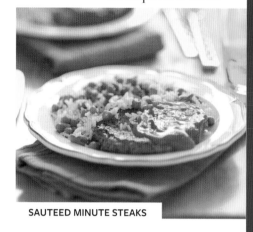

SAUTEED MINUTE STEAKS

Sauteed Minute Steaks

It only takes 20 minutes to get these steaks table-ready! The spicy sauce gives them a nice zip.

—INGE SCHERMERHORN KINGSTON, NH

START TO FINISH: 20 MIN.
MAKES: 2 SERVINGS

- ¼ cup all-purpose flour
- ½ teaspoon garlic salt
- ¼ teaspoon pepper
- 2 beef cubed steaks (5 ounces each)
- 1 tablespoon canola oil
- ⅓ cup ketchup
- 1 tablespoon lemon juice
- 1 teaspoon Worcestershire sauce
- ¾ teaspoon ground mustard

1. In a large resealable plastic bag, combine the flour, garlic salt and pepper. Add steaks, one at a time, and shake to coat.

2. In a large skillet coated with cooking spray, cook steaks in oil over medium heat for 3-4 minutes on each side or until no longer pink. Remove and keep warm. Stir in the remaining ingredients; heat through. Serve with the steaks.

PER SERVING *318 cal., 12 g fat (2 g sat. fat), 80 mg chol., 768 mg sodium, 18 g carb., 1 g fiber, 34 g pro.* **Diabetic Exchanges:** *4 lean meat, 1½ fat, 1 starch.*

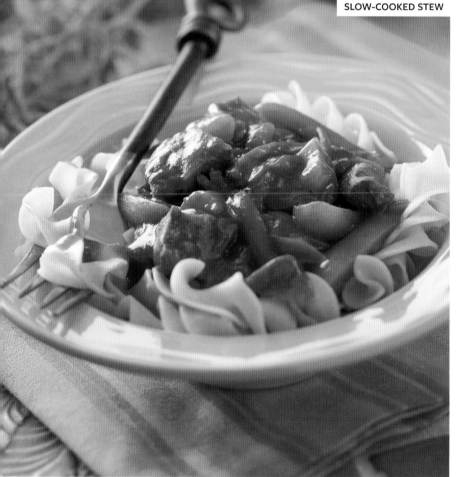

SLOW-COOKED STEW

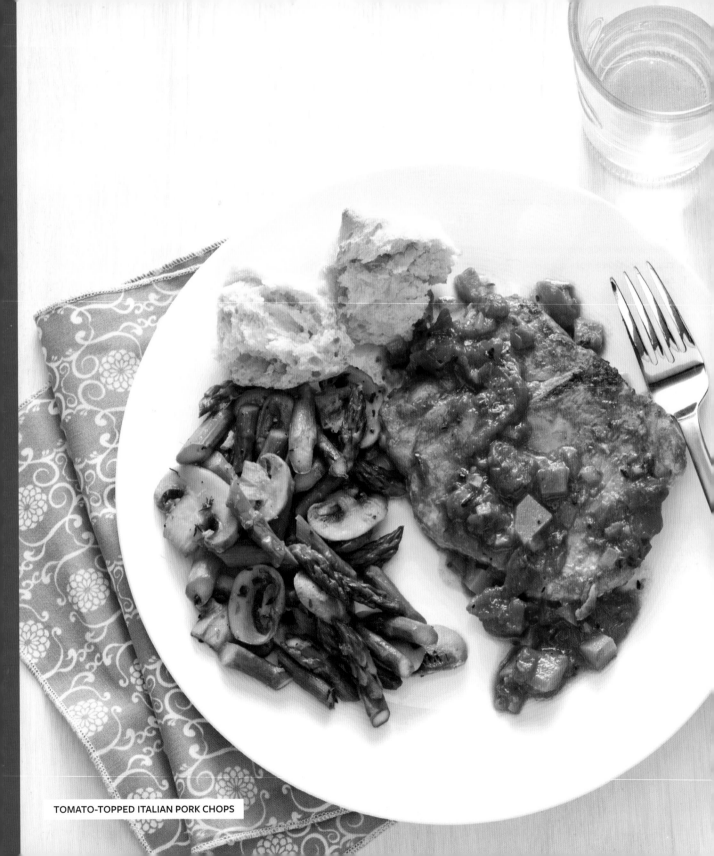

TOMATO-TOPPED ITALIAN PORK CHOPS

Tomato-Topped Italian Pork Chops

Time to bring out the slow cooker! You're only seven ingredients away from a nutritious yet delicious meal.

—KRYSTLE CHASSE RADIUM HOT SPRINGS, BC

PREP: 25 MIN. • **COOK:** 8 HOURS
MAKES: 6 SERVINGS

- 6 **bone-in pork loin chops (7 ounces each)**
- 1 **tablespoon canola oil**
- 1 **small onion, chopped**
- ½ **cup chopped carrot**
- 1 **can (14½ ounces) diced tomatoes, drained**
- ¼ **cup reduced-fat balsamic vinaigrette**
- 2 **teaspoons dried oregano**

1. In a large skillet, brown chops in oil in batches. Transfer to a 4- or 5-qt. slow cooker coated with cooking spray. Saute the onion and carrot in drippings until tender. Stir in the tomatoes, vinaigrette and oregano; pour over the chops.
2. Cover and cook on low for 8-10 hours or until the meat is tender.
PER SERVING *267 cal., 12 g fat (3 g sat. fat), 86 mg chol., 234 mg sodium, 7 g carb., 2 g fiber, 31 g pro.* **Diabetic Exchanges:** *4 lean meat, 1 vegetable, 1 fat.*

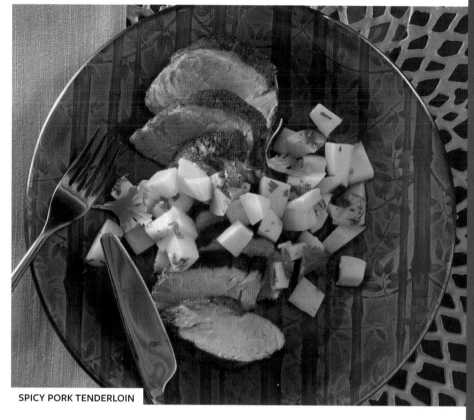

SPICY PORK TENDERLOIN

Spicy Pork Tenderloin

Cool, sweet mango salsa melds with the spicy rub on my pork tenderloin for a delicious, bold-flavored main dish.

—CAROLYN CARTELLI PARSIPPANY, NJ

PREP: 20 MIN. + CHILLING • **GRILL:** 25 MIN.
MAKES: 4 SERVINGS (2 CUPS SALSA)

- 1 **pork tenderloin (1 pound)**
- 1 **tablespoon olive oil**
- 2 **teaspoons coarsely ground pepper**
- 1½ **teaspoons paprika**
- ½ **teaspoon salt**
- ½ **teaspoon garlic powder**
- ½ **teaspoon chili powder**
- ½ **teaspoon ground cinnamon**
- ¼ **teaspoon cayenne pepper**

MANGO SALSA
- 1 **medium mango, peeled and cubed**
- 2 **tablespoons minced fresh cilantro**
- 2 **tablespoons lime juice**
- 1 **tablespoon honey**

1. Rub pork with oil. Combine the pepper, paprika, salt, garlic powder, chili powder, cinnamon and cayenne; rub over pork. Refrigerate for 30 minutes.
2. Using long-handled tongs, moisten a paper towel with cooking oil and lightly coat the grill rack. Prepare grill for indirect heat using a drip pan. Place pork over drip pan and grill, covered, over indirect medium-hot heat for 25-30 minutes or until a thermometer reads 160°. Let stand 5 minutes; slice. .
3. In a small bowl, combine mango, cilantro, lime juice and honey; serve with pork.
PER SERVING *3 ounces cooked pork with ½ cup salsa equals 222 cal., 8 g fat (2 g sat. fat), 63 mg chol., 345 mg sodium, 16 g carb., 2 g fiber, 23 g pro.* **Diabetic Exchanges:** *3 lean meat, ½ starch, ½ fruit, ½ fat.*

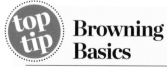

Browning Basics

Quickly browning meat in a skillet before simmering it in a slow cooker seals in the juices and gives the meat a deep, rich color.

Makeover Beef & Sausage Lasagna

My original version of this dish was higher in saturated fat. You'll love this healthy take.

—JACOB KITZMAN SEATTLE, WA

PREP: 45 MIN. • **BAKE:** 45 MIN. + STANDING
MAKES: 12 SERVINGS

- ¾ pound lean ground beef (90% lean)
- ¾ pound Italian turkey sausage links, casings removed
- 1 medium onion, chopped
- 1 medium green pepper, chopped
- 1 jar (26 ounces) spaghetti sauce
- 1 package (8 ounces) reduced-fat cream cheese, cubed
- 1 cup (8 ounces) 1% cottage cheese
- 1 egg, lightly beaten
- 1 tablespoon minced fresh parsley
- 6 whole wheat lasagna noodles, cooked and drained
- 1 cup (4 ounces) shredded reduced-fat Italian cheese blend
- 3 teaspoons Italian seasoning, divided
- 1 cup (4 ounces) shredded part-skim mozzarella cheese

1. In a large skillet, cook the beef, sausage, onion and green pepper over medium heat until meat is no longer pink; drain. Set aside 1 cup spaghetti sauce; stir remaining sauce into meat mixture. Bring to a boil. Reduce heat; simmer, uncovered, for 8-10 minutes or until thickened.

2. In a small saucepan, melt cream cheese over medium heat. Remove from the heat. Stir in the cottage cheese, egg and parsley.

3. Spread meat sauce into a 13x9-in. baking dish coated with cooking spray. Top with three noodles, Italian cheese blend, 1½ teaspoons Italian seasoning and cream cheese mixture. Layer with remaining noodles and reserved spaghetti sauce; sprinkle with mozzarella and remaining Italian seasoning.

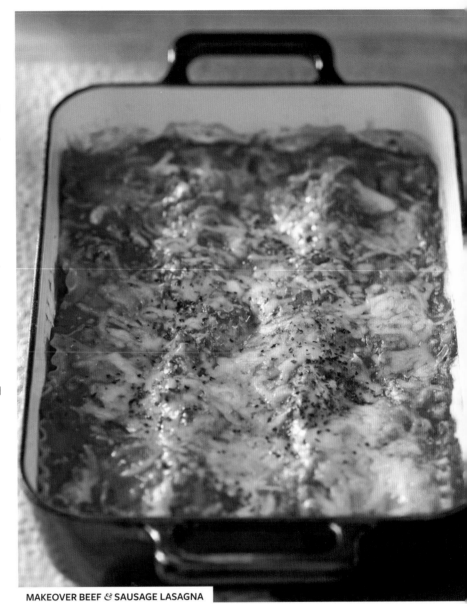

MAKEOVER BEEF & SAUSAGE LASAGNA

4. Cover and bake at 350° for 35 minutes. Bake, uncovered, for 10-15 minutes or until bubbly. Let stand for 15 minutes before cutting.

PER SERVING *298 cal., 15 g fat (7 g sat. fat), 78 mg chol., 772 mg sodium, 17 g carb., 3 g fiber, 23 g pro.* **Diabetic Exchanges:** *3 lean meat, 1½ fat, 1 starch.*

top tip Freezer Fix

Refrigerate leftover lasagna overnight. The next day, cut into individual servings, wrapping each in heavy duty foil. Store in the freezer for fast meals.

Slow-Cooked Caribbean Pot Roast

This dish is especially good in the fall and winter, but it's definitely an all-year-round recipe. What a tasty change of pace!

—**JENN TIDWELL** FAIR OAKS, CA

PREP: 30 MIN. • **COOK:** 6 HOURS
MAKES: 10 SERVINGS

- 2 medium sweet potatoes, cubed
- 2 large carrots, sliced
- ¼ cup chopped celery
- 1 boneless beef chuck roast (2½ pounds)
- 1 tablespoon canola oil
- 1 large onion, chopped
- 2 garlic cloves, minced
- 1 tablespoon all-purpose flour
- 1 tablespoon sugar
- 1 tablespoon brown sugar
- 1 teaspoon ground cumin
- ¾ teaspoon salt
- ¾ teaspoon ground coriander
- ¾ teaspoon chili powder
- ½ teaspoon dried oregano
- ⅛ teaspoon ground cinnamon
- ¾ teaspoon grated orange peel
- ¾ teaspoon baking cocoa
- 1 can (15 ounces) tomato sauce

1. Place potatoes, carrots and celery in a 5-qt. slow cooker. In a large skillet, brown meat in oil on all sides. Transfer meat to slow cooker.

2. In the same skillet, saute onion in drippings until tender. Add garlic; cook 1 minute longer. Combine flour, sugar, brown sugar, seasonings, orange peel and cocoa. Stir in tomato sauce; add to skillet and heat through. Pour over beef.

3. Cover and cook on low for 6-8 hours or until beef and vegetables are tender.

PER SERVING *3 ounces cooked beef with ½ cup vegetable mixture equals 278 cal., 12 g fat (4 g sat. fat), 74 mg chol., 453 mg sodium, 16 g carb., 3 g fiber, 25 g pro.* **Diabetic Exchanges:** *3 lean meat, 1 starch, 1 vegetable, ½ fat.*

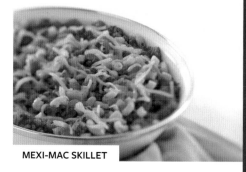

MEXI-MAC SKILLET

Mexi-Mac Skillet

My husband loves this recipe, and I love how simple it is to put together! You don't even need to precook the noodles.

—**MAURANE RAMSEY** FORT WAYNE, IN

START TO FINISH: 30 MIN.
MAKES: 5 SERVINGS

- 1 pound lean ground beef (90% lean)
- 1 large onion, chopped
- 1 can (14½ ounces) diced tomatoes, undrained
- 1 can (8 ounces) tomato sauce
- 1 cup fresh or frozen corn
- ½ cup water
- 1¼ teaspoons chili powder
- 1 teaspoon dried oregano
- ½ teaspoon salt
- ⅔ cup uncooked elbow macaroni
- ⅔ cup shredded reduced-fat cheddar cheese

1. In a large nonstick skillet over medium-high heat, cook beef and onion until meat is no longer pink; drain. Stir in the tomatoes, tomato sauce, corn, water, chili powder, oregano and salt.

2. Bring to a boil; stir in macaroni. Reduce heat; cover and simmer for 18-22 minutes or until macaroni is tender. Sprinkle with cheese.

PER SERVING *1 cup equals 283 cal., 11 g fat (5 g sat. fat), 55 mg chol., 716 mg sodium, 23 g carb., 4 g fiber, 25 g pro.* **Diabetic Exchanges:** *3 lean meat, 1 starch, 1 vegetable.*

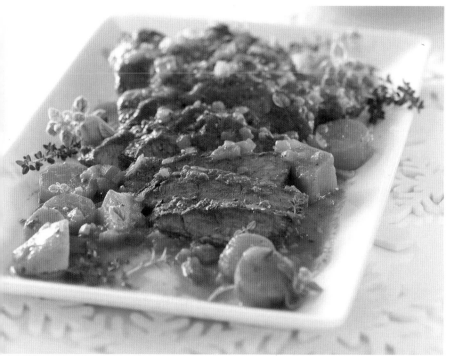

SLOW-COOKED CARIBBEAN POT ROAST

Southwest Steak

Lime juice tenderizes the steak, while garlic, chili powder and red pepper flakes kick things up. My husband and I came up with this recipe together when we wanted something lighter to make on the grill.

—CAROLINE SHIVELY C/O EVA SYNALOVSKI
NEW YORK, NY

PREP: 15 MIN. + MARINATING • **GRILL:** 10 MIN.
MAKES: 8 SERVINGS

- ¼ cup lime juice
- 6 garlic cloves, minced
- 4 teaspoons chili powder
- 4 teaspoons canola oil
- 1 teaspoon salt
- 1 teaspoon crushed red pepper flakes
- 1 teaspoon pepper
- 2 beef flank steaks (1 pound each)

1. In a large resealable plastic bag, combine the first seven ingredients; add beef. Seal bag and turn to coat; refrigerate for 4 hours or overnight.
2. Drain and discard marinade. Using long-handled tongs, moisten a paper towel with cooking oil and lightly coat the grill rack. Grill the beef, covered, over medium heat or broil 4 in. from the heat for 5-7 minutes on each side or until meat reaches desired doneness (for medium-rare, a thermometer should read 145°; medium, 160°; well-done, 170°).
3. Let stand for 5 minutes; thinly slice across the grain.

PER SERVING *3 ounces cooked beef equals 187 cal., 10 g fat (4 g sat. fat), 54 mg chol., 259 mg sodium, 2 g carb., trace fiber, 22 g pro.* **Diabetic Exchanges:** *3 lean meat, 1 fat.*

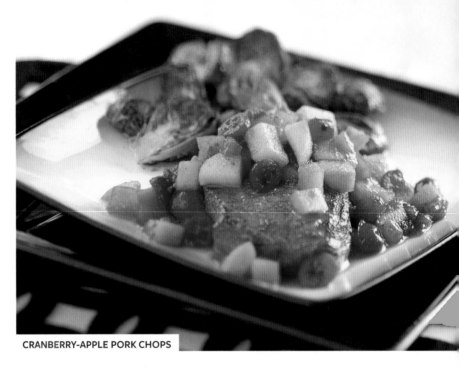

CRANBERRY-APPLE PORK CHOPS

Cranberry-Apple Pork Chops

These colorful, sweet-tart chops deliver a tasty punch with every bite!
—KATIE SHIREMAN AUDUBON, PA

PREP: 15 MIN. + MARINATING • **COOK:** 15 MIN.
MAKES: 2 SERVINGS

- 3 teaspoons ground cinnamon
- 1½ teaspoons ground nutmeg
- ½ teaspoon pumpkin pie spice
- 2 boneless pork loin chops (4 ounces each)
- ½ cup plus 2 tablespoons unsweetened apple juice, divided
- ½ cup plus 2 tablespoons cranberry juice, divided
- 1 teaspoon canola oil
- 1 medium apple, peeled and finely chopped
- 1 cup chopped fresh cranberries
- ⅛ teaspoon salt

1. Mix cinnamon, nutmeg and pie spice; rub over chops. Place pork in a large resealable plastic bag; add ½ cup each of apple and cranberry juices. Seal bag and turn to coat; refrigerate 8 hours or overnight.
2. Drain chops, discarding marinade. In a large nonstick skillet coated with cooking spray, heat oil over medium heat; brown chops on both sides.
3. Add apple, cranberries, salt and remaining juices; bring to a boil. Reduce the heat; simmer, covered, 7-10 minutes or until a thermometer inserted in the pork reads 145° and the apple is tender, turning once. Let stand 5 minutes before serving.

PER SERVING *254 cal., 9 g fat (3 g sat. fat), 55 mg chol., 181 mg sodium, 21 g carb., 4 g fiber, 22 g pro.* **Diabetic Exchanges:** *3 lean meat, 1½ fruit.*

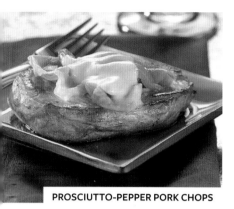

PROSCIUTTO-PEPPER PORK CHOPS

Prosciutto-Pepper Pork Chops

It's easy to adjust this meal to feed anywhere from two to eight people. Serve the chops with pasta salad for a satisfying, light meal.

—DONNA PRISCO RANDOLPH, NJ

START TO FINISH: 20 MIN.
MAKES: 4 SERVINGS

- 4 boneless pork loin chops (4 ounces each)
- ⅛ teaspoon garlic powder
- ⅛ teaspoon pepper
- 2 teaspoons canola oil
- 4 thin slices prosciutto or deli ham
- ½ cup julienned roasted sweet red peppers
- 2 slices reduced-fat provolone cheese, cut in half

1. Sprinkle pork chops with garlic powder and pepper. In a large nonstick skillet, cook chops in oil over medium heat for 4-5 minutes on each side or until a thermometer reads 145°.

2. Top each pork chop with prosciutto, red peppers and cheese. Cover and cook for 1-2 minutes or until the cheese is melted. Let stand for 5 minutes before serving.

PER SERVING *237 cal., 12 g fat (4 g sat. fat), 72 mg chol., 483 mg sodium, 1 g carb., trace fiber, 28 g pro.* **Diabetic Exchanges:** *4 lean meat, ½ fat.*

Linguine with Ham & Swiss Cheese

This version of my old linguine casserole recipe eliminates nearly half the saturated fat without losing the creamy texture or the distinctive Swiss cheese flavor.

—MIKE TCHOU PEPPER PIKE, OH

PREP: 15 MIN. • BAKE: 45 MIN.
MAKES: 8 SERVINGS

- 8 ounces uncooked whole wheat linguine, broken in half
- 2 cups cubed fully cooked lean ham
- 1¾ cups (7 ounces) shredded Swiss cheese, divided
- 1 can (10¾ ounces) reduced-fat reduced-sodium condensed cream of mushroom soup, undiluted
- 1 cup (8 ounces) reduced-fat sour cream
- 1 medium onion, chopped
- 1 small green pepper, finely chopped

1. Cook linguine according to package directions. Meanwhile, in a large bowl, combine the ham, 1½ cups of cheese, soup, sour cream, onion and green pepper. Drain pasta; add to the ham mixture and stir to coat.

2. Transfer to a 13x9-in. baking dish coated with cooking spray. Cover and bake at 350° for 35 minutes. Uncover; sprinkle with the remaining cheese. Bake 10-15 minutes longer or until cheese is melted.

PER SERVING *1 cup equals 293 cal., 12 g fat (7 g sat. fat), 47 mg chol., 665 mg sodium, 29 g carb., 4 g fiber, 19 g pro.* **Diabetic Exchanges:** *2 starch, 2 lean meat, 1 fat.*

LINGUINE WITH HAM & SWISS CHEESE

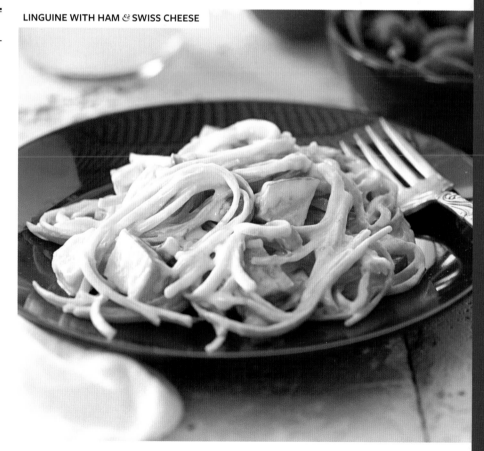

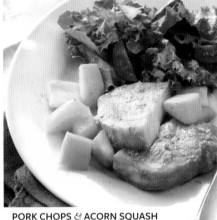

PORK CHOPS & ACORN SQUASH

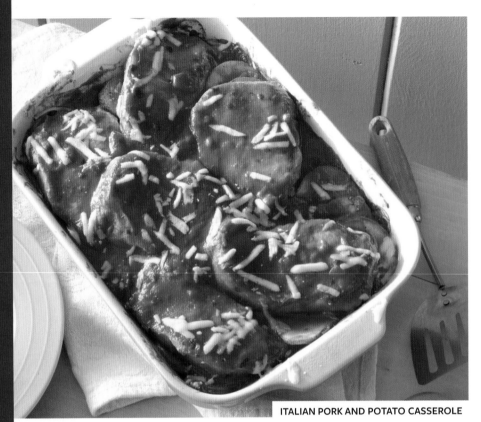

ITALIAN PORK AND POTATO CASSEROLE

Italian Pork and Potato Casserole

Three generations of my family have cherished this recipe. My mother concocted it years ago using a few ingredients she had on hand. When the casserole starts cooking in the oven, it brings back so many memories of home.

—THERESA KREYCHE TUSTIN, CA

PREP: 10 MIN. • **BAKE:** 45 MIN.
MAKES: 6 SERVINGS

- 6 **cups sliced red potatoes**
- 3 **tablespoons water**
- 1 **garlic clove, minced**
- ½ **teaspoon salt**
- ⅛ **teaspoon pepper**
- 6 **boneless pork loin chops (6 ounces each)**
- 1 **jar (24 ounces) marinara sauce**
- ¼ **cup shredded Parmesan cheese**

1. Place potatoes and water in a microwave-safe dish. Cover and microwave on high for 5 minutes or until almost tender; drain.
2. Place potatoes in a 13x9-in. baking dish coated with cooking spray. Sprinkle with garlic, salt and pepper. Top with pork chops and marinara sauce. Cover and bake at 350° for 40-45 minutes or until a thermometer inserted in the pork reads 145° and the potatoes are tender.
3. Sprinkle with cheese. Bake, uncovered, 3-5 minutes longer or until cheese is melted. Let stand 5 minutes before serving.
NOTE *This recipe was tested in a 1,100-watt microwave.*
PER SERVING *412 cal., 11 g fat (4 g sat. fat), 84 mg chol., 506 mg sodium, 38 g carb., 4 g fiber, 39 g pro.* **Diabetic Exchanges:** *5 lean meat, 2½ starch.*

Pork Chops & Acorn Squash

My husband and I can never get enough of the fresh acorn squash from our garden, so we added them to this recipe. We put our slow cooker to good use when we throw in these tasty chops.

—MARY JOHNSON COLOMA, WI

PREP: 15 MIN. • **COOK:** 4 HOURS
MAKES: 6 SERVINGS

- 6 **boneless pork loin chops (4 ounces each)**
- 2 **medium acorn squash, peeled and cubed**
- ½ **cup packed brown sugar**
- 2 **tablespoons butter, melted**
- 1 **tablespoon orange juice**
- ¾ **teaspoon salt**
- ½ **teaspoon grated orange peel**
- ¾ **teaspoon browning sauce, optional**

1. Place pork chops in a 5-qt. slow cooker; add squash. In a small bowl, combine the brown sugar, butter, orange juice, salt, orange peel and browning sauce if desired; pour over squash. Cover and cook on low for 4-6 hours or until meat is tender.
PER SERVING *317 cal., 10 g fat (5 g sat. fat), 65 mg chol., 365 mg sodium, 34 g carb., 2 g fiber, 23 g pro.* **Diabetic Exchanges:** *3 lean meat, 2 starch, 1 fat.*

Horseradish-Encrusted Beef Tenderloin

Wow friends and family with this tender beef in a golden horseradish crust.

—**LAURA BAGOZZI** DUBLIN, OH

PREP: 30 MIN. + COOLING
BAKE: 45 MIN. + STANDING
MAKES: 8 SERVINGS

- 1 **whole garlic bulb**
- 1 **teaspoon olive oil**
- ⅓ **cup prepared horseradish**
- ¼ **teaspoon salt**
- ¼ **teaspoon dried basil**
- ¼ **teaspoon dried thyme**
- ¼ **teaspoon pepper**
- ⅓ **cup soft bread crumbs**
- 1 **beef tenderloin roast (3 pounds)**

1. Remove papery outer skin from garlic (do not peel or separate cloves). Cut top off garlic bulb; brush with oil. Wrap in heavy-duty foil. Bake at 425° for 30-35 minutes or until softened. Cool for 10-15 minutes.

2. Squeeze softened garlic into a small bowl; stir in the horseradish, salt, basil, thyme and pepper. Add bread crumbs; toss to coat. Spread over top of tenderloin. Place on a rack in a large shallow roasting pan.

3. Bake at 400° for 45-55 minutes or until meat reaches desired doneness (for medium-rare, a thermometer should read 145°; medium, 160°; well-done, 170°). Let stand for about 10 minutes before slicing.

PER SERVING *5 ounces cooked beef equals 268 cal., 11 g fat (4 g sat. fat), 75 mg chol., 119 mg sodium, 4 g carb., 1 g fiber, 37 g pro.* **Diabetic Exchange:** *5 lean meat.*

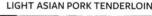

HORSERADISH-ENCRUSTED BEEF TENDERLOIN

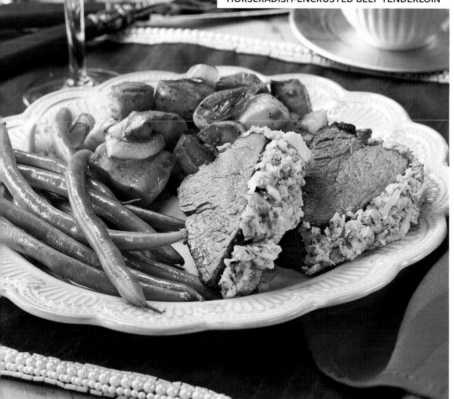

Light Asian Pork Tenderloin

I serve this light dish with jasmine rice and broccoli as a special dinner for two.

—**ANNEMARIE HARRIS** HADDONFIELD, NJ

PREP: 10 MIN. + MARINATING • **BAKE:** 20 MIN.
MAKES: 2 SERVINGS

- ½ **cup reduced-sodium soy sauce**
- 1 **tablespoon minced fresh gingerroot**
- 1½ **teaspoons sesame oil**
- 2 **whole cloves**
- 1 **pork tenderloin (¾ pound)**
- ¼ **cup sesame seeds**
- 1 **tablespoon honey**
- 1 **tablespoon brown sugar**

1. In a large resealable plastic bag, combine the soy sauce, ginger, sesame oil and cloves. Add the pork; seal bag and turn to coat. Refrigerate for 8 hours or overnight.

2. Drain and discard marinade. Place sesame seeds in a shallow dish. Roll pork in sesame seeds and place in a 13x9-in. baking dish coated with cooking spray. Drizzle with honey; sprinkle with brown sugar.

3. Bake, uncovered, at 425° for 20-30 minutes or until a meat thermometer reads 160°.

PER SERVING *324 cal., 12 g fat (2 g sat. fat), 95 mg chol., 437 mg sodium, 19 g carb., trace fiber, 37 g pro.* **Diabetic Exchanges:** *5 lean meat, 1 starch, 1 fat.*

LIGHT ASIAN PORK TENDERLOIN

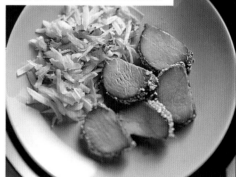

Pot Roast with Vegetables

This classic recipe uses an economical cut of beef that's simmered to perfection.

— NATIONAL LIVESTOCK AND MEAT BOARD

PREP: 10 MIN.
BAKE: 2¼ HOURS + STANDING
MAKES: 8 SERVINGS

- 1 **garlic clove, minced**
- 1 **teaspoon dried oregano**
- ½ **teaspoon lemon-pepper seasoning**
- 1 **boneless beef chuck pot roast (3 pounds)**
- 1 **tablespoon canola oil**
- ¾ **cup plus 1 tablespoon water, divided**
- 16 **small new potatoes, halved**
- 4 **medium carrots, cut into 2½ inch pieces**
- 4 **medium parsnips, cut into 2½ inch pieces**
- 2 **small leeks, cut into 1½ inch pieces**
- 2 **teaspoons cornstarch**

1. Combine the garlic, oregano and lemon-pepper; rub over roast. In a Dutch oven, brown roast in oil on all sides; drain. Add ¾ cup water; bring to a boil. Reduce heat; cover and simmer for 1¾ hours.

2. Add vegetables; cover and simmer for 30-35 minutes longer or until the beef is tender. Remove to a serving platter and keep warm. Let stand for 10 minutes before slicing.

3. Strain cooking liquid; skim off fat. Return 1 cup liquid to pan and bring to a boil over medium-high heat.

4. Combine cornstarch and remaining water until smooth; add to pan. Cook and stir for 1 minute or until gravy is thickened and bubbly. Serve with roast and vegetables.

PER SERVING *287 cal., 7 g fat (0 sat. fat), 64 mg chol., 48 mg sodium, 28 g carb., 0 fiber, 27 g pro.* **Diabetic Exchanges:** *4 lean meat, 1½ starch, 1 vegetable.*

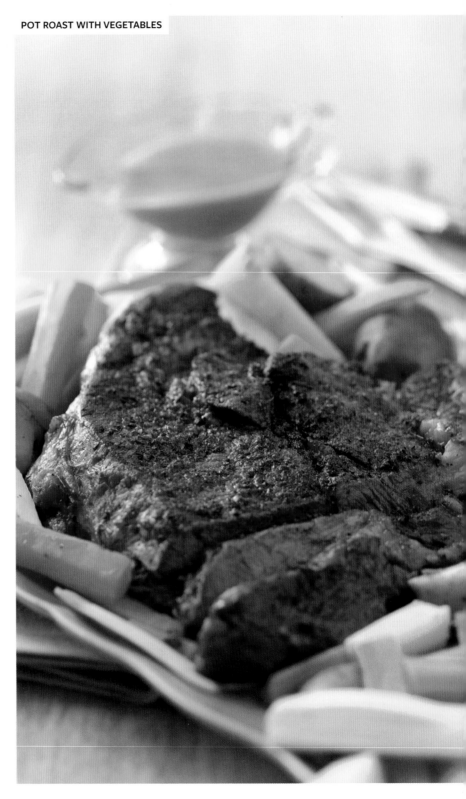

POT ROAST WITH VEGETABLES

Christmas Carol Ham

Supper is so simple when you prepare this slow-cooked entree. My family loves it! Simmered in pineapple juice, the ham slices are really flavorful.

—**JULIE WILLIQUETTE** HARTSELLE, AL

PREP: 10 MIN. • **COOK:** 2 HOURS
MAKES: 8 SERVINGS

- 2 **pounds fully cooked boneless ham, cut into eight slices**
- ½ **cup packed brown sugar**
- ¼ **cup unsweetened pineapple juice**
- 1½ **teaspoons white vinegar**
- ¼ **teaspoon ground mustard**

Place ham slices in a 3-qt. slow cooker. In a small bowl, combine the brown sugar, pineapple juice, vinegar and mustard; pour over ham. Cover and cook on low for 2-3 hours or until heated through.

PER SERVING *186 cal., 5 g fat (2 g sat. fat), 83 mg chol., 1,237 mg sodium, 15 g carb., trace fiber, 21 g pro.* **Diabetic Exchanges:** *3 lean meat, 1 starch.*

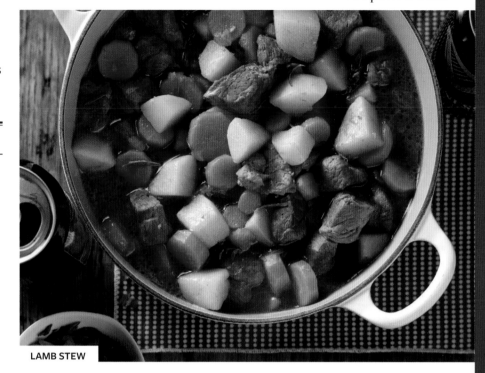

LAMB STEW

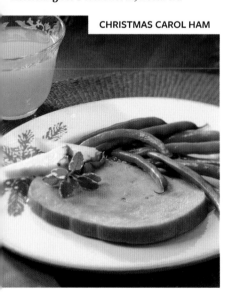

CHRISTMAS CAROL HAM

Lamb Stew

My grandmother used to make this stew as a special Sunday meal. It's also a memorable treat from Ireland. If you like your stew thick and rich, you've got to try this one!

—**VICKIE DESOURDY** WASHINGTON, NC

PREP: 40 MIN. • **BAKE:** 1½ HOURS
MAKES: 8 SERVINGS (2½ QUARTS)

- 2 **pounds lamb stew meat, cut into 1-inch cubes**
- 1 **tablespoon butter**
- 1 **tablespoon olive oil**
- 1 **pound carrots, sliced**
- 2 **medium onions, thinly sliced**
- 2 **garlic cloves, minced**
- 1½ **cups reduced-sodium chicken broth**
- 1 **bottle (12 ounces) Guinness stout or additional reduced-sodium chicken broth**
- 6 **medium red potatoes, peeled and cut into 1-inch cubes**
- 4 **bay leaves**
- 2 **fresh thyme sprigs**
- 2 **fresh rosemary sprigs**
- 2 **teaspoons salt**
- 1½ **teaspoons pepper**
- ¼ **cup heavy whipping cream**

1. Preheat oven to 325°. In an ovenproof Dutch oven, brown lamb in butter and oil in batches. Remove and keep warm. In the same pan, saute carrots and onions in drippings until crisp-tender. Add garlic; cook 1 minute. Gradually add broth and beer. Stir in lamb, potatoes, bay leaves, thyme, rosemary, salt and pepper.

2. Cover and bake 1½ to 2 hours or until meat and vegetables are tender, stirring every 30 minutes. Discard bay leaves, thyme and rosemary. Stir in the cream; heat through.

PER SERVING *1¼ cups equals 311 cal., 12 g fat (5 g sat. fat), 88 mg chol., 829 mg sodium, 23 g carb., 4 g fiber, 26 g pro.* **Diabetic Exchanges:** *3 lean meat, 2 vegetable, 1 starch, 1 fat.*

Glazed Pork Roast

Featuring a hint of orange, my roast doesn't last long once I set it out. I usually take it along to potlucks and get-togethers.

—RADELLE KNAPPENBERGER OVIEDO, FL

PREP: 30 MIN. • **COOK:** 4 HOURS
MAKES: 16 SERVINGS

- 1 **boneless pork loin roast (4 pounds), trimmed**
- 1 **tablespoon olive oil**
- 1 **tablespoon butter, melted**
- ⅔ **cup thawed orange juice concentrate**
- ⅓ **cup water**
- 3 **garlic cloves, minced**
- 1½ **teaspoons salt**
- ½ **teaspoon pepper**

GLAZE
- ¼ **cup packed brown sugar**
- 2 **tablespoons balsamic vinegar**
- 1 **tablespoon thawed orange juice concentrate**
- 1 **garlic clove, minced**
- 1 **can (11 ounces) mandarin oranges, drained, optional**

1. Cut roast in half. In a large skillet, brown roast in oil and butter on all sides.

2. Transfer to a 5-qt. slow cooker. Add the orange juice concentrate, water, garlic, salt and pepper. Cover and cook on low for 4-6 hours or until the meat is tender.

3. For glaze, in a small saucepan, combine the brown sugar, vinegar, orange juice concentrate and garlic. Bring to a boil. Reduce heat; simmer, uncovered, for 3-5 minutes or until reduced to about ¼ cup. Brush over roast. Garnish with oranges if desired.

PER SERVING *3 ounces equals 190 cal., 7 g fat (2 g sat. fat), 58 mg chol., 263 mg sodium, 9 g carb., trace fiber, 22 g pro.* **Diabetic Exchanges:** *3 lean meat, ½ starch.*

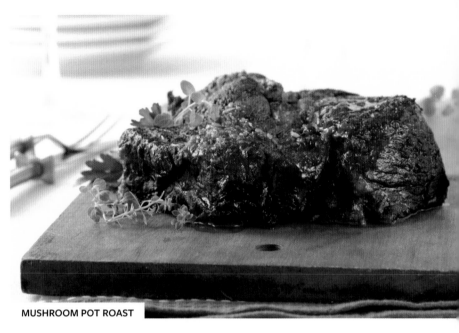

MUSHROOM POT ROAST

Mushroom Pot Roast

Packed with wholesome veggies and tender beef, this is one company-special dish that everyone will like—whether following a special diet or not.

—ANGIE STEWART TOPEKA, KS

PREP: 25 MIN. • **COOK:** 6 HOURS
MAKES: 10 SERVINGS

- 1 **boneless beef chuck roast (3 to 4 pounds)**
- ½ **teaspoon salt**
- ¼ **teaspoon pepper**
- 1 **tablespoon canola oil**
- 1½ **pounds sliced fresh shiitake mushrooms**
- 2½ **cups thinly sliced onions**
- 1½ **cups reduced-sodium beef broth**
- 1½ **cups dry red wine or additional reduced-sodium beef broth**
- 1 **can (8 ounces) tomato sauce**
- ¾ **cup chopped peeled parsnips**
- ¾ **cup chopped celery**
- ¾ **cup chopped carrots**
- 8 **garlic cloves, minced**
- 2 **bay leaves**
- 1½ **teaspoons dried thyme**
- 1 **teaspoon chili powder**
- ¼ **cup cornstarch**
- ¼ **cup water**
  Mashed potatoes

1. Sprinkle roast with salt and pepper. In a Dutch oven, brown roast in oil on all sides. Transfer to a 6-qt. slow cooker. Add the mushrooms, onions, broth, wine, tomato sauce, parsnips, celery, carrots, garlic, bay leaves, thyme and chili powder. Cover and cook on low for 6-8 hours or until the meat is tender.

2. Remove meat and vegetables to a serving platter; keep warm. Discard bay leaves. Skim fat from cooking juices; transfer to a small saucepan. Bring liquid to a boil. Combine cornstarch and water until smooth; gradually stir into the pan. Bring to a boil; cook and stir for 2 minutes or until thickened. Serve with mashed potatoes, meat and vegetables.

PER SERVING *4 ounces cooked beef with ⅔ cup vegetables and ½ cup gravy equals 310 cal., 14 g fat (5 g sat. fat), 89 mg chol., 363 mg sodium, 14 g carb., 3 g fiber, 30 g pro.* **Diabetic Exchanges:** *4 lean meat, 2 vegetable, 1½ fat.*

Easy Burgundy Stew

This satisfying stew has almost two-thirds less sodium than similar convenience products. To lower it even further, replace the diced tomatoes with the no-salt variety.

—COLEEN BALCH CLAY, NY

PREP: 20 MIN. • **BAKE:** 3 HOURS
MAKES: 7 SERVINGS

- 1 boneless beef chuck roast (2 pounds), cut into 1-inch cubes
- 1 can (14½ ounces) diced tomatoes, undrained
- ½ pound sliced fresh mushrooms
- 4 medium carrots, sliced
- 2 medium onions, sliced
- 2 celery ribs, chopped
- 1 cup Burgundy wine or reduced-sodium beef broth
- 1 tablespoon minced fresh thyme or 1 teaspoon dried thyme
- ½ teaspoon salt
- ½ teaspoon ground mustard
- ¼ teaspoon pepper
- 3 tablespoons all-purpose flour
- 1 cup water

In an ovenproof Dutch oven, combine the first 11 ingredients. Combine flour and water until smooth. Gradually stir into stew. Cover and bake at 325° for 3 hours or until meat and vegetables are tender, stirring every 30 minutes.
PER SERVING *1 cup equals 287 cal., 13 g fat (5 g sat. fat), 84 mg chol., 332 mg sodium, 15 g carb., 4 g fiber, 28 g pro.* **Diabetic Exchanges:** *3 lean meat, 2 vegetable, 1 fat.*

CHILI PORK TENDERLOIN

Chili Pork Tenderloin

Just because a dish is good for you doesn't mean it has to be tough and without flavor. My family can't get enough of this tender pork meal.

—RENEE BARFIELD THOMASTON, GA

PREP: 10 MIN. • **BAKE:** 25 MIN.
MAKES: 3 SERVINGS

- 1 tablespoon lime juice
- 1 teaspoon chili powder
- 1 teaspoon reduced-sodium soy sauce
- ½ teaspoon sugar
- ½ teaspoon salt
- ¼ teaspoon pepper
- 1 pork tenderloin (1 pound)
- 1 tablespoon canola oil

1. In a small bowl, combine the first six ingredients; brush over pork. In a large ovenproof skillet, brown pork in oil on all sides.
2. Bake at 375° for 25-30 minutes or until a thermometer reads 145°. Let stand for 5 minutes before slicing.
PER SERVING *224 cal., 10 g fat (2 g sat. fat), 84 mg chol., 529 mg sodium, 2 g carb., trace fiber, 30 g pro.* **Diabetic Exchanges:** *4 lean meat, 1 fat.*

EASY BURGUNDY STEW

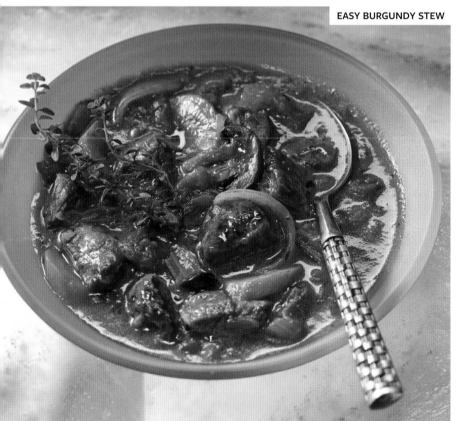

Stovetop Beef 'n' Shells

I fix this supper when I'm pressed for time. Pair it with salad, bread and fruit for a simple but comforting meal.

—**DONNA ROBERTS** MANHATTAN, KS

START TO FINISH: 30 MIN.
MAKES: 4 SERVINGS

- 1½ **cups uncooked medium pasta shells**
- 1 **pound lean ground beef (90% lean)**
- 1 **medium onion, chopped**
- 1 **garlic clove, minced**
- 1 **can (15 ounces) crushed tomatoes**
- 1 **can (8 ounces) tomato sauce**
- 1 **teaspoon sugar**
- ½ **teaspoon salt**
- ½ **teaspoon pepper**

1. Cook pasta according to package directions. Meanwhile, in a large saucepan, cook beef and onion over medium heat until meat is no longer pink. Add the garlic; cook 1 minute longer. Drain.

2. Stir in the tomatoes, tomato sauce, sugar, salt and pepper. Bring to a boil. Reduce heat; simmer, uncovered, for 10-15 minutes. Drain pasta; stir into beef mixture and heat through.

PER SERVING *1¼ cups equals 339 cal., 9 g fat (4 g sat. fat), 56 mg chol., 772 mg sodium, 36 g carb., 4 g fiber, 29 g pro.* **Diabetic Exchange:** *3 lean meat, 3 vegetable, 1½ starch.*

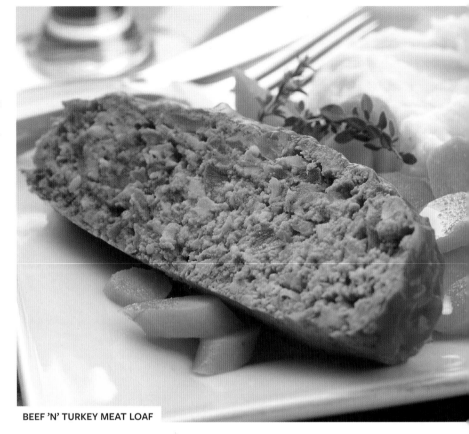

BEEF 'N' TURKEY MEAT LOAF

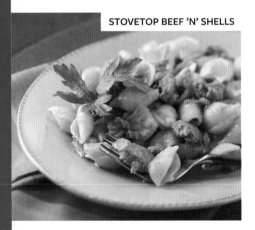

STOVETOP BEEF 'N' SHELLS

Beef 'n' Turkey Meat Loaf

Shredded potatoes bulk up my meat loaf, seasoned with garlic and thyme.

—**FERN NEAD** FLORENCE, KY

PREP: 15 MIN. • **BAKE:** 50 MIN. + STANDING
MAKES: 6 SERVINGS

- 2 **egg whites, beaten**
- ⅔ **cup ketchup, divided**
- 1 **medium potato, peeled and finely shredded**
- 1 **medium green pepper, finely chopped**
- 1 **small onion, grated**
- 3 **garlic cloves, minced**
- 1 **teaspoon salt**
- 1 **teaspoon dried thyme**
- ½ **teaspoon pepper**
- ¾ **pound lean ground beef (90% lean)**
- ¾ **pound lean ground turkey**

1. In a large bowl, combine egg whites and ⅓ cup ketchup. Stir in the potato, green pepper, onion, garlic, salt, thyme and pepper. Crumble beef and turkey over mixture and mix well. Shape into a 10x 4-in. loaf.

2. Line a 15x10x1-in. baking pan with heavy-duty foil and coat the foil with cooking spray. Place loaf in pan. Bake, uncovered, at 375° for 45 minutes; drain. Brush with remaining ketchup. Bake 5-10 minutes longer or until no pink remains and a thermometer reads 165°. Let meat loaf stand for 10 minutes before slicing.

PER SERVING *240 cal., 9 g fat (3 g sat. fat), 79 mg chol., 808 mg sodium, 16 g carb., 2 g fiber, 23 g pro.* **Diabetic Exchanges:** *3 lean meat, 1 starch.*

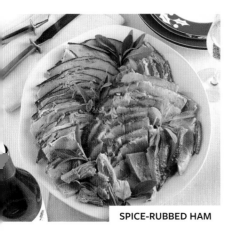

SPICE-RUBBED HAM

Spice-Rubbed Ham

Now this is a ham! It's sweet and smoky, with just the right amount of clove and ginger...and it serves a crowd!

—**SHARON TIPTON** WINTER GARDEN, FL

PREP: 15 MIN.
BAKE: 3¼ HOURS + STANDING
MAKES: 24 SERVINGS

- 1 fully cooked semi-boneless ham (8 to 10 pounds)
- ½ cup spicy brown mustard
- ¼ cup packed brown sugar
- ¼ teaspoon ground ginger
- ¼ teaspoon ground cinnamon
  Whole cloves

1. Place ham on a rack in a shallow roasting pan. Score the surface of the ham, making diamond shapes ½ in. deep. Combine the mustard, brown sugar, ginger and cinnamon; rub over surface of ham. Insert a clove into each diamond.
2. Bake, uncovered, at 325° for 1½ hours. Cover and bake for 1¾ to 2 hours longer or until a thermometer reads 140°. Cover loosely with foil if ham browns too quickly. Discard cloves. Let stand for 10 minutes before slicing.
PER SERVING *3 ounces equals 139 cal., 4 g fat (1 g sat. fat), 66 mg chol., 858 mg sodium, 3 g carb., trace fiber, 22 g pro. Diabetic Exchange: 3 lean meat.*

Black Bean and Beef Tostadas

All you need are a handful of ingredients to whip up one of my family's all-time favorites. You can also easily double the recipe for company or extra guests.

—**SUSAN BROWN** KANSAS CITY, KS

START TO FINISH: 30 MIN.
MAKES: 4 SERVINGS

- 8 ounces lean ground beef (90% lean)
- 1 can (10 ounces) diced tomatoes and green chilies, undrained
- 1 can (15 ounces) black beans, rinsed and drained
- 1 can (16 ounces) refried beans
- 8 tostada shells

Optional toppings: shredded lettuce, shredded reduced-fat Mexican cheese blend, sour cream and/or salsa

1. In a large skillet, cook beef over medium heat until no longer pink; drain. Stir in tomatoes. Bring to a boil. Reduce heat; simmer, uncovered, for 6-8 minutes or until liquid is reduced to 2 tablespoons. Stir in black beans; heat through.
2. Spread refried beans over tostada shells. Top with beef mixture. Serve with toppings of your choice.
PER SERVING *390 cal., 11 g fat (3 g sat. fat), 44 mg chol., 944 mg sodium, 49 g carb., 12 g fiber, 24 g pro. Diabetic Exchanges: 3 starch, 3 lean meat.*

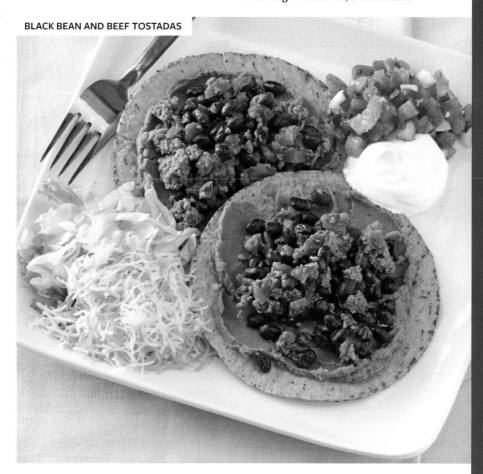

BLACK BEAN AND BEEF TOSTADAS

Asian Beef Strips

For a more ethnic version of this recipe, soak the beef strips in Japanese rice wine (sake). The beef also can be grilled for a little change-of-pace flavor. This is one recipe that's ideal for small households.

—**JOE VARGA** COLLINGSWOOD, NJ

PREP: 15 MIN. + MARINATING • **BROIL:** 5 MIN.
MAKES: 2 SERVINGS

- ½ pound beef top sirloin steak, cut into ¼-inch strips
- 2 green onions, thinly sliced
- ¼ cup reduced-sodium soy sauce
- 3 tablespoons sugar
- 2 tablespoons white wine or unsweetened apple juice
- 4 garlic cloves, minced
- 1 tablespoon sesame seeds
- 1 teaspoon sesame oil
- ¼ teaspoon pepper
  Hot cooked rice, optional

1. Flatten each strip of steak to ⅛-in. thickness.
2. In a large resealable plastic bag, combine the onions, soy sauce, sugar, wine, garlic, sesame seeds, oil and pepper; add the beef. Seal bag and turn to coat; refrigerate for at least 1 hour. Drain and discard marinade.
3. Place beef on a small broiler pan. Broil 3-4 in. from the heat for 2-3 minutes on each side or until meat reaches desired doneness. Serve with rice if desired.
PER SERVING *195 cal., 7 g fat (2 g sat. fat), 63 mg chol., 436 mg sodium, 8 g carb., trace fiber, 23 g pro.* **Diabetic Exchanges:** *3 lean meat, ½ starch.*

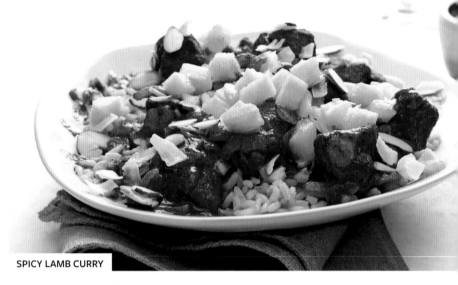
SPICY LAMB CURRY

Spicy Lamb Curry

I've tweaked this curry over the years using a blend of aromatic spices. Fenugreek seeds can be found in specialty spice stores and are common in Middle Eastern curries and chutneys, but you can leave them out of this recipe if you desire.

—**JANIS KRACHT** WINDSOR, NY

PREP: 25 MIN. + MARINATING
COOK: 1 HOUR
MAKES: 6 SERVINGS

- 3 tablespoons ground cumin
- 2 tablespoons ground ginger
- 1 tablespoon ground coriander
- 1 tablespoon ground fenugreek
- 4 garlic cloves, minced
- 1 teaspoon ground cloves
- ½ teaspoon ground cinnamon
- 2 pounds lamb stew meat, cut into ¾-inch pieces
- 1 tablespoon olive oil
- 2 large onions, chopped
- ½ cup water
- 2 tablespoons paprika
- 2 tablespoons tomato paste
- 1 teaspoon salt
- 1 teaspoon ground mustard
- 1 teaspoon chili powder
- 1 cup (8 ounces) plain yogurt
- 3 cups hot cooked brown rice
  Optional toppings: cubed fresh pineapple, flaked coconut and toasted sliced almonds

1. In a large resealable plastic bag, combine the first seven ingredients. Add the lamb; seal bag and turn to coat. Refrigerate for 8 hours or overnight.
2. In a Dutch oven, brown meat in oil in batches; remove and keep warm. In the same pan, cook onions in drippings until tender. Add the water, paprika, tomato paste, salt, mustard and the chili powder.
3. Return lamb to pan. Bring to a boil. Reduce heat; cover and simmer for 1 to 1½ hours or until meat is tender. Remove from the heat; stir in yogurt. Serve with rice. Top with pineapple, coconut and almonds if desired.
NOTE *Fenugreek is available from Penzeys Spices. Call 800-741-7787 or visit penzeys.com.*
PER SERVING *¾ cup curry with ½ cup rice equals 419 cal., 14 g fat (4 g sat. fat), 104 mg chol., 534 mg sodium, 36 g carb., 6 g fiber, 37 g pro.* **Diabetic Exchanges:** *4 lean meat, 2 starch, 1 vegetable, 1 fat.*

Italian Beef Tortellini Stew

This was the first recipe I created on my own—it turned out to be a keeper! You'll enjoy the rich stew, full of veggies, tender beef and a splash of red wine.

—TAMMY MUNYON WICHITA, KS

PREP: 25 MIN. • **COOK:** 1¾ HOURS
MAKES: 6 SERVINGS (2¼ QUARTS)

- ⅓ **cup all-purpose flour**
- 1 **teaspoon pepper, divided**
- 1 **pound beef stew meat, cut into 1-inch cubes**
- 3 **tablespoons olive oil, divided**
- 2 **medium zucchini, cut into ½-inch pieces**
- 1 **large onion, chopped**
- 2 **celery ribs, sliced**
- 3 **small carrots, sliced**
- 3 **garlic cloves, minced**
- 1½ **teaspoons each dried oregano, basil and marjoram**
- ½ **cup dry red wine or reduced-sodium beef broth**
- 1 **can (28 ounces) crushed tomatoes**
- 3 **cups reduced-sodium beef broth**
- 1 **teaspoon sugar**
- 1 **package (9 ounces) refrigerated cheese tortellini**
- 1 **package (6 ounces) fresh baby spinach**

1. In a large resealable plastic bag, combine flour and ½ teaspoon pepper. Add beef, a few pieces at a time, and shake to coat.

2. In a Dutch oven, brown beef in 2 tablespoons oil; drain. Remove and set aside. In the same pan, saute the zucchini, onion, celery and carrots in remaining oil until tender. Add the garlic, oregano, basil and marjoram; cook 1 minute longer.

3. Add wine, stirring to loosen browned bits from pan. Return beef to pan; add the tomatoes, broth, sugar and remaining pepper. Bring to a boil. Reduce heat; cover and simmer for 1½ hours or until beef is tender. Add tortellini and spinach. Return to a boil. Cook, uncovered, for 7-9 minutes or until tortellini is tender.

PER SERVING *1½ cups equals 416 cal., 16 g fat (5 g sat. fat), 68 mg chol., 642 mg sodium, 43 g carb., 7 g fiber, 26 g pro. Diabetic Exchanges: 3 starch, 2 lean meat, 1½ fat.*

Corn Bread Casserole

Creamy mushroom stuffing tucked inside moist chops makes this dish special enough to serve company. Although the recipe serves just two, it can be doubled or tripled.

—LADONNA REED PONCA CITY, OK

PREP: 15 MIN. • **BAKE:** 35 MIN.
MAKES: 2 SERVINGS

- 2 **boneless pork loin chops (4 ounces each)**
- ½ **pound sliced fresh mushrooms**
- 2 **tablespoons all-purpose flour**
- ½ **cup reduced-sodium chicken broth**
- ½ **cup reduced-fat sour cream**
- 1 **tablespoon shredded Parmesan cheese**
- 2 **garlic cloves, minced**
  Pepper to taste
- ½ **cup crushed corn bread stuffing**

1. In a large skillet coated with cooking spray, brown pork chops on both sides; set aside. In the same skillet, saute mushrooms until tender. Transfer mushrooms to a 1½-qt. baking dish coated with cooking spray.

2. In a small bowl, combine flour and broth until smooth. Stir in the sour cream, cheese, garlic and pepper; pour over mushrooms. Top with pork chops.

3. Cover and bake at 350° for about 25 minutes. Sprinkle with stuffing. Bake 10 minutes longer or until a thermometer reads 160°.

PER SERVING *363 cal., 13 g fat (7 g sat. fat), 76 mg chol., 434 mg sodium, 27 g carb., 2 g fiber, 33 g pro. Diabetic Exchanges: 3 lean meat, 1½ starch, 1 vegetable, 1 fat.*

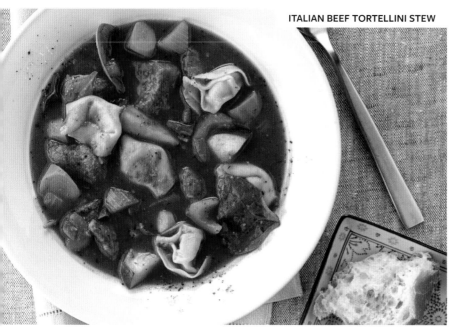

ITALIAN BEEF TORTELLINI STEW

Berry Barbecued Pork Roast

Moist and tender, this elegant pork roast topped with a thick, ruby-red cranberry barbecue sauce is sure to hit the spot at special dinners and holiday meals.

—DORIS HEATH FRANKLIN, NC

PREP: 15 MIN. • **BAKE:** 1 HOUR + STANDING
MAKES: 12 SERVINGS

- 1 **boneless rolled pork loin roast (3 pounds)**
- ¼ **teaspoon salt**
- ¼ **teaspoon pepper**
- 4 **cups fresh or frozen cranberries**
- 1 **cup sugar**
- ½ **cup orange juice**
- ½ **cup barbecue sauce**

1. Sprinkle roast with salt and pepper. Place with fat side up on a rack in a shallow roasting pan. Bake, uncovered, at 350° for 45 minutes.

2. Meanwhile, in a saucepan, combine the cranberries, sugar, orange juice and barbecue sauce. Bring to a boil. Reduce heat to medium-low; cook and stir for 10-12 minutes or until cranberries pop and sauce is thickened.

3. Brush some of the sauce over roast. Bake 15-20 minutes longer or until a thermometer reads 145°, brushing often with sauce. Let meat stand for 10 minutes before slicing. Serve with remaining sauce.

PER SERVING *3 ounces equals 262 cal., 8 g fat (3 g sat. fat), 67 mg chol., 190 mg sodium, 23 g carb., 1 g fiber, 24 g pro.* *Diabetic Exchanges:: 3 lean meat, 1 starch, ½ fruit.*

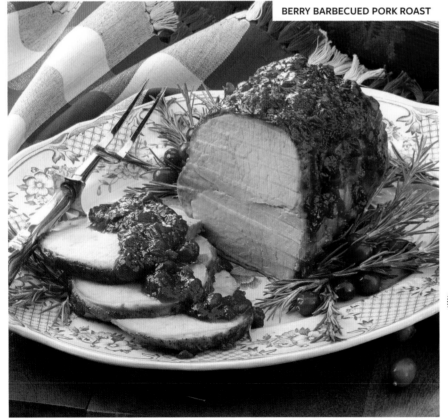

BERRY BARBECUED PORK ROAST

Chipotle-Rubbed Beef Tenderloin

Go ahead, rub it in! Coating traditional tenderloin with lively, peppery seasonings gives it a south-of-the-border twist. Your family or dinner guests will be impressed.

—TASTE OF HOME TEST KITCHEN

PREP: 10 MIN. + CHILLING
BAKE: 45 MIN. + STANDING
MAKES: 8 SERVINGS

- 1 **beef tenderloin roast (2 pounds)**
- 2 **teaspoons canola oil**
- 3 **teaspoons coarsely ground pepper**
- 3 **garlic cloves, minced**
- 2½ **teaspoons brown sugar**
- 1 **teaspoon salt**
- 1 **teaspoon ground coriander**
- ½ **teaspoon ground chipotle pepper**
- ¼ **teaspoon cayenne pepper**

1. Brush beef with oil. Combine the remaining ingredients; rub over meat. Cover and refrigerate for 2 hours.

2. Place on a rack coated with cooking spray in a shallow roasting pan. Bake, uncovered, at 400° for 45-55 minutes or until meat reaches desired doneness (for medium-rare, a thermometer should read 145°; medium, 160°; well-done, 170°). Let meat stand for 10 minutes before slicing.

PER SERVING *3 ounces equals 195 cal., 9 g fat (3 g sat. fat), 71 mg chol., 351 mg sodium, 2 g carb., trace fiber, 24 g pro.* *Diabetic Exchange: 3 lean meat.*

top tip Peeling Pointers

It's easy to peel fresh garlic. Using the blade of a chef's knife, crush garlic clove. Peel away skin. Chop or mince as directed in the recipe.

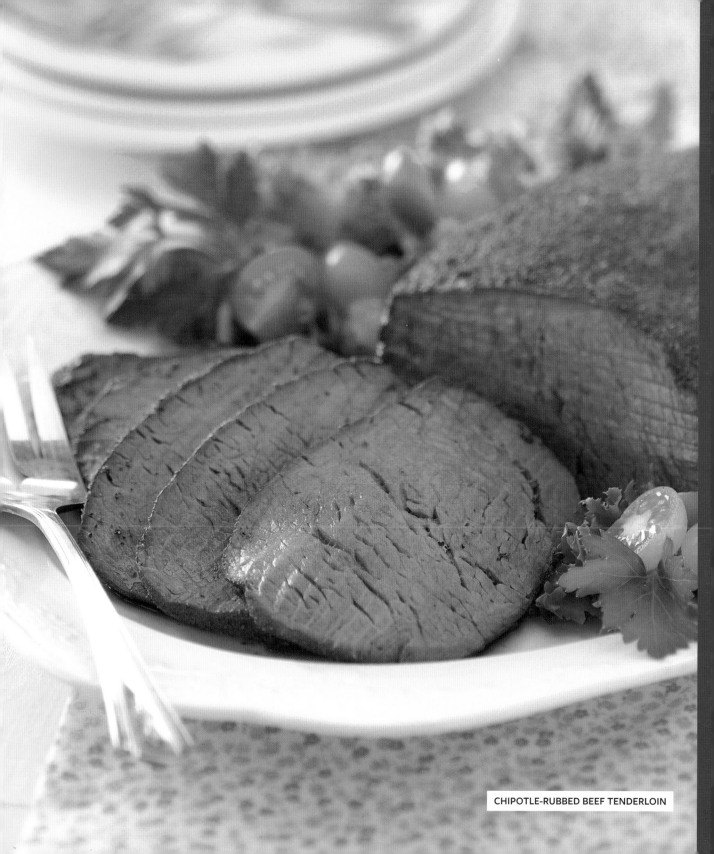

CHIPOTLE-RUBBED BEEF TENDERLOIN

Pork 'n' Pineapple Stir-Fry

A light sweet-and-sour sauce gently coats lean pork and mixed vegetables in this colorful stir-fry. Ginger and garlic give it zip, while pineapple adds a touch of the tropics.

—**REBECCA BAIRD** SALT LAKE CITY, UT

PREP: 20 MIN. + MARINATING
COOK: 15 MIN.
MAKES: 6 SERVINGS

- 4½ teaspoons all-purpose flour
- 5 tablespoons reduced-sodium soy sauce, divided
- 1 pork tenderloin (1 pound), cut into ½-inch cubes
- 2 tablespoons plus 1 teaspoon cornstarch
- 1 cup reduced-sodium chicken broth
- ¼ cup packed brown sugar
- ¼ cup rice vinegar
- ¼ cup sherry or additional reduced-sodium chicken broth
- 1 teaspoon sesame oil
- ¼ teaspoon white pepper
- 2 teaspoons canola oil, divided
- 1 large onion, chopped
- 2 medium carrots, thinly sliced
- 1 tablespoon minced fresh gingerroot
- 2 garlic cloves, minced
- 1 cup cubed fresh pineapple
- 1 large sweet red pepper, cut into ¾-inch pieces
- ½ cup thinly sliced green onions
  Hot cooked rice, optional

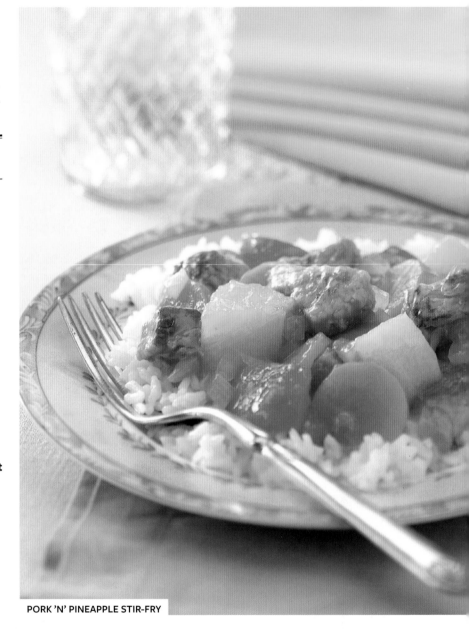

PORK 'N' PINEAPPLE STIR-FRY

1. Place flour and 1 tablespoon soy sauce in a large resealable plastic bag; add pork. Seal bag and turn to coat; refrigerate for 30 minutes.
2. In a small bowl, combine the cornstarch, broth, brown sugar, vinegar, sherry, sesame oil, white pepper and remaining soy sauce until smooth; set aside.
3. In a large skillet or wok, stir-fry pork in 1 teaspoon canola oil for 4-8 minutes or until meat is tender. Remove with a slotted spoon and keep warm.
4. Stir-fry the onion, carrots and ginger in remaining oil for 3-4 minutes. Add garlic; cook 1 minute longer. Add the pineapple, red pepper and green onions; stir-fry for 3-4 minutes or until vegetables are crisp-tender.
5. Stir cornstarch mixture and add to the pan. Bring to a boil; cook and stir for 2 minutes or until thickened. Return pork to the pan; heat through. Serve with rice if desired.
PER SERVING ⅔ cup equals 227 cal., 5 g fat (1 g sat. fat), 42 mg chol., 652 mg sodium, 26 g carb., 2 g fiber, 18 g pro. *Diabetic Exchanges: 2 lean meat, 1 starch, 1 vegetable, ½ fat.*

Glazed Pork with Strawberry Couscous

I like making this dish when mint and strawberries are plentiful in my garden. It adds a homey touch to the recipe.

—**BERNICE JANOWSKI** STEVENS POINT, WI

PREP: 15 MIN.
BAKE: 1 HOUR 20 MIN. + STANDING
MAKES: 10 SERVINGS

- 2 teaspoons dried marjoram
- 1 teaspoon salt
- 1 teaspoon seasoned pepper
- 1 bone-in pork loin roast (5 pounds)
- ½ cup seedless strawberry jam
- ½ cup orange juice, divided
- 1 can (14½ ounces) chicken broth
- 1 package (10 ounces) plain couscous
- 1 cup fresh strawberries, quartered
- ¼ cup minced fresh mint
- 2 teaspoons grated orange peel

1. Line the bottom of a large shallow roasting pan with foil; set aside. Combine the marjoram, salt and pepper; rub over roast. Place in pan. Bake, uncovered, at 350° for 1 hour.
2. Combine jam and ¼ cup orange juice; brush half over pork. Bake 20-30 minutes longer or until a meat thermometer reads 160°, basting with remaining jam mixture every 10 minutes. Let stand for 10 minutes before slicing.
3. Meanwhile, in a small saucepan, bring broth to a boil. Stir in couscous. Cover and remove from the heat; let stand for 5 minutes or until liquid is absorbed. Fluff with a fork; stir in the strawberries, mint, orange peel and remaining orange juice. Serve with the pork.
PER SERVING *4 ounces cooked meat with ½ cup couscous mixture equals 383 cal., 11 g fat (4 g sat. fat), 92 mg chol., 493 mg sodium, 35 g carb., 2 g fiber, 36 g pro.* **Diabetic Exchanges:** *4 lean meat, 2 starch, 1 fat.*

Bean Beef Burgers

When it comes to healthy eating, it's easy to boost your fiber intake with something as simple as eating more whole grains. So if you still want to enjoy a burger without all the fat—and also sneak in more fiber, these sizzling patties are your answer.

—**JENNIFER KUNZ** AUSTIN, TX

START TO FINISH: 30 MIN.
MAKES: 6 SERVINGS

- 1 cup water
- ½ cup bulgur
- 1 can (15 ounces) black beans, rinsed and drained
- 3 green onions, sliced
- 1 tablespoon stone-ground mustard
- 1 garlic clove, halved
- ¼ teaspoon salt
- ¼ teaspoon pepper
- 1 egg, lightly beaten
- ½ pound lean ground beef (90% lean)
- 1 tablespoon canola oil
- 6 whole wheat hamburger buns, split
  Spinach leaves, sliced red onion and tomato

1. In a small saucepan, bring water to a boil. Stir in bulgur. Reduce heat; cover and simmer for 15-20 minutes or until tender. In a food processor, combine the beans, onions, mustard and garlic. Cover and pulse until blended. Stir in salt and pepper.
2. In a large bowl, combine the egg and the bulgur and bean mixture. Crumble beef over mixture and mix well. Shape into six patties.
3. In a large nonstick skillet, cook patties in oil in batches for 4-5 minutes on each side or until a thermometer reads 160° and juices run clear. Serve on buns with spinach, onion and tomato.
PER SERVING *307 cal., 8 g fat (2 g sat. fat), 54 mg chol., 517 mg sodium, 42 g carb., 9 g fiber, 17 g pro.* **Diabetic Exchanges:** *2 starch, 2 lean meat, 1 fat.*

BEAN BEEF BURGERS

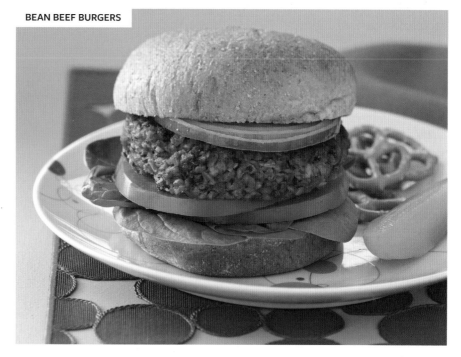

Slow-Cooked Sirloin

My family of five likes to eat beef, so I make this dish often. I usually serve it with homemade bread or rolls to soak up the savory gravy.

—**VICKI TORMASCHY** DICKINSON, ND

PREP: 20 MIN. • **COOK:** 3½ HOURS
MAKES: 6 SERVINGS

- 1 beef top sirloin steak (1½ pounds)
- 1 medium onion, cut into 1-inch chunks
- 1 medium green pepper, cut into 1-inch chunks
- 1 can (14½ ounces) reduced-sodium beef broth
- ¼ cup Worcestershire sauce
- ¼ teaspoon dill weed
- ¼ teaspoon dried thyme
- ¼ teaspoon pepper
  Dash crushed red pepper flakes
- 2 tablespoons cornstarch
- 2 tablespoons water

1. In a large nonstick skillet coated with cooking spray, brown beef on both sides. Place onion and green pepper in a 3-qt. slow cooker. Top with beef. Combine the broth, Worcestershire sauce, dill, thyme, pepper and pepper flakes; pour over beef. Cover and cook on high for 3-4 hours or until meat reaches desired doneness and the vegetables are crisp-tender.

2. Remove beef and keep warm. Combine cornstarch and water until smooth; gradually stir into cooking juices. Cover and cook on high for 30 minutes or until slightly thickened. Return the beef to the slow cooker; heat through.

PER SERVING *199 cal., 6 g fat (2 g sat. fat), 68 mg chol., 305 mg sodium, 8 g carb., 1 g fiber, 26 g pro.* **Diabetic Exchanges:** *3 lean meat, 1 vegetable.*

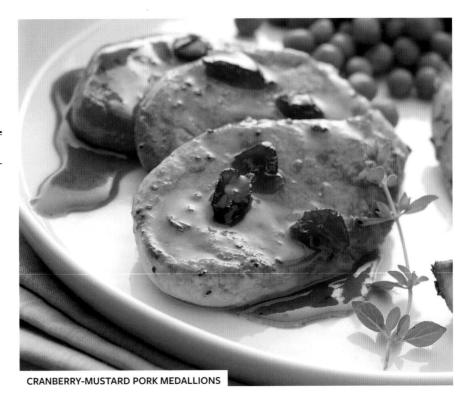

CRANBERRY-MUSTARD PORK MEDALLIONS

Cranberry-Mustard Pork Medallions

Topped with cranberry sauce, my pork medallions are both lean and filling. Guests will probably think you fussed!

—**TAMI MORRISON** KENT, WA

PREP: 15 MIN. • **COOK:** 20 MIN.
MAKES: 4 SERVINGS

- ⅔ cup water
- ⅓ cup thawed unsweetened apple juice concentrate
- ⅓ cup thawed cranberry juice concentrate
- ⅓ cup port wine or 1 tablespoon additional cranberry juice concentrate plus ¼ cup water
- 1 pork tenderloin (1 pound)
- ¼ teaspoon garlic salt
- ⅛ teaspoon pepper
- 1 tablespoon olive oil
- 1 tablespoon butter
- 2 to 3 tablespoons Dijon mustard
- ⅓ cup dried cranberries

1. In a bowl, combine the first four ingredients; set aside. Cut pork into 1-in. slices; flatten to ¼-in. thickness. Sprinkle with garlic salt and pepper.

2. In a large nonstick skillet, saute pork in oil and butter in batches for 2-3 minutes on each side or until the juices run clear. Remove and keep warm.

3. Add reserved juice mixture to the skillet; bring to a boil. Reduce heat; simmer for 3 minutes. Stir in mustard; cook and stir for 6-8 minutes or until slightly thickened. Add cranberries. Return the pork to the pan; cover and simmer for 5 minutes or until heated through.

PER SERVING *332 cal., 11 g fat (4 g sat. fat), 71 mg chol., 419 mg sodium, 34 g carb., 1 g fiber, 23 g pro.* **Diabetic Exchanges:** *3 lean meat, 1 starch, 1 fruit, 1 fat.*

Elegant Pork Marsala

Wine and fresh mushrooms lend a touch of sophistication to this reinvention of an Italian classic.

—KIM GILLIS HIGH FALLS, NY

START TO FINISH: 30 MIN.
MAKES: 6 SERVINGS

- ⅓ cup whole wheat flour
- ½ teaspoon pepper
- 6 boneless pork loin chops (4 ounces each)
- 1 tablespoon olive oil
- 2 cups sliced fresh mushrooms
- ⅓ cup chopped onion
- 2 turkey bacon strips, chopped
- ¼ teaspoon minced garlic
- 1 cup Marsala wine or additional reduced-sodium chicken broth
- 5 teaspoons cornstarch
- ⅔ cup reduced-sodium chicken broth

1. In a shallow bowl, mix flour and pepper. Dip pork chops in flour mixture to coat both sides; shake off excess.
2. In a large nonstick skillet coated with cooking spray, heat oil over medium heat. Add pork chops; cook 4-5 minutes on each side or until a thermometer reads 145°. Remove from pan; keep warm.
3. In same skillet, add mushrooms, onion and bacon to drippings; cook and stir 2-3 minutes or until mushrooms are tender. Add garlic; cook 1 minute longer. Add wine; increase heat to medium-high. Cook, stirring to loosen browned bits from pan.
4. In a small bowl, mix cornstarch and broth until smooth; add to pan. Bring to a boil; cook and stir 2 minutes or until slightly thickened. Serve with pork.

PER SERVING *1 pork chop with ⅓ cup sauce equals 232 cal., 10 g fat (3 g sat. fat), 60 mg chol., 161 mg sodium, 7 g carb., 1 g fiber, 24 g pro.* **Diabetic Exchanges:** *3 lean meat, ½ starch, ½ fat.*

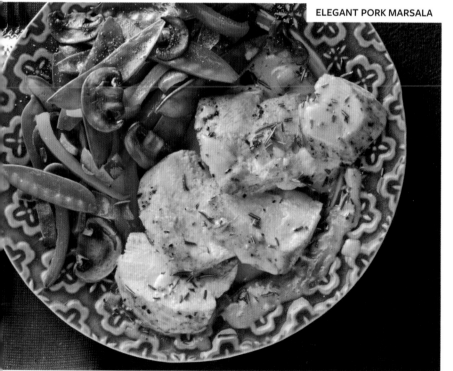
ELEGANT PORK MARSALA

Pork Chops with Orange Sauce

Tangy orange marinade gives these chops a citrusy twist. Add mashed potatoes or rice and a simple side salad for a fuss-free supper that everyone will enjoy.

—MARY CHANDLER GRAND TOWER, IL

PREP: 15 MIN. + MARINATING
BROIL: 10 MIN.
MAKES: 4 SERVINGS

- 1 cup orange juice
- ½ cup unsweetened pineapple juice
- ¼ cup reduced-sodium soy sauce
- 2 tablespoons honey
- 2 garlic cloves, minced
- ½ teaspoon grated orange peel
- ¼ teaspoon pepper
- 4 bone-in pork loin chops (7 ounces each)
- 1 tablespoon cornstarch

1. In a small bowl, combine the first seven ingredients. Pour a scant 1 cup into a large resealable plastic bag; add pork chops. Seal bag and turn to coat; refrigerate for 8 hours or overnight. Cover and refrigerate remaining marinade for sauce.
2. Drain chops and discard marinade. Using long-handled tongs, moisten a paper towel with cooking oil and lightly coat the grill rack.
3. Grill chops, covered, over medium heat or broil 4-5 in. from the heat for 4-5 minutes on each side or until a thermometer reads 145°. Let stand for 5 minutes before serving.
4. Meanwhile, in a small saucepan, combine cornstarch and reserved marinade. Bring to a boil; cook and stir for 2 minutes or until thickened. Serve with chops.

PER SERVING *269 cal., 8 g fat (3 g sat. fat), 86 mg chol., 451 mg sodium, 15 g carb., trace fiber, 31 g pro.* **Diabetic Exchanges:** *4 lean meat, 1 starch.*

Hungarian Goulash

My grandmother used to make this goulash for my mother. Paprika and caraway add wonderful flavor and the sour cream gives it a creamy richness.

—MARCIA DOYLE POMPANO, FL

PREP: 20 MIN. • **COOK:** 7 HOURS
MAKES: 12 SERVINGS

- 3 medium onions, chopped
- 2 medium carrots, chopped
- 2 medium green peppers, chopped
- 3 pounds beef stew meat, cut into 1-inch cubes
- ½ teaspoon plus ¼ teaspoon salt, divided
- ½ teaspoon plus ¼ teaspoon pepper, divided
- 2 tablespoons olive oil
- 1½ cups reduced-sodium beef broth
- ¼ cup all-purpose flour
- 3 tablespoons paprika
- 2 tablespoons tomato paste
- 1 teaspoon caraway seeds
- 1 garlic clove, minced
   Dash sugar
- 12 cups uncooked whole wheat egg noodles
- 1 cup (8 ounces) reduced-fat sour cream

1. Place the onions, carrots and green peppers in a 5-qt. slow cooker. Sprinkle the meat with ½ teaspoon salt and ½ teaspoon pepper. In a large skillet, brown meat in oil in batches. Transfer to slow cooker.

2. Add broth to skillet, stirring to loosen browned bits from pan. Combine the flour, paprika, tomato paste, caraway seeds, garlic, sugar and remaining salt and pepper; stir into skillet. Bring to a boil; cook and stir for 2 minutes or until thickened. Pour over meat. Cover and cook on low for 7-9 hours or until meat is tender.

3. Meanwhile, cook noodles according to package directions. Stir sour cream into slow cooker. Drain noodles; serve with goulash.

PER SERVING ⅔ cup goulash with 1 cup noodles equals 388 cal., 13 g fat (4 g sat. fat), 78 mg chol., 285 mg sodium, 41 g carb., 7 g fiber, 31 g pro. **Diabetic Exchanges:** 3 lean meat, 2 starch, 1 vegetable, 1 fat.

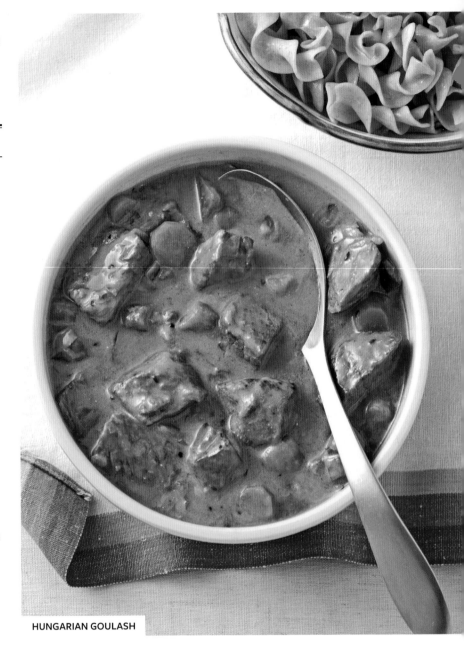

HUNGARIAN GOULASH

top tip Fresh Scent

After chopping onions, sprinkle your hands with salt, rub them together, then wash them. No more smelly hands!

Pineapple Pork

You'll need just a few ingredients to pull off this special entree of juicy grilled pineapple slices and ginger-flavored tenderloin.

—DONNA NOEL GRAY, ME

PREP: 10 MIN. + MARINATING • **GRILL:** 30 MIN.
MAKES: 4 SERVINGS

- 1 cup unsweetened pineapple juice
- ¼ cup minced fresh gingerroot
- ¼ cup reduced-sodium soy sauce
- 4 garlic cloves, minced
- 1 teaspoon ground mustard
- 2 pork tenderloins (¾ pound each)
- 1 fresh pineapple, cut into 12 slices

1. In a small bowl, combine the first five ingredients. Pour ⅔ cup marinade into a large resealable plastic bag. Add the pork; seal bag and turn to coat. Refrigerate for 8 hours or overnight. Cover and refrigerate the remaining marinade.

2. Drain and discard the marinade. Moisten a paper towel with cooking oil; using long-handled tongs, lightly coat the grill rack.

3. Prepare grill for indirect heat, using a drip pan. Place pork over drip pan and grill, covered, over indirect medium-hot heat for 25-30 minutes or until a thermometer reads 160°, basting occasionally with reserved marinade. Let stand for 5 minutes before slicing.

4. Meanwhile, grill pineapple slices for 2-3 minutes on each side or until heated through; serve with pork.

PER SERVING *295 cal., 6 g fat (2 g sat. fat), 95 mg chol., 523 mg sodium, 23 g carb., 2 g fiber, 36 g pro.* **Diabetic Exchanges:** *5 lean meat, 1 fruit.*

Herb Grilled Pork Tenderloin

A flavorful herb marinade turns this tenderloin into a mouthwatering creation. The marinade is also great on chicken.

—JUDY NEIL ROYAL OAK, MI

PREP: 10 MIN. + MARINATING • **GRILL:** 25 MIN.
MAKES: 6 SERVINGS

- ½ cup sherry or reduced-sodium chicken broth
- 3 tablespoons lemon juice
- 3 tablespoons reduced-sodium soy sauce
- 3 tablespoons honey
- 1 tablespoon canola oil
- 3 garlic cloves, minced
- 4½ teaspoons minced fresh sage or 1½ teaspoons rubbed sage
- 1 tablespoon minced fresh thyme or 1 teaspoon dried thyme
- 1 bay leaf
- 2 pork tenderloins (1 pound each)

1. In a small bowl, combine the first nine ingredients. Pour ¾ cup marinade into a large resealable plastic bag; add pork. Seal bag and turn to coat; refrigerate for at least 4 hours. Cover and refrigerate remaining marinade.

2. Drain pork and discard marinade. Using long-handled tongs, moisten a paper towel with cooking oil and lightly coat the grill rack. Prepare grill for indirect heat using a drip pan.

3. Place pork over drip pan and grill, covered, over indirect medium-hot heat for 25-40 minutes or until a thermometer reads 160°, basting occasionally with reserved marinade. Let stand for 5 minutes before slicing.

PER SERVING *226 cal., 7 g fat (2 g sat. fat), 84 mg chol., 261 mg sodium, 7 g carb., trace fiber, 30 g pro.* **Diabetic Exchanges:** *4 lean meat, ½ starch.*

HERB GRILLED PORK TENDERLOIN

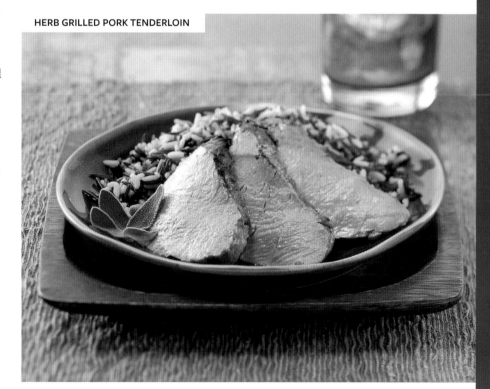

Pork with Blueberry Herb Sauce

Showcase blueberries in a whole new way! Mixing the berries with balsamic vinegar results in a sweet-savory sauce that would also go well with chicken.

—**LIBBY WALP** CHICAGO, IL

PREP: 15 MIN. • **COOK:** 20 MIN.
MAKES: 4 SERVINGS

- 1 garlic clove, minced
- 1 teaspoon pepper
- ½ teaspoon salt
- ⅛ teaspoon cayenne pepper
- 4 boneless pork loin chops (6 ounces each)
- 2 cups fresh blueberries
- ¼ cup packed brown sugar
- 2 tablespoons minced fresh parsley
- 1 tablespoon balsamic vinegar
- 2 teaspoons butter
- 1 teaspoon minced fresh thyme or ¼ teaspoon dried thyme
- 1 teaspoon fresh sage or ¼ teaspoon dried sage leaves

1. In a small bowl, combine the garlic, pepper, salt and cayenne; sprinkle over the pork.

2. In a large ovenproof skillet coated with cooking spray, brown pork chops. Bake, uncovered at 350° for 10-15 minutes or until a thermometer reads 160°. Remove pork and keep warm.

3. Add remaining ingredients to the pan. Cook and stir over medium heat until thickened, about 8 minutes. Serve with pork.

PER SERVING *343 cal., 12 g fat (5 g sat. fat), 87 mg chol., 364 mg sodium, 25 g carb., 2 g fiber, 33 g pro.* **Diabetic Exchanges:** *5 lean meat, 1 starch, ½ fruit.*

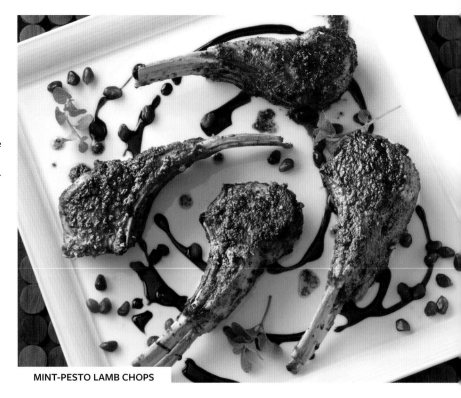

MINT-PESTO LAMB CHOPS

Mint-Pesto Lamb Chops

The simple mint-cilantro pesto marries well with lamb, while the pomegranate-balsamic reduction adds the perfect balance to finish off the dish. This entree is easy to prepare and sure to impress.

—**MELANIE STEVENSON** READING, PA

PREP: 40 MIN. • **COOK:** 20 MIN.
MAKES: 8 SERVINGS

- 2 cups pomegranate juice
- 1 cup balsamic vinegar

PESTO
- ¼ cup fresh mint leaves
- ¼ cup fresh cilantro leaves
- 8 garlic cloves, peeled
- 1 teaspoon salt
- 1 teaspoon pepper
- ¼ cup olive oil

LAMB
- 8 double-cut lamb rib chops (2 inches thick and 4 ounces each)
- 1 tablespoon olive oil

1. In a large saucepan, bring the pomegranate juice and vinegar to a boil over medium heat; cook until reduced to ½ cup.

2. Meanwhile, for pesto, place the mint, cilantro, garlic, salt and pepper in a small food processor; cover and pulse until chopped. While processing, gradually add oil in a steady stream.

3. Coat chops with pesto. In a large ovenproof skillet, brown lamb in oil on all sides.

4. Bake, uncovered, at 450° in oven for 15-20 minutes or until meat reaches desired doneness (for medium-rare, a thermometer should read 145°; medium, 160°; well-done, 170°). Drizzle with pomegranate sauce.

PER SERVING *2 lamb chops with 1 tablespoon sauce equals 238 cal., 13 g fat (3 g sat. fat), 45 mg chol., 352 mg sodium, 15 g carb., trace fiber, 15 g pro.* **Diabetic Exchanges:** *2 lean meat, 1½ fat, 1 starch.*

South of the Border Sirloin

Marinated in beer and jalapenos, these steaks have a mild kick that folks are sure to love! They're topped with veggies, bread crumbs and cheese for a fussed-over appearance and a special taste.

—**GILDA LESTER** MILLSBORO, DE

PREP: 15 MIN. + MARINATING • **BROIL:** 5 MIN.
MAKES: 4 SERVINGS

- 1 **bottle (12 ounces) light or nonalcoholic beer**
- 1 **medium onion, chopped**
- 3 **garlic cloves, minced**
- 1 **tablespoon chili powder**
- 1 **teaspoon salt**
- 1 **teaspoon pepper**
- 1 **beef top sirloin steak (1 pound)**

TOPPING

- 2 **large onions, thinly sliced**
- 5 **teaspoons olive oil, divided**
- 2 **jalapeno peppers, seeded and minced**
- 1 **medium sweet red pepper, julienned**
- 3 **garlic cloves, minced**
- 3 **tablespoons dry bread crumbs**
- 3 **tablespoons shredded reduced-fat cheddar cheese**

1. In a large resealable plastic bag, combine the first six ingredients. Cut steak into four serving-size pieces; place in bag. Seal bag and turn to coat; refrigerate for up to 2 hours.

2. Meanwhile, in a large ovenproof skillet, cook onions in 2 teaspoons oil over medium heat for 15-20 minutes or until onions are golden brown, stirring occasionally. Add peppers and garlic; cook 4 minutes longer. Remove and keep warm.

3. Drain and discard marinade. In the same skillet over medium heat, cook steak in 2 teaspoons oil for 3-4 minutes on each side or until meat reaches desired doneness (for medium-rare, a meat thermometer should read 145°; medium, 160°; well-done, 170°).

4. Spoon onion mixture over steaks. In a small bowl, combine the bread crumbs, cheese and remaining oil; sprinkle over tops. Broil 3-4 in. from the heat for 2-3 minutes or until golden brown.

NOTE *Wear disposable gloves when cutting hot peppers; the oils can burn skin. Avoid touching your face.*

PER SERVING *280 cal., 12 g fat (3 g sat. fat), 50 mg chol., 228 mg sodium, 15 g carb., 3 g fiber, 28 g pro.* **Diabetic Exchanges:** *3 lean meat, 2 vegetable, 1 fat.*

Pork Satay with Rice Noodles

I love adding peanut butter to savory recipes. Intensify the flavor in this one by sprinkling minced fresh cilantro and chopped peanuts on top.

—**STEPHANIE ANDERSON** HORSEHEADS, NY

PREP: 20 MIN. • **COOK:** 4 HOURS
MAKES: 6 SERVINGS

- 1½ **pounds boneless pork loin chops, cut into 2-inch pieces**
- ¼ **teaspoon pepper**
- 1 **medium onion, halved and sliced**
- ⅓ **cup creamy peanut butter**
- ¼ **cup reduced-sodium soy sauce**
- ½ **teaspoon onion powder**
- ½ **teaspoon garlic powder**
- ½ **teaspoon hot pepper sauce**
- 1 **can (14½ ounces) reduced-sodium chicken broth**
- 3 **tablespoons cornstarch**
- 3 **tablespoons water**
- 9 **ounces uncooked thick rice noodles Minced fresh cilantro and chopped peanuts, optional**

1. Sprinkle pork with pepper. Place in a 3-qt. slow cooker; top with onion. In a small bowl, mix peanut butter, soy sauce, onion powder, garlic powder and pepper sauce; gradually add broth. Pour over onion. Cook, covered, on low for 4-6 hours or until pork is tender.

2. Remove pork from slow cooker and keep warm. Skim fat from cooking juices; transfer cooking juices to a large skillet. Bring to a boil. In a small bowl, mix cornstarch and water until smooth and add to pan. Return to a boil; cook and stir 2 minutes or until thickened. Add pork; heat through.

3. Meanwhile, cook noodles according to package directions; drain. Serve with pork mixture. If desired, sprinkle with cilantro and peanuts.

NOTE *Reduced-fat peanut butter is not recommended for this recipe.*

PER SERVING *411 cal., 14 g fat (4 g sat. fat), 55 mg chol., 700 mg sodium, 41 g carb., 2 g fiber, 30 g pro.* **Diabetic Exchanges:** *3 lean meat, 2½ starch, 1 fat.*

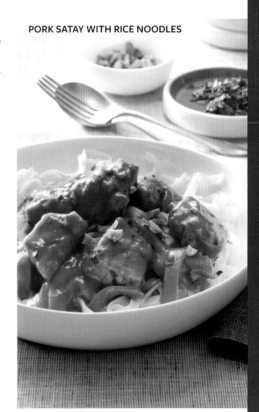

PORK SATAY WITH RICE NOODLES

chicken & turkey

Eating healthy doesn't have to be boring. Take your pick of any of these good-for-you options that don't sacrifice flavor. Your **whole family** is sure to spoon out second helpings!

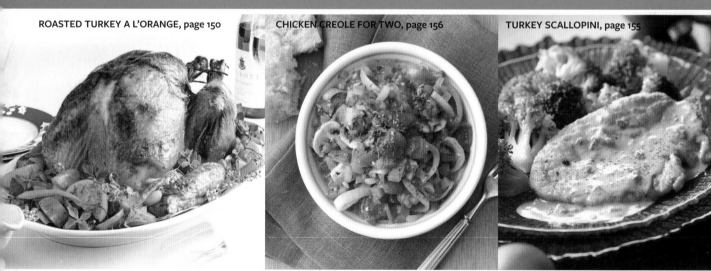

ROASTED TURKEY A L'ORANGE, page 150   CHICKEN CREOLE FOR TWO, page 156   TURKEY SCALLOPINI, page 155

4. Bake, uncovered, at 350° for 1½ to 1¾ hours or until chicken juices run clear and a thermometer reads 180° (cover loosely with foil if browning too quickly). Baste with the pan drippings if desired.

5. Cover and let stand for 15 minutes. Remove and discard skin, garlic, lemon and herbs from cavity before carving.

PER SERVING *3 ounces equals 163 cal., 6 g fat (2 g sat. fat), 67 mg chol., 289 mg sodium, 3 g carb., trace fiber, 23 g pro.* **Diabetic Exchange:** *3 lean meat.*

Mini Chicken Loaves

Have a delicious entree ready in only 15 minutes! These loaves are perfect any time of the year.

—**LORRAINE CALAND** SHUNIAH, IN

START TO FINISH: 15 MIN.
MAKES: 4 SERVINGS

- 1 **cup salsa, divided**
- ¾ **cup fresh or frozen corn, thawed**
- ⅓ **cup dry bread crumbs**
- 2 **teaspoons chili powder**
- ⅛ **teaspoon salt**
- ⅛ **teaspoon pepper**
- 1 **pound ground chicken**

1. In a large bowl, combine ¾ cup salsa, corn, bread crumbs, chili powder, salt and pepper. Crumble chicken over mixture and mix well. Shape into four loaves; place in an 11-in. x 7-in. microwave-safe dish coated with cooking spray.

2. Cover and microwave on high for 5-6 minutes or until a thermometer reads 165° and juices run clear. Serve with remaining salsa.

NOTE *This recipe was tested in a 1,100-watt microwave.*

PER SERVING *235 cal., 10 g fat (3 g sat. fat), 75 mg chol., 514 mg sodium, 15 g carb., 3 g fiber, 20 g pro.* **Diabetic Exchanges:** *3 lean meat, 1 starch.*

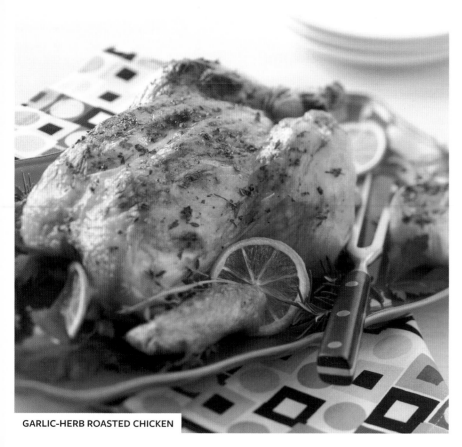

GARLIC-HERB ROASTED CHICKEN

Garlic-Herb Roasted Chicken

Since the garlic and herbs make this roasted chicken so flavorful, you can eliminate the salt from the recipe if you like.

—**CINDY STEFFEN** CEDARBURG, WI

PREP: 10 MIN. • **BAKE:** 1½ HOURS
MAKES: 8 SERVINGS

- 1 **roasting chicken (4 to 5 pounds)**
- 2 **teaspoons each minced fresh parsley, rosemary, sage and thyme**
- ¾ **teaspoon salt**
- ¼ **teaspoon pepper**
- 20 **garlic cloves, peeled and sliced**
- 1 **medium lemon, halved**
- 1 **large whole garlic bulb**
- 1 **sprig each fresh parsley, rosemary, sage and thyme**

1. With fingers, carefully loosen skin around the chicken breast, leg and thigh. Combine minced parsley, rosemary, sage, thyme, salt and pepper; rub half under skin. Place sliced garlic cloves under skin. Squeeze half of the lemon into the cavity and place the squeezed half in the cavity.

2. Remove papery outer skin from whole garlic bulb (do not peel or separate cloves). Cut top off garlic bulb. Place garlic bulb and herb sprigs in the cavity. Skewer chicken openings; tie the drumsticks together with kitchen string.

3. Place chicken breast side up on a rack in a roasting pan. Squeeze the remaining lemon half over chicken; rub remaining herb mixture over chicken.

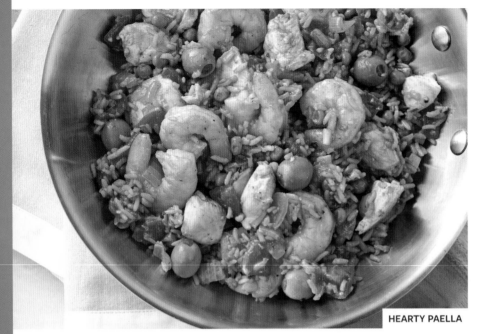

HEARTY PAELLA

Hearty Paella

I had paella for the first time in Spain. And it was so good, I've been on the quest to re-create the rich flavors of that dish ever since. We love the shrimp, chicken, veggies and olives in this easy, delicious make-at-home version.

—LIBBY WALP CHICAGO, IL

PREP: 25 MIN. • **COOK:** 30 MIN.
MAKES: 6 SERVINGS

- 1¼ pounds boneless skinless chicken breasts, cut into 1-inch cubes
- 1 tablespoon olive oil
- 1 cup uncooked long grain rice
- 1 medium onion, chopped
- 2 garlic cloves, minced
- 2¼ cups reduced-sodium chicken broth
- 1 can (14½ ounces) diced tomatoes, undrained
- 1 teaspoon dried oregano
- ½ teaspoon paprika
- ¼ teaspoon salt
- ¼ teaspoon pepper
- ⅛ teaspoon saffron threads
- ⅛ teaspoon ground turmeric
- 1 pound uncooked medium shrimp, peeled and deveined
- ¾ cup frozen peas
- 12 pimiento-stuffed olives
- 1 medium lemon, cut into six wedges

1. In a large skillet over medium heat, cook chicken in oil until no longer pink. Remove and keep warm. Add rice and onion to the pan; cook until rice is lightly browned and onion is tender, stirring frequently. Add garlic; cook 1 minute longer.

2. Stir in the broth, tomatoes, oregano, paprika, salt, pepper, saffron and turmeric. Bring to a boil. Reduce heat to low; cover and cook for 10 minutes.

3. Add the shrimp, peas and olives. Cover and cook 10 minutes longer or until rice is tender, shrimp turn pink and liquid is absorbed. Add chicken; heat through. Serve with lemon wedges.

PER SERVING *1⅓ cups equals 367 cal., 8 g fat (1 g sat. fat), 144 mg chol., 778 mg sodium, 36 g carb., 3 g fiber, 37 g pro. Diabetic Exchanges: 5 lean meat, 2 starch, 1 vegetable, 1 fat.*

Cran-Apple Turkey Skillet

You'll need only one skillet to pull off this meal. Talk about simple!

—LISA RENSHAW KANSAS CITY, MO

START TO FINISH: 20 MIN.
MAKES: 6 SERVINGS

- 2 medium apples, peeled and thinly sliced
- ¾ cup apple cider or unsweetened apple juice
- ¾ cup reduced-sodium chicken broth
- ⅓ cup dried cranberries
- ⅛ teaspoon ground nutmeg
- 3 cups cubed cooked turkey breast
- 1 package (6 ounces) corn bread stuffing mix

1. In a large skillet, combine the apples, apple cider, broth, cranberries and nutmeg. Bring to a boil. Reduce heat; cover and simmer for 4-5 minutes or until the apples are tender, stirring occasionally.

2. Stir in the turkey and stuffing mix. Cover and cook for 2-3 minutes or until heated through.

PER SERVING *1 cup equals 267 cal., 2 g fat (trace sat. fat), 60 mg chol., 630 mg sodium, 36 g carb., 2 g fiber, 25 g pro. Diabetic Exchanges: 3 lean meat, 1 starch, 1 fruit.*

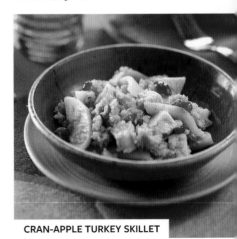

CRAN-APPLE TURKEY SKILLET

Crispy Asian Chicken Salad

Asian flavor, crunchy almonds and crispy breaded chicken make this a salad you'll turn to time and again.

—**BETH DAUENHAUER** PUEBLO, CO

START TO FINISH: 30 MIN.
MAKES: 2 SERVINGS

- 2 boneless skinless chicken breast halves (4 ounces each)
- 2 teaspoons hoisin sauce
- 1 teaspoon sesame oil
- ½ cup panko (Japanese) bread crumbs
- 4 teaspoons sesame seeds
- 2 teaspoons canola oil
- 4 cups spring mix salad greens
- 1 small green pepper, julienned
- 1 small sweet red pepper, julienned
- 1 medium carrot, julienned
- ½ cup sliced fresh mushrooms
- 2 tablespoons thinly sliced onion
- 2 tablespoons sliced almonds, toasted
- ¼ cup reduced-fat sesame ginger salad dressing

1. Flatten chicken breasts to ½-in. thickness. Combine hoisin sauce and sesame oil; brush over chicken. In a shallow bowl, combine panko and sesame seeds; dip chicken in mixture.

2. In a large nonstick skillet coated with cooking spray, cook chicken in oil for 5-6 minutes on each side or until no longer pink.

3. Meanwhile, divide salad greens between two plates. Top with peppers, carrot, mushrooms and onion. Slice chicken; place on top. Sprinkle with almonds and drizzle with dressing.

PER SERVING *386 cal., 17 g fat (2 g sat. fat), 63 mg chol., 620 mg sodium, 29 g carb., 6 g fiber, 30 g pro.* **Diabetic Exchanges:** *3 lean meat, 2 vegetable, 2 fat, 1 starch.*

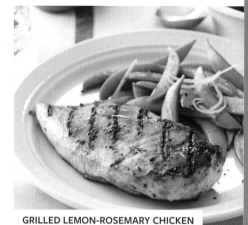

GRILLED LEMON-ROSEMARY CHICKEN

Grilled Lemon-Rosemary Chicken

Broiled or grilled, this chicken recipe has been a favorite for years. Switch it up with herbs you have on hand.

—**REBECCA SODERGREN** CENTERVILLE, OH

PREP: 10 MIN. + MARINATING • **GRILL:** 15 MIN.
MAKES: 6 SERVINGS

- ¼ cup lemon juice
- 3 tablespoons honey
- 2 teaspoons canola oil
- 1 teaspoon dried rosemary, crushed
- ½ teaspoon salt
- ⅛ teaspoon pepper
- 6 boneless skinless chicken breast halves (6 ounces each)

1. In a large resealable plastic bag, combine the first six ingredients. Add the chicken; seal bag and turn to coat. Refrigerate for 2 hours.

2. Drain and discard marinade. Moisten a paper towel with cooking oil; using long-handled tongs, lightly coat the grill rack. Grill chicken, covered, over medium heat or broil 4 in. from the heat for 6-8 minutes on each side or until a thermometer reads 170°.

PER SERVING *187 cal., 4 g fat (1 g sat. fat), 94 mg chol., 102 mg sodium, 1 g carb., trace fiber, 34 g pro.* **Diabetic Exchange:** *5 lean meat.*

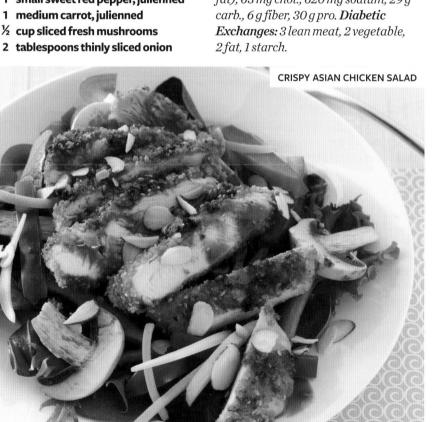

CRISPY ASIAN CHICKEN SALAD

Parmesan Chicken Couscous

Spruce up leftover chicken in this innovative dish. I like to serve it with a side of fruit.

—LISA ABBOTT NEW BERLIN, WI

START TO FINISH: 20 MIN.
MAKES: 4 SERVINGS

- ½ cup chopped walnuts
- 2 teaspoons olive oil, divided
- 3 garlic cloves, minced
- 2 cups chopped fresh spinach
- 1½ cups cubed cooked chicken
- 1¼ cups water
- 2 teaspoons dried basil
- ¼ teaspoon pepper
- 1 package (5.9 ounces) Parmesan couscous
- ¼ cup grated Parmesan cheese

1. In a large saucepan, cook walnuts over medium heat in 1 teaspoon oil for 2-3 minutes or until toasted. Remove and set aside.

2. In the same pan, saute garlic in remaining oil for 1 minute. Add the spinach, chicken, water, basil and pepper. Bring to a boil. Stir in couscous. Remove from the heat; cover and let stand for 5-10 minutes or until water is absorbed. Fluff with a fork.

3. Stir in the walnuts and sprinkle with Parmesan cheese.

PER SERVING *391 cal., 18 g fat (3 g sat. fat), 51 mg chol., 490 mg sodium, 34 g carb., 3 g fiber, 25 g pro.* **Diabetic Exchanges:** *3 lean meat, 2 starch, 2 fat.*

PARMESAN CHICKEN COUSCOUS

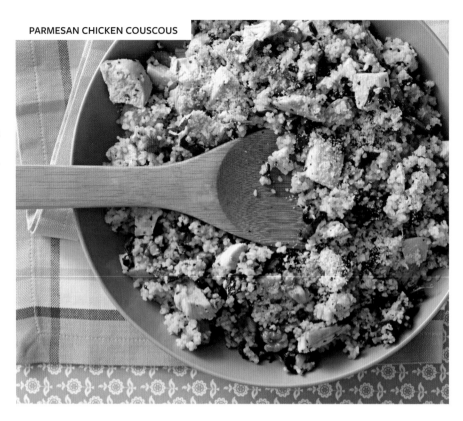

Honey-Mustard Turkey Breast

If you don't have honey mustard, use ¼ cup each of honey and brown mustard.

—TASTE OF HOME TEST KITCHEN

PREP: 10 MIN.
BAKE: 1¾ HOURS + STANDING
MAKES: 10-12 SERVINGS

- 1 bone-in turkey breast (5 to 6 pounds)
- ½ cup honey mustard
- ¾ teaspoon dried rosemary, crushed
- ½ teaspoon onion powder
- ¼ teaspoon salt
- ⅛ teaspoon garlic powder
- ⅛ teaspoon pepper

1. Place the turkey breast, skin side up, on a rack in a foil-lined shallow roasting pan. In a small bowl, combine the remaining ingredients. Spoon over the turkey.

2. Bake, uncovered, at 325° for 1¾ to 2½ hours or until a thermometer reads 170°, basting every 30 minutes. Cover and let stand for 10 minutes before slicing.

HONEY-APPLE TURKEY BREAST *Omit honey mustard and seasonings. Heat ¾ cup thawed apple juice concentrate, ⅓ cup honey and 1 tablespoon ground mustard over low heat for 2-3 minutes or just until blended, stirring occasionally. Prepare the turkey as directed in a foil-lined pan. Pour honey mixture over turkey. Proceed as directed, basting with pan juices every 30 minutes. (Cover loosely with foil if turkey browns too quickly.)*

PER SERVING *5 ounces equals 283 cal., 11 g fat (3 g sat. fat), 102 mg chol., 221 mg sodium, 5 g carb., trace fiber, 40 g pro.* **Diabetic Exchange:** *5 medium-fat meat.*

Garden Vegetable & Chicken Skillet

Toss together bright vegetables, rice and chicken for this perfect one-dish supper.

—**TASTE OF HOME TEST KITCHEN**

PREP: 20 MIN. • **COOK:** 20 MIN.
MAKES: 4 SERVINGS

- 1½ **pounds boneless skinless chicken breasts, cut into ½-inch cubes**
- 1 **medium yellow summer squash, chopped**
- 1 **medium onion, chopped**
- 1 **medium carrot, chopped**
- 2 **tablespoons butter**
- 3 **cups fresh baby spinach**
- 1 **garlic clove, minced**
- ½ **teaspoon salt**
- ½ **teaspoon dried thyme**
- ¼ **teaspoon pepper**
- 1 **cup uncooked instant brown rice**
- 1¼ **cups water**
- 1 **tablespoon lemon juice**

1. In a large skillet, saute the chicken, squash, onion and carrot in butter for 5-6 minutes or until chicken is no longer pink; drain. Add the spinach, garlic, salt, thyme and pepper; cook 2 minutes longer.

2. Stir in rice and water. Bring to a boil. Reduce heat; cover and simmer for 10-15 minutes or until rice is tender. Stir in lemon juice.

PER SERVING *1½ cups equals 355 cal., 11 g fat (5 g sat. fat), 109 mg chol., 453 mg sodium, 25 g carb., 3 g fiber, 38 g pro.* **Diabetic Exchanges:** *5 lean meat, 1 starch, 1 vegetable, 1 fat.*

Mediterranean Chicken with Spaghetti Squash

Brimming with classic Mediterranean ingredients, this restaurant-quality dish will be an instant hit. Serve it with a quick salad for a complete meal.

—**JAYNE MARTIN** STRATHCLAIR, MB

PREP: 35 MIN. • **COOK:** 35 MIN.
MAKES: 6 SERVINGS

- 1 **medium spaghetti squash**
- 1½ **pounds boneless skinless chicken breasts, cut into ½-inch cubes**
- 5 **center-cut bacon strips, chopped**
- 1 **medium leek (white portion only), coarsely chopped**
- 4 **garlic cloves, minced**
- 3 **tablespoons all-purpose flour**
- 1 **cup reduced-sodium chicken broth**
- ½ **cup white wine or additional reduced-sodium chicken broth**
- ⅓ **cup half-and-half cream**
- 2 **plum tomatoes, chopped**
- 1 **can (2¼ ounces) sliced ripe olives, drained**
- ⅓ **cup grated Parmesan cheese**
- 1½ **teaspoons minced fresh sage or ½ teaspoon rubbed sage**
- 1 **teaspoon minced fresh thyme or ¼ teaspoon dried thyme**
- ½ **teaspoon salt**
- ⅛ **teaspoon pepper**

1. Cut squash in half lengthwise; discard seeds. Place squash cut side down on a microwave-safe plate. Microwave, uncovered, on high for 15-18 minutes or until tender.

2. Meanwhile, in a large nonstick skillet coated with cooking spray, cook chicken over medium heat until no longer pink; drain. Remove from the skillet.

3. In the same skillet, cook bacon and leek over medium heat until bacon is crisp. Using a slotted spoon, remove bacon mixture to paper towels. Add garlic; cook for 1 minute. Stir in flour until blended; gradually add the broth, wine and cream. Bring to a boil; cook and stir for 1-2 minutes or until thickened. Stir in the remaining ingredients. Add chicken and bacon mixture; heat through.

4. When squash is cool enough to handle, use a fork to separate strands. Serve with chicken mixture.

PER SERVING *1¾ cups equals 340 cal., 12 g fat (4 g sat. fat), 82 mg chol., 656 mg sodium, 27 g carb., 5 g fiber, 30 g pro.* **Diabetic Exchanges:** *4 lean meat, 2 fat, 1½ starch.*

MEDITERRANEAN CHICKEN WITH SPAGHETTI SQUASH

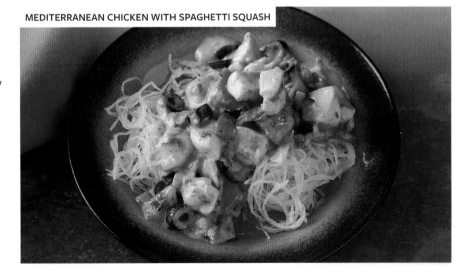

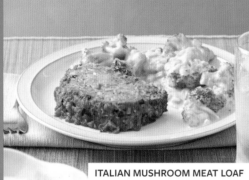

ITALIAN MUSHROOM MEAT LOAF

Italian Mushroom Meat Loaf

Healthful oats and flaxseed amp up the nutrition in this tasty Italian meat loaf.

—**KYLIE(PETRULIA) WERNING** CANDLER, NC

PREP: 30 MIN. • **BAKE:** 1 HOUR
MAKES: 8 SERVINGS

- 1 **egg, lightly beaten**
- ¼ **pound fresh mushrooms, chopped**
- ½ **cup old-fashioned oats**
- ½ **cup chopped red onion**
- ¼ **cup ground flaxseed**
- ½ **teaspoon pepper**
- 1 **package (19½ ounces) Italian turkey sausage links, casings removed, crumbled**
- 1 **pound lean ground beef (90% lean)**
- 1 **cup marinara or spaghetti sauce**

1. In a large bowl, combine the egg, mushrooms, oats, onion, flax and pepper. Crumble turkey and beef over mixture and mix well.

2. Shape into a 10-in. x 4-in. loaf. Place in a 13-in. x 9-in. baking dish coated with cooking spray. Bake, uncovered, at 350° for 50 minutes; drain. Top with marinara sauce. Bake 10-15 minutes longer or until no pink remains and a thermometer reads 165°.

PER SERVING *361 cal., 14 g fat (3 g sat. fat), 103 mg chol., 509 mg sodium, 10 g carb., 2 g fiber, 25 g pro.* **Diabetic Exchanges:** *3 lean meat, ½ starch.*

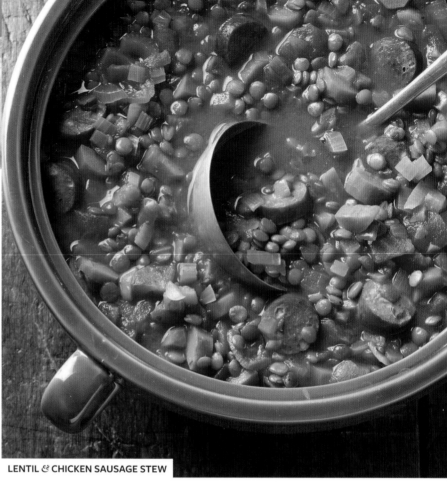

LENTIL & CHICKEN SAUSAGE STEW

Lentil & Chicken Sausage Stew

This hearty stew will warm your family right down to their toes! Serve with corn bread or rolls to soak up every last morsel.

—**JAN VALDEZ** CHICAGO, IL

PREP: 15 MIN. • **COOK:** 8 HOURS
MAKES: 6 SERVINGS

- 1 **carton (32 ounces) reduced-sodium chicken broth**
- 1 **can (28 ounces) diced tomatoes, undrained**
- 3 **fully cooked spicy chicken sausage links (3 ounces each), cut into ½-inch slices**
- 1 **cup dried lentils, rinsed**
- 1 **medium onion, chopped**
- 1 **medium carrot, chopped**
- 1 **celery rib, chopped**
- 2 **garlic cloves, minced**
- ½ **teaspoon dried thyme**

In a 4- or 5-qt. slow cooker, combine all ingredients. Cover and cook on low for 8-10 hours or until lentils are tender.

PER SERVING *1½ cups equals 231 cal., 4 g fat (1 g sat. fat), 33 mg chol., 803 mg sodium, 31 g carb., 13 g fiber, 19 g pro.* **Diabetic Exchanges:** *2 lean meat, 2 vegetable, 1 starch.*

Garlic-Mushroom Turkey Slices

My daughter is a picky eater, but she loves this! Plus, it's low in fat.

—RICK FLEISHMAN BEVERLY HILLS, CA

START TO FINISH: 30 MIN.
MAKES: 4 SERVINGS

- ½ **cup all-purpose flour**
- ½ **teaspoon dried oregano**
- ½ **teaspoon paprika**
- ¾ **teaspoon salt, divided**
- ¼ **teaspoon pepper, divided**
- 1 **package (17.6 ounces) turkey breast cutlets**
- 1 **tablespoon olive oil**
- ¾ **cup reduced-sodium chicken broth**
- ¼ **cup white wine or additional reduced-sodium chicken broth**
- ½ **pound sliced fresh mushrooms**
- 2 **garlic cloves, minced**

1. In a large resealable plastic bag, combine the flour, oregano, paprika, ½ teaspoon salt and ⅛ teaspoon pepper. Add turkey, a few pieces at a time, and shake to coat.

2. In a large nonstick skillet coated with cooking spray, cook turkey in oil in batches over medium heat for 1-2 minutes on each side or until no longer pink. Remove and keep warm.

3. Add broth and wine to the skillet; stir in mushrooms and remaining salt and pepper. Cook and stir for 4-6 minutes or until mushrooms are tender. Add garlic; cook 1 minute longer. Return turkey to the pan; heat through.

PER SERVING *218 cal., 4 g fat (1 g sat. fat), 77 mg chol., 440 mg sodium, 8 g carb., 1 g fiber, 34 g pro.* **Diabetic Exchanges:** *4 lean meat, ½ starch, ½ fat.*

Mexicali Chicken

My family has clamored for this recipe at dinner for years. Fresh cilantro may be added to the salsa, if desired.

—AVANELL HEWITT

NORTH RICHLAND HILLS, TX

START TO FINISH: 30 MIN.
MAKES: 4 SERVINGS

- 1 **medium tomato, finely chopped**
- 1 **small onion, finely chopped**
- 2 **jalapeno peppers, seeded and chopped**
- 2 **tablespoons lime juice**
- 1 **garlic clove, minced**
- ¼ **teaspoon salt**
- ⅛ **teaspoon pepper**
- 4 **boneless skinless chicken breast halves (4 ounces each)**
- 1 **to 2 teaspoons reduced-sodium taco seasoning**
- 4 **bacon strips, halved**
- 4 **slices reduced-fat provolone cheese**
- 1 **medium lime, cut into four wedges**

1. In a small bowl, combine the tomato, onion, jalapenos, lime juice, garlic, salt and pepper. Chill until serving.

2. Sprinkle chicken with taco seasoning; set aside. In a large skillet, cook bacon over medium heat until crisp. Remove to paper towels; drain.

3. If grilling the chicken, moisten a paper towel with cooking oil; using long-handled tongs, rub on grill rack to coat lightly. Grill chicken, covered, over medium heat or broil 4 in. from the heat for 4-7 minutes on each side or until a thermometer reads 165°.

4. Top with bacon and cheese; cook 1 minute longer or until cheese is melted. Serve with salsa; squeeze lime wedges over top.

NOTE *Wear disposable gloves when cutting hot peppers; the oils can burn skin. Avoid touching your face.*

PER SERVING *227 cal., 9 g fat (4 g sat. fat), 80 mg chol., 532 mg sodium, 5 g carb., 1 g fiber, 31 g pro.* **Diabetic Exchanges:** *4 lean meat, 1 vegetable, ½ fat.*

MEXICALI CHICKEN

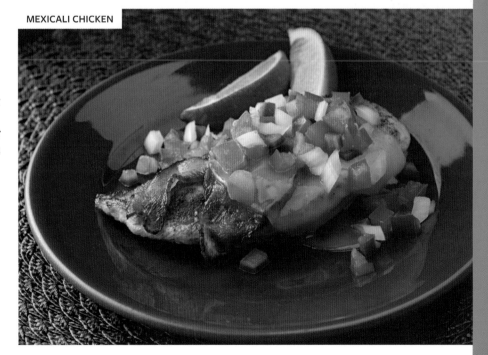

Simple Sesame Chicken

When I returned home after 20 years as a missionary in the Philippines, I started experimenting to make food like we had enjoyed there. These flavorful chicken strips come really close!

—**LYNN JONAS** MADISON, WI

PREP: 15 MIN. • **COOK:** 10 MIN./BATCH
MAKES: 6 SERVINGS

- ⅓ cup all-purpose flour
- ½ teaspoon salt
- ¼ teaspoon pepper
- 1⅔ cups Caesar salad croutons, crushed
- ¼ cup sesame seeds
- 2 eggs, lightly beaten
- 1½ pounds boneless skinless chicken breasts, cut into 1-inch strips
- 2 teaspoons butter
- 2 teaspoons canola oil

1. In a shallow bowl, combine the flour, salt and pepper. In another shallow bowl, combine crushed croutons and sesame seeds. Place eggs in a third shallow bowl. Coat chicken with flour mixture, then dip in eggs and coat with crouton mixture.

2. In a large nonstick skillet coated with cooking spray, cook chicken in butter and oil in batches over medium heat for 4-6 minutes on each side or until no longer pink.

PER SERVING *255 cal., 11 g fat (3 g sat. fat), 120 mg chol., 319 mg sodium, 11 g carb., 1 g fiber, 27 g pro.* **Diabetic Exchanges:** *3 lean meat, 1 starch, 1 fat.*

Thai Chicken Thighs

Thanks to the slow cooker, a traditional Thai dish with peanut butter, jalapeno peppers and chili sauce becomes incredibly easy to prepare. If you want to crank up the spice a bit, use more jalapeno peppers.

—**TASTE OF HOME TEST KITCHEN**

PREP: 25 MIN. • **COOK:** 5 HOURS
MAKES: 8 SERVINGS

- 8 bone-in chicken thighs (about 3 pounds), skin removed
- ½ cup salsa
- ¼ cup creamy peanut butter
- 2 tablespoons lemon juice
- 2 tablespoons reduced-sodium soy sauce
- 1 tablespoon chopped seeded jalapeno pepper
- 2 teaspoons Thai chili sauce
- 1 garlic clove, minced
- 1 teaspoon minced fresh gingerroot
- 2 green onions, sliced
- 2 tablespoons sesame seeds, toasted
  Hot cooked basmati rice, optional

1. Place chicken in a 3-qt. slow cooker. In a small bowl, combine the salsa, peanut butter, lemon juice, soy sauce, jalapeno, Thai chili sauce, garlic and ginger; pour over chicken.

2. Cover and cook on low for 5-6 hours or until chicken is tender. Sprinkle with green onions and sesame seeds. Serve with rice if desired.

NOTE *Wear disposable gloves when cutting hot peppers; the oils can burn skin. Avoid touching your face.*

PER SERVING *1 thigh with ¼ cup sauce equals 261 cal., 15 g fat (4 g sat. fat), 87 mg chol., 350 mg sodium, 5 g carb., 1 g fiber, 27 g pro.* **Diabetic Exchanges:** *4 lean meat, 1 fat, ½ starch.*

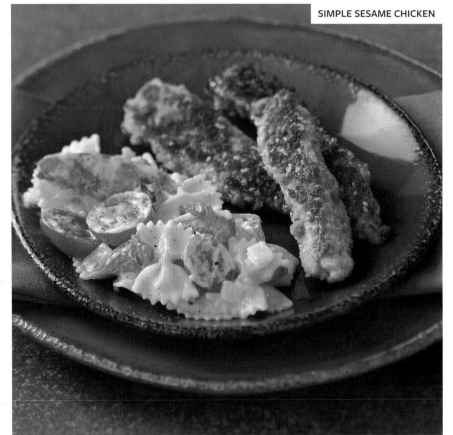

SIMPLE SESAME CHICKEN

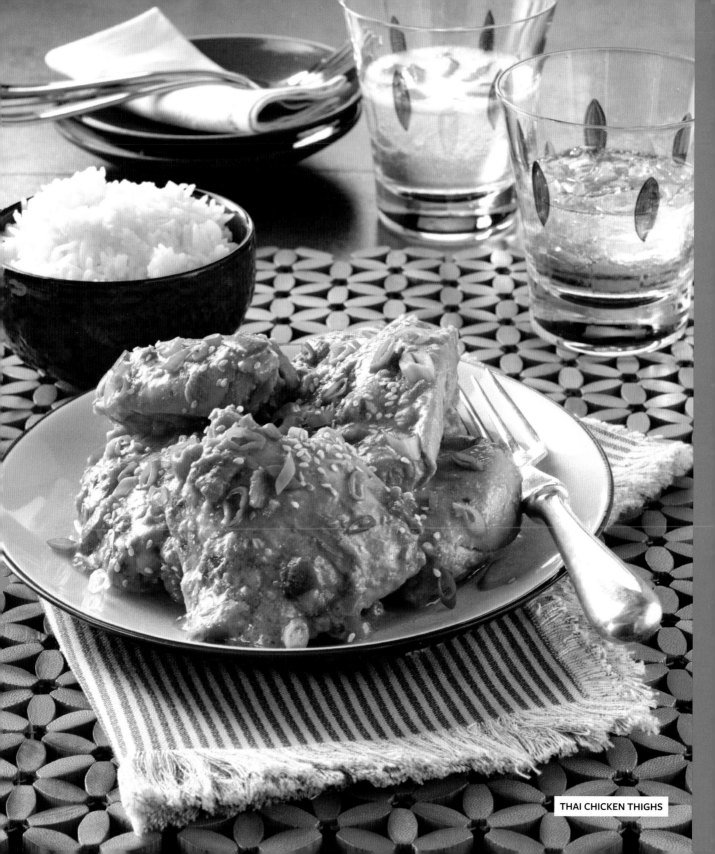

THAI CHICKEN THIGHS

Makeover Swiss Chicken Supreme

Enjoy this lighter take on my original recipe. This version has 560 fewer calories, 81% less fat and nearly 75% less sodium.
—**STEPHANIE BELL** KAYSVILLE, UT

PREP: 15 MIN. • **BAKE:** 30 MIN.
MAKES: 4 SERVINGS

- 4 **boneless skinless chicken breast halves (4 ounces each)**
- 1 **tablespoon dried minced onion**
- ½ **teaspoon garlic powder**
- ¼ **teaspoon salt**
- ⅛ **teaspoon pepper**
- 4 **slices (¾ ounce each) reduced-fat Swiss cheese**
- 1 **can (10¾ ounces) reduced-fat reduced-sodium condensed cream of chicken soup, undiluted**
- ⅓ **cup reduced-fat sour cream**
- ½ **cup fat-free milk**
- ⅓ **cup crushed reduced-fat butter-flavored crackers (about 8 crackers)**
- 1 **teaspoon butter, melted**

1. Place the chicken in a 13-in. x 9-in. baking dish coated with cooking spray. Sprinkle with minced onion, garlic powder, salt and pepper. Top each chicken piece with a slice of cheese.
2. In a small bowl, combine soup, sour cream and milk; pour over chicken. Toss the cracker crumbs and butter; sprinkle over chicken. Bake, uncovered, at 350° for 30-40 minutes or until a thermometer reads 170°.
PER SERVING *310 cal., 11 g fat (5 g sat. fat), 89 mg chol., 567 mg sodium, 17 g carb., trace fiber, 34 g pro. Diabetic Exchanges: 3 lean meat, 2 fat, 1 starch.*

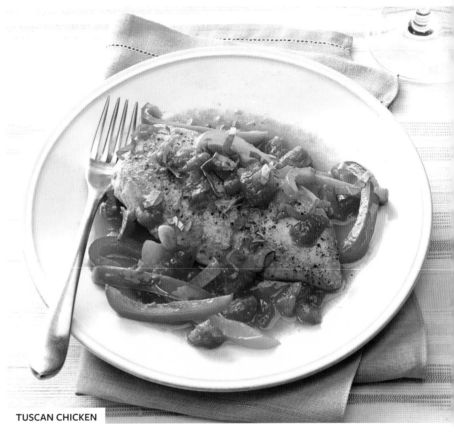

TUSCAN CHICKEN

Tuscan Chicken

I created this recipe one night when I was looking for a new lighter way to prepare chicken. I recently lost about 30 pounds, and this is one dish I prepare often.
—**CARLA WELLS** SOMERSET, KY

PREP: 25 MIN. • **COOK:** 15 MIN.
MAKES: 4 SERVINGS

- 4 **boneless skinless chicken breast halves (6 ounces each)**
- ¼ **teaspoon pepper**
- 2 **tablespoons olive oil**
- 1 **each medium green, sweet red and yellow peppers, julienned**
- 2 **thin slices prosciutto or deli ham, chopped**
- 2 **garlic cloves, minced**
- 1 **can (14½ ounces) diced tomatoes, undrained**
- ¼ **cup reduced-sodium chicken broth**
- 2 **tablespoons minced fresh basil or 2 teaspoons dried basil**
- 1 **teaspoon minced fresh oregano or ¼ teaspoon dried oregano**

1. Sprinkle chicken with pepper. In a large nonstick skillet, brown chicken in oil. Remove and keep warm. In the same skillet, saute peppers and prosciutto until peppers are tender. Add garlic; cook 1 minute longer.
2. Add the tomatoes, broth, basil, oregano and chicken. Bring to a boil. Reduce heat; cover and simmer for 12-15 minutes or until a thermometer reads 170°.
PER SERVING *304 cal., 12 g fat (2 g sat. fat), 100 mg chol., 389 mg sodium, 11 g carb., 3 g fiber, 38 g pro. Diabetic Exchanges: 5 lean meat, 2 vegetable, 1 fat.*

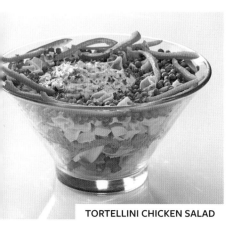

TORTELLINI CHICKEN SALAD

Tortellini Chicken Salad

If you like pesto, you'll love it even more mixed into this good-for-you salad.

—**EDIE DESPAIN** LOGAN, UT

PREP: 25 MIN. • **COOK:** 15 MIN. + CHILLING
MAKES: 6 SERVINGS

- 1 **package (9 ounces) refrigerated cheese tortellini**
- 1 **cup frozen peas**
- 5 **cups torn romaine**
- 1½ **cups shredded carrots**
- 2 **cups cubed cooked chicken breast**
- ½ **cup julienned sweet red pepper**
- ½ **cup fat-free mayonnaise**
- 1 **jar (3 ounces) prepared pesto**
- ¼ **cup buttermilk**
- 2 **tablespoons minced fresh parsley**

1. Cook tortellini according to package directions, adding peas during the last 4-5 minutes of cooking. Drain and rinse in cold water.
2. In a large glass bowl, layer romaine, carrots, chicken, tortellini and peas, and red pepper. In a small bowl, mix mayonnaise, pesto and buttermilk. Spread over top. Sprinkle with parsley. Refrigerate until chilled.
PER SERVING 1½ cups equals 337 cal., 13 g fat (4 g sat. fat), 62 mg chol., 525 mg sodium, 32 g carb., 5 g fiber, 25 g pro. **Diabetic Exchanges:** 3 lean meat, 2 starch, 1 fat.

Chicken Tacos with Avocado Salsa

I make these tacos to accommodate various diets in our family. Served with a simple green salad, it's a meal we can dig into together.

—**CHRISTINE SCHENHER** EXETER, CA

START TO FINISH: 30 MIN.
MAKES: 4 SERVINGS

- 1 **pound boneless skinless chicken breasts, cut into ½-inch strips**
- ⅓ **cup water**
- 1 **tablespoon chili powder**
- 1 **teaspoon sugar**
- 1 **teaspoon onion powder**
- 1 **teaspoon paprika**
- 1 **teaspoon ground cumin**
- 1 **teaspoon dried oregano**
- ½ **teaspoon salt**
- ½ **teaspoon garlic powder**
- 1 **medium ripe avocado, peeled and cubed**
- 1 **cup fresh or frozen corn**
- 1 **cup cherry tomatoes, quartered**
- 2 **teaspoons lime juice**
- 8 **taco shells, warmed**

1. In a large nonstick skillet coated with cooking spray, brown chicken. Add the water, chili powder, sugar, onion powder, paprika, cumin, oregano, salt and garlic powder. Cook over medium heat for 5-6 minutes or until chicken is no longer pink, stirring occasionally.
2. Meanwhile, in a small bowl, gently combine the avocado, corn, tomatoes and lime juice. Spoon chicken mixture into taco shells; top with avocado salsa.
PER SERVING 354 cal., 15 g fat (3 g sat. fat), 63 mg chol., 474 mg sodium, 30 g carb., 6 g fiber, 27 g pro. **Diabetic Exchanges:** 3 lean meat, 2 starch, 1 fat.

CHICKEN TACOS WITH AVOCADO SALSA

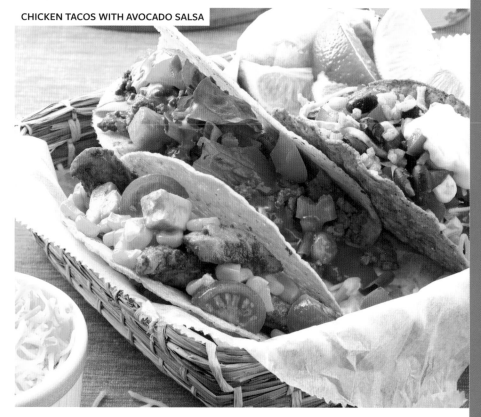

Chicken Pasta Skillet

My husband (a very picky eater) loves mac and cheese, but I was trying to come up with a healthier noodle dish that would include some fiber and vegetables. He ended up loving this!

—**HEATHER MCCLINTOCK** COLUMBUS, OH

START TO FINISH: 30 MIN.
MAKES: 6 SERVINGS

- 3 **cups uncooked whole wheat spiral pasta**
- 2 **cups fresh broccoli florets**
- 2 **tablespoons plus 1 teaspoon all-purpose flour**
- 1¼ **cups reduced-sodium chicken broth**
- 2 **tablespoons butter**
- ½ **cup fat-free half-and-half**
- 4 **ounces reduced-fat process cheese (Velveeta), cubed**
- 1 **teaspoon garlic-herb seasoning blend**
- ¼ **teaspoon salt**
- 2½ **cups cubed cooked chicken breast**
- ½ **cup shredded cheddar cheese**

1. In a large saucepan, cook pasta according to package directions, adding broccoli during the last 2 minutes of cooking; drain.

2. Meanwhile, in a small bowl, whisk flour and broth until smooth. In a large skillet, melt butter over medium heat; stir in broth mixture. Add half-and-half. Bring to a boil; cook and stir 1 minute or until thickened. Add the process cheese, seasoning blend and salt; stir until smooth.

3. Add chicken and pasta mixture; heat through, stirring occasionally. Remove from heat; sprinkle with cheddar cheese. Let stand, covered, for 5-10 minutes or until cheese is melted.

PER SERVING *335 cal., 11 g fat (6 g sat. fat), 72 mg chol., 671 mg sodium, 29 g carb., 4 g fiber, 29 g pro.* **Diabetic Exchanges:** *3 lean meat, 2 starch, 1 fat.*

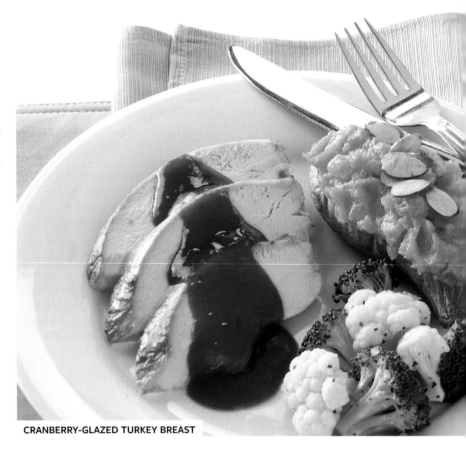

CRANBERRY-GLAZED TURKEY BREAST

Cranberry-Glazed Turkey Breast

This golden-brown turkey breast is just four ingredients away!

—**AUDREY PETTERSON** MAIDSTONE, SK

PREP: 20 MIN.
BAKE: 1½ HOURS + STANDING
MAKES: 12 SERVINGS

- 1¼ **cups jellied cranberry sauce**
- ⅔ **cup thawed unsweetened apple juice concentrate**
- 2 **tablespoons butter**
- 1 **bone-in turkey breast (5 to 6 pounds)**

1. In a small saucepan, bring the cranberry sauce, apple juice concentrate and butter to a boil. Remove from the heat; cool.

2. Carefully loosen skin of turkey breast. Set aside ½ cup sauce for basting and ¾ cup for serving. Spoon remaining sauce onto the turkey, rubbing mixture under and over skin.

3. Place turkey on a rack in a shallow roasting pan. Bake, uncovered, at 325° for 1½ to 2 hours or until a thermometer reads 170°, basting occasionally with reserved sauce. Cover and let stand for 10 minutes before carving. Warm reserved ¾ cup of sauce; serve with turkey.

PER SERVING *5 ounces cooked turkey (without skin) equals 244 cal., 3 g fat (1 g sat. fat), 103 mg chol., 91 mg sodium, 17 g carb., trace fiber, 36 g pro.* **Diabetic Exchanges:** *5 lean meat, 1 starch.*

Chicken Chow Mein

When we go out for Chinese food, my husband always orders chicken chow mein. So I created this recipe for a homemade take on his favorite.

—BETH DAUENHAUER PUEBLO, CO

START TO FINISH: 30 MIN.
MAKES: 2 SERVINGS

- 1 tablespoon cornstarch
- ⅔ cup reduced-sodium chicken broth
- 1 teaspoon reduced-sodium soy sauce
- ½ teaspoon salt
- ¼ teaspoon ground ginger
- ¼ pound sliced fresh mushrooms
- ⅔ cup thinly sliced celery
- ¼ cup sliced onion
- ¼ cup thinly sliced green pepper
- 2 tablespoons julienned carrot
- 1 teaspoon canola oil
- 1 garlic clove, minced
- 1 cup cubed cooked chicken breast
- 1 cup cooked brown rice
- 2 tablespoons chow mein noodles

1. In a small bowl, combine the cornstarch, broth, soy sauce, salt and ginger until smooth; set aside.

2. In a large skillet or wok, stir-fry the mushrooms, celery, onion, pepper and carrot in oil for 5 minutes. Add garlic; stir-fry for 1-2 minutes longer or until vegetables are crisp-tender.

3. Stir cornstarch mixture and add to the pan. Bring to a boil; cook and stir for 2 minutes or until thickened. Add chicken; heat through. Serve with rice; sprinkle with chow mein noodles.

PER SERVING *307 cal., 7 g fat (1 g sat. fat), 54 mg chol., 984 mg sodium, 35 g carb., 4 g fiber, 27 g pro. **Diabetic Exchanges:** 3 lean meat, 2 starch, 1 vegetable, ½ fat.*

Sausage Spinach Pasta Bake

I've sometimes swapped in other meats, such as chicken sausage, veal or ground pork, and added in summer squash, zucchini, green beans and mushrooms, depending on what's in season. Also, fresh herbs add a lot to this dish.

—KIM FORNI CLAREMONT, NH

PREP: 35 MIN. • **BAKE:** 25 MIN.
MAKES: 10 SERVINGS

- 1 package (16 ounces) whole wheat spiral pasta
- 1 pound Italian turkey sausage links, casings removed
- 1 medium onion, chopped
- 5 garlic cloves, minced
- 1 can (28 ounces) crushed tomatoes
- 1 can (14½ ounces) diced tomatoes, undrained
- 1 teaspoon dried oregano
- 1 teaspoon dried basil
- ¼ teaspoon pepper
- 1 package (10 ounces) frozen chopped spinach, thawed and squeezed dry
- ½ cup half-and-half cream
- 2 cups (8 ounces) shredded part-skim mozzarella cheese
- ½ cup grated Parmesan cheese

1. Cook pasta according to package directions.

2. Meanwhile, in a large skillet, cook turkey and onion over medium heat until meat is no longer pink. Add garlic. Cook 1 minute longer; drain. Stir in the tomatoes, oregano, basil and pepper. Bring to a boil. Reduce heat; simmer, uncovered, for 10 minutes.

3. Drain pasta; stir into turkey mixture. Add the spinach and cream; heat through. Transfer to a 13-in. x 9-in. baking dish coated with cooking spray. Sprinkle with cheeses. Bake, uncovered, at 350° for 25-30 minutes or until golden brown.

PER SERVING *1⅓ cup equals 377 cal., 11 g fat (5 g sat. fat), 50 mg chol., 622 mg sodium, 45 g carb., 8 g fiber, 25 g pro. **Diabetic Exchanges:** 3 lean meat, 2 starch, 2 vegetable, ½ fat.*

SAUSAGE SPINACH PASTA BAKE

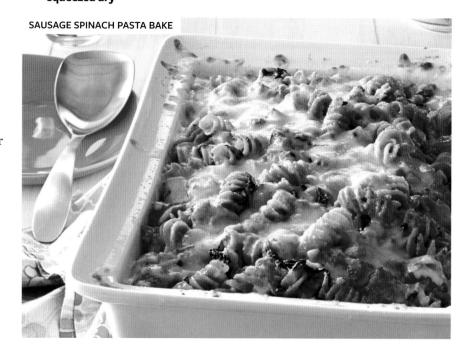

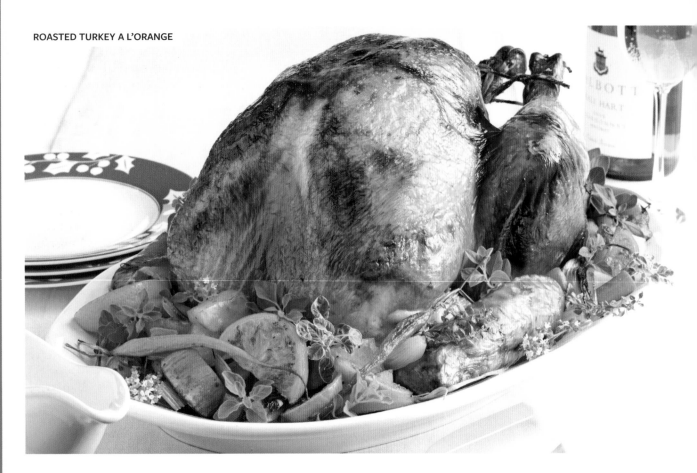

Roasted Turkey a l'Orange

My niece says this is the best turkey she's ever had—she even requests it in the middle of summer!

—ROBIN HAAS CRANSTON, RI

PREP: 40 MIN.
BAKE: 3½ HOURS + STANDING
MAKES: 28 SERVINGS

- 1 **whole garlic bulb, cloves separated and peeled**
- 1 **large navel orange**
- ¼ **cup orange marmalade**
- 2 **tablespoons lemon juice**
- 1 **tablespoon honey**
- 2 **teaspoons dried parsley flakes**
- 1 **teaspoon paprika**
- 1 **teaspoon dried oregano**
- ½ **teaspoon salt**
- ½ **teaspoon dried thyme**
- ½ **teaspoon pepper**
- 1 **turkey (14 pounds)**
- 4 **celery ribs, quartered**
- 4 **large carrots, quartered**
- 1 **large onion, quartered**
- 1 **large potato, peeled and cut into 2-inch cubes**
- 1 **large sweet potato, peeled and cut into 2-inch cubes**

1. Mince four garlic cloves; transfer to a small bowl. Juice half of the orange; add to bowl. Stir in the marmalade, lemon juice, honey, parsley, paprika, oregano, salt, thyme and pepper. With fingers, carefully loosen skin from the turkey; rub ½ cup marmalade mixture under the skin.

2. Thinly slice remaining orange half; place under the skin. Brush turkey with remaining marmalade mixture. Place remaining garlic cloves inside the cavity. Tuck wings under turkey; tie drumsticks together.

3. Combine the celery, carrots, onion and potatoes in a roasting pan. Place turkey, breast side up, over vegetables.

4. Bake at 325° for 3½ to 4 hours or until a thermometer reads 180°, basting occasionally with pan drippings. Cover loosely with foil if turkey browns too quickly. Cover and let stand for 20 minutes before carving.

PER SERVING *4 ounces cooked turkey (calculated without skin and vegetables) equals 207 cal., 6 g fat (2 g sat. fat), 86 mg chol., 123 mg sodium, 4 g carb., trace fiber, 33 g pro.* **Diabetic Exchange:** *4 lean meat.*

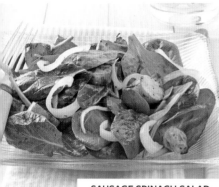

SAUSAGE SPINACH SALAD

Sausage Spinach Salad

Turn a tangy salad into a hearty meal just by adding sausage. I use chicken sausage, but you can use different varieties and flavors. The mustard dressing is also nice with smoked salmon or chicken.

—**DEBORAH WILLIAMS** PEORIA, AZ

START TO FINISH: 20 MIN.
MAKES: 2 SERVINGS

- 4 **teaspoons olive oil, divided**
- 2 **fully cooked Italian chicken sausage links (3 ounces each), cut into ¼-inch slices**
- ½ **medium onion, halved and sliced**
- 4 **cups fresh baby spinach**
- 1½ **teaspoons balsamic vinegar**
- 1 **teaspoon stone-ground mustard**

1. In a large nonstick skillet coated with cooking spray, heat 1 teaspoon oil over medium heat. Add the sausage and onion; cook and stir until sausage is lightly browned and the onion is crisp-tender.

2. Place spinach in a large bowl. In a small bowl, whisk vinegar, mustard and remaining oil. Drizzle over spinach; toss to coat. Add sausage mixture; serve immediately.

PER SERVING *244 cal., 16 g fat (3 g sat. fat), 65 mg chol., 581 mg sodium, 8 g carb., 2 g fiber, 17 g pro.* **Diabetic Exchanges:** *2 lean meat, 2 vegetable, 2 fat.*

Hearty Chicken Casserole

Bring the flavors of the Southwest to your table with this delectable high-fiber dish. The cheesy topping and creamy consistency are sure to win 'em over!

—**JENNY EBERT** EAU CLAIRE, WI

PREP: 15 MIN. • **BAKE:** 25 MIN.
MAKES: 6 SERVINGS

- 2 **celery ribs, chopped**
- 1 **small onion, chopped**
- 1½ **teaspoons olive oil**
- 3 **cups cubed cooked chicken breast**
- 1 **can (16 ounces) kidney beans, rinsed and drained**
- 1 **can (15 ounces) black beans, rinsed and drained**
- 1 **tablespoon chili powder**
- 2 **teaspoons ground cumin**
- 1 **can (14½ ounces) no-salt-added diced tomatoes, undrained**
- 1 **can (10¾ ounces) reduced-fat reduced-sodium condensed cream of mushroom soup, undiluted**
- 1 **cup (4 ounces) shredded reduced-fat cheddar cheese**

HEARTY CHICKEN CASSEROLE

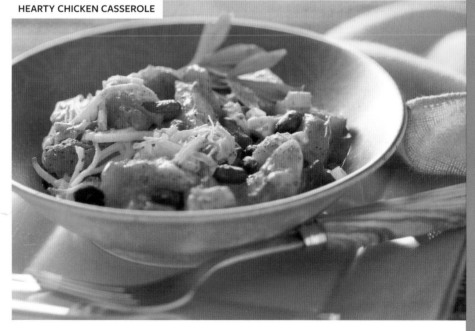

1. In a large nonstick skillet coated with cooking spray, saute celery and onion in oil until tender. Stir in the chicken, beans, chili powder and cumin; heat through.

2. Transfer to a shallow 2½-qt. baking dish coated with cooking spray. Combine tomatoes and soup; pour over chicken mixture.

3. Bake, uncovered, at 350° for 20 minutes. Sprinkle with cheese. Bake 5-10 minutes longer or until heated through and cheese is melted.

4. Serve immediately or before baking, cover and freeze casserole for up to 3 months.

TO USE FROZEN CASSEROLE *Thaw in the refrigerator overnight. Remove from the refrigerator 30 minutes before baking. Bake according to directions.*
PER SERVING *1½ cups equals 346 cal., 9 g fat (4 g sat. fat), 71 mg chol., 670 mg sodium, 32 g carb., 9 g fiber, 35 g pro.* **Diabetic Exchanges:** *4 lean meat, 2 starch, 1 vegetable, 1 fat.*

Pronto Penne Pasta

My four boys don't have a problem eating healthy whenever I make this!

—**TOMISSA HUART** UNION, IL

START TO FINISH: 30 MIN.
MAKES: 6 SERVINGS

- 2¼ cups uncooked whole wheat penne pasta
- 1 pound Italian turkey sausage links, casings removed
- 1 medium red onion, chopped
- 1 medium green pepper, chopped
- 1 can (14½ ounces) no-salt-added diced tomatoes, undrained
- 1 can (14½ ounces) reduced-sodium chicken broth
- 2 garlic cloves, minced
- 2 teaspoons dried tarragon
- 2 teaspoons dried basil
- ¼ teaspoon cayenne pepper
- ¼ cup all-purpose flour
- ½ cup fat-free milk
- ½ cup shredded reduced-fat cheddar cheese
- ¼ cup grated Parmesan cheese

1. Cook pasta according to package directions. Meanwhile, crumble sausage into a large nonstick skillet coated with cooking spray. Add onion and green pepper; cook and stir over medium heat until meat is no longer pink. Drain. Stir in the tomatoes, broth, garlic, tarragon, basil and cayenne.
2. In a small bowl, combine flour and milk until smooth; stir into sausage mixture. Bring to a boil; cook and stir for 2 minutes or until thickened.
3. Remove from heat. Stir in cheddar cheese until melted. Drain pasta; toss with sausage mix. Sprinkle each serving with 2 teaspoons Parmesan cheese.
PER SERVING *1 cup equals 373 cal., 11 g fat (3 g sat. fat), 55 mg chol., 800 mg sodium, 45 g carb., 4 g fiber, 24 g pro. Diabetic Exchanges: 2½ starch, 2 medium-fat meat, 1 vegetable.*

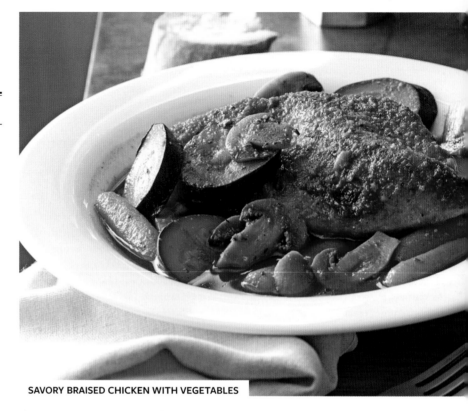

SAVORY BRAISED CHICKEN WITH VEGETABLES

Savory Braised Chicken with Vegetables

Folks will think you worked all day on this masterpiece, but it can be your little secret when it comes to how easy it is.

—**MICHELLE COLLINS** LAKE ORION, MI

PREP: 15 MIN. • **COOK:** 40 MIN.
MAKES: 6 SERVINGS

- ½ cup seasoned bread crumbs
- 6 boneless skinless chicken breast halves (4 ounces each)
- 2 tablespoons olive oil
- 1 can (14½ ounces) beef broth
- 2 tablespoons tomato paste
- 1 teaspoon poultry seasoning
- ½ teaspoon salt
- ½ teaspoon pepper
- 1 pound fresh baby carrots
- 1 pound sliced fresh mushrooms
- 2 medium zucchini, sliced
  Sliced French bread baguette, optional

1. Place bread crumbs in a shallow bowl. Dip chicken breasts in bread crumbs to coat both sides; shake off the excess.
2. In a Dutch oven, heat oil over medium heat. Add chicken in batches; cook 2-4 minutes on each side or until browned. Remove chicken from pan.
3. Add broth, tomato paste and seasonings to same pan; cook over medium-high heat, stirring to loosen browned bits from pan. Add vegetables and chicken; bring to a boil. Reduce heat; simmer, covered, 25-30 minutes or until vegetables are tender and a thermometer inserted in chicken reads 165°. If desired, serve with a baguette.
PER SERVING *1 chicken breast half with 1 cup vegetable mixture equals 247 cal., 8 g fat (1 g sat. fat), 63 mg chol., 703 mg sodium, 16 g carb., 3 g fiber, 28 g pro. Diabetic Exchanges: 3 lean meat, 2 vegetable, 1 fat, ½ starch.*

Slow Cooker Turkey Breast

If you're craving turkey but don't have time to tend to it in the oven, this recipe makes an ideal solution.

—**MARIA JUCO** MILWAUKEE, WI

PREP: 10 MIN. • **COOK:** 5 HOURS
MAKES: 14 SERVINGS

- 1 **bone-in turkey breast (6 to 7 pounds), skin removed**
- 1 **tablespoon olive oil**
- 1 **teaspoon dried minced garlic**
- 1 **teaspoon seasoned salt**
- 1 **teaspoon paprika**
- 1 **teaspoon Italian seasoning**
- 1 **teaspoon pepper**
- ½ **cup water**

Brush turkey with oil. Combine the garlic, seasoned salt, paprika, Italian seasoning and pepper; rub over turkey. Transfer to a 6-qt. slow cooker; add water. Cover and cook on low for 5-6 hours or until tender.

PER SERVING *4 ounces equals 174 cal., 2 g fat (trace sat. fat), 101 mg chol., 172 mg sodium, trace carb., trace fiber, 37 g pro.* **Diabetic Exchange:** *4 lean meat.*

Smokey Sausage & Apple Pizza

This good-for-you pizza combines savory chicken sausage with fresh fruit and vegetables. It makes for a unique dinner that won't sabotage your waistline.

—**LINDSAY WILLIAMS** HASTINGS, MN

PREP: 40 MIN. + STANDING • **BAKE:** 15 MIN.
MAKES: 4 SERVINGS

- ½ **cup all-purpose flour**
- ½ to ¾ **cup whole wheat flour**
- 1 **teaspoon quick-rise yeast**
- ½ **teaspoon salt**
  Dash sugar
- ½ **cup warm water (120° to 130°)**
- 4½ **teaspoons olive oil**
- 1 **tablespoon honey**

TOPPINGS
- 1 **small onion, chopped**
- 3 **teaspoons cider vinegar, divided**
- 2 **teaspoons maple syrup, divided**
  Dash salt
  Dash cayenne pepper
- 2 **teaspoons olive oil**
- 1½ **teaspoons chopped fresh sage**
- 1 **teaspoon Dijon mustard**
- 1 **tablespoon cornmeal**
- 2 **cups chopped beet greens or fresh spinach**
- ½ **cup chopped apple**
- 2 **fully cooked apple chicken sausage links or flavor of your choice (3 ounces each), sliced**
- ¾ **cup shredded smoked cheddar cheese**

1. In a small bowl, combine the all-purpose flour, ½ cup whole wheat flour, yeast, salt and sugar. Stir in the water, oil and honey; beat just until moistened. Stir in enough remaining whole wheat flour to form a soft dough (dough will be sticky).

2. Turn onto a floured surface; knead until smooth and elastic, about 6-8 minutes. Cover dough and let rest for 30 minutes.

3. Meanwhile, in a large skillet, saute the onion, 2 teaspoons vinegar, 1 teaspoon syrup, salt and cayenne in oil until onion is tender. Remove from the heat; stir in the sage, mustard and remaining vinegar and syrup.

4. Grease a 12-in. pizza pan; sprinkle with cornmeal. Roll out the dough to fit prepared pan; prick thoroughly with a fork.

5. Bake at 450° for 5-8 minutes or until edges are lightly browned.

6. Arrange the onion mixture, beet greens, apple, sausages and cheese over top. Bake 5-7 minutes longer or until crust is golden and cheese is melted.

PER SERVING *388 cal., 17 g fat (6 g sat. fat), 48 mg chol., 836 mg sodium, 41 g carb., 4 g fiber, 20 g pro.* **Diabetic Exchanges:** *3 lean meat, 2½ starch, 1½ fat.*

SLOW COOKER TURKEY BREAST

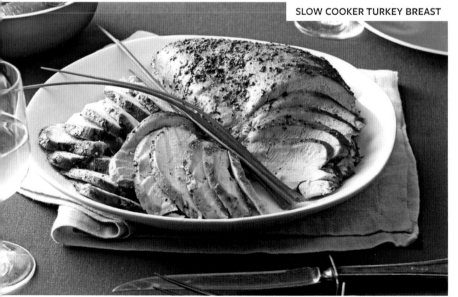

Chipotle Apricot Chicken

Although chipotle peppers may be unfamiliar to some home cooks, they're worth exploring! Their flavor really complements the apricots in this main course for an absolutely wonderful meal.

—TRISHA KRUSE EAGLE, ID

START TO FINISH: 30 MIN.
MAKES: 4 SERVINGS

- 4 boneless skinless chicken breast halves (6 ounces each)
- 2 tablespoons butter
- 2 fresh apricots, thinly sliced
- ½ cup chicken broth
- ⅓ cup apricot preserves
- 2 tablespoons chopped chipotle pepper in adobo sauce
- ½ teaspoon salt
  Hot cooked rice, optional

1. In a large skillet, brown chicken in butter on both sides. Combine the apricots, broth, preserves, chipotle pepper and salt; pour over chicken.
2. Bring to a boil. Reduce heat; simmer, uncovered, for 15-20 minutes or until a thermometer reads 170° and sauce is thickened. Serve with rice if desired.

PER SERVING *312 cal., 10 g fat (5 g sat. fat), 109 mg chol., 612 mg sodium, 20 g carb., 1 g fiber, 35 g pro. Diabetic Exchanges: 5 lean meat, 1 starch, 1 fat.*

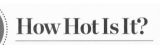

How Hot Is It?

A chipotle pepper, which is a smoked jalapeno, is hotter than a jalapeno, but it's not as hot as a serrano, cayenne or habanero pepper.

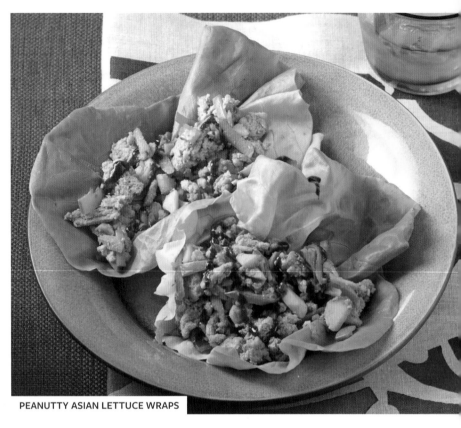

PEANUTTY ASIAN LETTUCE WRAPS

Peanutty Asian Lettuce Wraps

This recipe packs so much punch into a beautiful, healthy presentation. I usually serve it with a little extra hoisin on the side.

—MANDY RIVERS LEXINGTON, SC

START TO FINISH: 30 MIN.
MAKES: 6 SERVINGS

- 1½ pounds lean ground turkey
- ½ cup shredded carrot
- 2 tablespoons minced fresh gingerroot
- 4 garlic cloves, minced
- 1 can (8 ounces) whole water chestnuts, drained and chopped
- 4 green onions, chopped
- ½ cup chopped fresh snow peas
- ⅓ cup reduced-sodium teriyaki sauce
- ¼ cup hoisin sauce
- 3 tablespoons creamy peanut butter
- 1 tablespoon rice vinegar
- 1 tablespoon sesame oil
- 12 Bibb lettuce leaves
  Additional hoisin sauce, optional

1. In a large skillet, cook turkey and carrot over medium heat until meat is no longer pink and carrot is tender; drain. Add ginger and garlic; cook 1 minute longer.
2. Stir in the chestnuts, onions, snow peas, teriyaki sauce, hoisin sauce, peanut butter, vinegar and oil; heat through. Divide among lettuce leaves; drizzle with additional hoisin sauce if desired. Fold lettuce over filling.

PER SERVING *2 wraps equals 313 cal., 16 g fat (4 g sat. fat), 90 mg chol., 613 mg sodium, 18 g carb., 3 g fiber, 24 g pro. Diabetic Exchanges: 3 lean meat, 2 vegetable, 2 fat, ½ starch.*

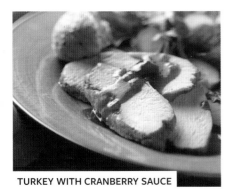

TURKEY WITH CRANBERRY SAUCE

Turkey with Cranberry Sauce

Turkey in the slow cooker? Believe it! You can also freeze leftovers for up to 3 months.

—**MARIE RAMSDEN** FAIRGROVE, MI

PREP: 15 MIN. • **COOK:** 4 HOURS
MAKES: 15 SERVINGS

- 2 **boneless skinless turkey breast halves (3 pounds each)**
- 1 **can (14 ounces) jellied cranberry sauce**
- ½ **cup plus 2 tablespoons water, divided**
- 1 **envelope onion soup mix**
- 2 **tablespoons cornstarch**

1. Place turkey breasts in a 5-qt. slow cooker. In a large bowl, combine the cranberry sauce, ½ cup water and soup mix. Pour over turkey. Cover and cook on low for 4-6 hours or meat is tender. Remove turkey and keep warm.

2. Transfer cooking juices to a large saucepan. Combine the cornstarch and remaining water until smooth. Bring cranberry mixture to a boil; gradually stir in cornstarch mixture until smooth. Cook and stir for 2 minutes or until thickened. Slice turkey; serve with cranberry sauce.

PER SERVING *6 ounces turkey equals 248 cal., 1 g fat (trace sat. fat), 112 mg chol., 259 mg sodium, 12 g carb., trace fiber, 45 g pro.* **Diabetic Exchanges:** *5 lean meat, ½ starch.*

Turkey Scallopini

Go ahead and double this recipe for a family gathering. A splash of white wine and spicy mustard add pizzazz to this classic favorite.

—**SUSAN WARREN** NORTH MANCHESTER, IN

START TO FINISH: 25 MIN.
MAKES: 4 SERVINGS

- ⅓ **cup all-purpose flour**
- ¼ **teaspoon dried rosemary, crushed**
- ¼ **teaspoon dried thyme**
- ⅛ **teaspoon white pepper**
- 1 **package (17.6 ounces) turkey breast cutlets**
- 4 **teaspoons canola oil**
- ¼ **cup white wine or reduced-sodium chicken broth**
- ½ **teaspoon cornstarch**
- ⅓ **cup reduced-sodium chicken broth**
- ½ **cup reduced-fat sour cream**
- 1 **teaspoon spicy brown mustard**
  Paprika, optional

1. In a shallow bowl, mix flour and seasonings. Dip cutlets in flour mixture to coat both sides; shake off excess. In a large nonstick skillet coated with cooking spray, heat oil over medium heat. Add turkey in batches and cook 2-4 minutes on each side or until meat is no longer pink. Remove to a serving plate; keep warm.

2. Add wine to pan; increase heat to medium-high. Cook 30 seconds, stirring to loosen browned bits from pan. In a small bowl, mix cornstarch and broth until smooth; stir into skillet. Bring to a boil; cook and stir 1-2 minutes or until slightly thickened.

3. Stir in sour cream and mustard; heat through. Pour over turkey. If desired, sprinkle with paprika.

PER SERVING *263 cal., 8 g fat (2 g sat. fat), 88 mg chol., 194 mg sodium, 11 g carb., trace fiber, 34 g pro.* **Diabetic Exchanges:** *4 lean meat, 1 starch, 1 fat.*

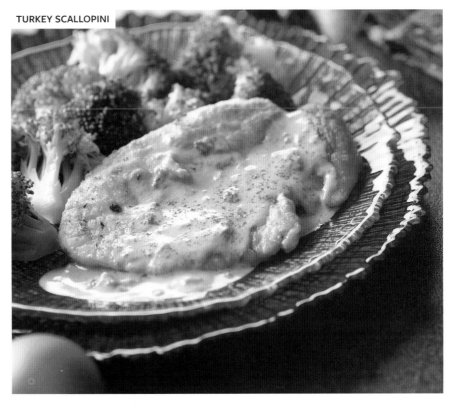

TURKEY SCALLOPINI

Pretzel-Crusted Chicken

Make extras of this so that you can enjoy leftovers the next day. It's delicious served either hot or cold, so go ahead and try it both ways to discover your preference.

—**EILEEN KORECKO** HOT SPRINGS VILLAGE, AR

PREP: 20 MIN. • **BAKE:** 40 MIN.
MAKES: 6 SERVINGS

- 4 cups miniature pretzels
- 5 cooked bacon strips, coarsely chopped
- ½ cup grated Parmesan cheese
- 1 tablespoon dried parsley flakes
- 1 egg
- ½ cup light or nonalcoholic beer
- ⅓ cup all-purpose flour
- 1 teaspoon paprika
- ¼ teaspoon ground ginger
- ¼ teaspoon pepper
- 1 broiler/fryer chicken (3 pounds), cut up and skin removed

1. Place the pretzels, bacon, cheese and parsley in a food processor; cover and process until coarsely chopped. Transfer to a shallow bowl.

2. In another shallow bowl, whisk the egg, beer, flour and spices. Dip a few pieces of chicken at a time in beer mixture, then pretzel mixture. Place chicken in a 13-in. x 9-in. baking dish coated with cooking spray. Bake at 350° for 40-50 minutes or until chicken juices run clear.

PER SERVING *6 ounces cooked chicken equals 283 cal., 9 g fat (3 g sat. fat), 98 mg chol., 498 mg sodium, 19 g carb., 1 g fiber, 30 g pro.* **Diabetic Exchanges:** *4 lean meat, 1 starch, ½ fat.*

PRETZEL-CRUSTED CHICKEN

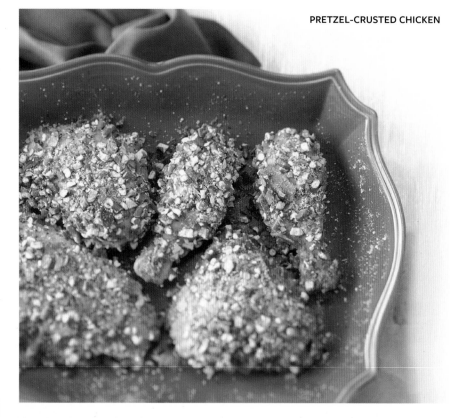

Chicken Creole for Two

I ladle this vegetable-packed chicken dish over jasmine rice, a long-grain rice that is not as sticky as most.

—**VIRGINIA CROWELL** LYONS, OR

PREP: 20 MIN. • **COOK:** 30 MIN.
MAKES: 2 SERVINGS

- ½ cup chopped green pepper
- ¼ cup thinly sliced onion
- ¼ cup chopped celery
- 1 garlic clove, minced
- 1 teaspoon canola oil, divided
- ¾ cup sliced fresh mushrooms
- ¾ cup undrained diced tomatoes
- 2 tablespoons chicken broth
- 1½ teaspoons minced fresh oregano or ½ teaspoon dried oregano
- 1½ teaspoons lemon juice
- ¾ teaspoon minced fresh basil or ¼ teaspoon dried basil
- ⅛ teaspoon each salt and pepper
- ⅛ teaspoon crushed red pepper flakes
- ½ pound boneless skinless chicken breasts, cubed
  Hot cooked rice
  Minced fresh parsley, optional

1. In a large saucepan, saute the green pepper, onion, celery and garlic in ½ teaspoon oil until tender. Add mushrooms; cook until liquid has evaporated. Stir in the tomatoes, broth, oregano, lemon juice, basil and spices. Bring to a boil. Reduce heat; cover and simmer 5-10 minutes or until slightly thickened and flavors are blended.

2. Meanwhile, in a Dutch oven, saute chicken in remaining oil until no longer pink. Return chicken to pan; stir in sauce. Heat through, stirring to loosen browned bits from pan. Serve over rice; garnish with parsley if desired.

PER SERVING *189 cal., 5 g fat (1 g sat. fat), 63 mg chol., 398 mg sodium, 10 g carb., 3 g fiber, 25 g pro.* **Diabetic Exchanges:** *3 lean meat, 2 vegetable, ½ fat.*

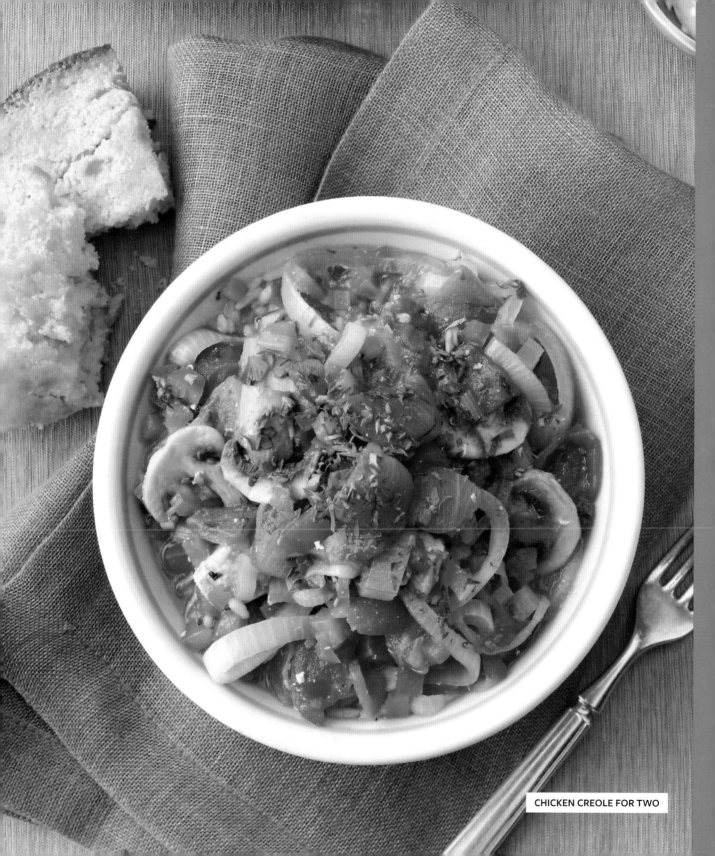

CHICKEN CREOLE FOR TWO

Two-Cheese Turkey Enchiladas

Sour cream and cream cheese create a rich filling for these turkey enchiladas. The entree is so popular in my house.

—SHELLY PLATTEN AMHERST, WI

PREP: 25 MIN. • **BAKE:** 20 MIN.
MAKES: 8 SERVINGS

- 1 **pound extra-lean ground turkey**
- 1 **large onion, chopped**
- ½ **cup chopped green pepper**
- 1 **teaspoon brown sugar**
- 1 **teaspoon garlic powder**
- 1 **teaspoon ground cumin**
- 1 **teaspoon chili powder**
- 1 **can (28 ounces) crushed tomatoes, divided**
- 1 **package (8 ounces) reduced-fat cream cheese**
- ¼ **cup fat-free sour cream**
- 1 **can (4 ounces) chopped green chilies**
- 1 **cup salsa**
- 8 **fat-free flour tortillas (8 inches), warmed**
- ½ **cup shredded reduced-fat cheddar cheese**

1. Crumble turkey into a large nonstick skillet; add the onion, green pepper, brown sugar and seasonings. Cook and stir over medium heat until turkey is no longer pink. Stir in 1 cup crushed tomatoes. Reduce heat; simmer, uncovered, for 10 minutes, stirring occasionally.

2. In a small bowl, beat the cream cheese, sour cream and chilies until blended; set aside. Combine salsa and remaining tomatoes; spread 1 cup into a 13-in. x 9-in. baking dish coated with cooking spray.

3. Spoon about 3 tablespoons cream cheese mixture and ⅓ cup turkey mixture down the center of each tortilla. Roll up and place seam side down in baking dish. Top with remaining salsa mixture; sprinkle with cheddar cheese.

4. Bake, uncovered, at 350° for 20-25 minutes or until bubbly.

PER SERVING *329 cal., 9 g fat (5 g sat. fat), 49 mg chol., 776 mg sodium, 39 g carb., 5 g fiber, 24 g pro.* **Diabetic Exchanges:** *2 starch, 2 lean meat, 2 vegetable.*

Sausage and Pumpkin Pasta

Flavored with pumpkin and white wine, this delightful pasta with Italian turkey sausage will have people talking.

—KATIE WOLLGAST FLORISSANT, MO

PREP: 20 MIN. • **COOK:** 15 MIN.
MAKES: 4 SERVINGS

- 2 **cups uncooked multigrain bow tie pasta**
- ½ **pound Italian turkey sausage links, casings removed**
- ½ **pound sliced fresh mushrooms**
- 1 **medium onion, chopped**
- 4 **garlic cloves, minced**
- 1 **cup reduced-sodium chicken broth**
- 1 **cup canned pumpkin**
- ½ **cup white wine or additional reduced-sodium chicken broth**
- ½ **teaspoon rubbed sage**
- ¼ **teaspoon salt**
- ¼ **teaspoon garlic powder**
- ¼ **teaspoon pepper**
- ¼ **cup grated Parmesan cheese**
- 1 **tablespoon dried parsley flakes**

1. Cook pasta according to package directions.

2. Meanwhile, in a large nonstick skillet coated with cooking spray, cook the sausage, mushrooms and onion over medium heat until meat is no longer pink. Add garlic; cook 1 minute longer. Stir in the broth, pumpkin, wine, sage, salt, garlic powder and pepper. Bring to a boil. Reduce heat; simmer, uncovered, for 5-6 minutes or until slightly thickened.

3. Drain pasta; add to the skillet and heat through. Just before serving, sprinkle with cheese and parsley.

PER SERVING *348 cal., 9 g fat (2 g sat. fat), 38 mg chol., 733 mg sodium, 42 g carb., 7 g fiber, 23 g pro.* **Diabetic Exchanges:** *2½ starch, 2 lean meat, 1 vegetable, ½ fat.*

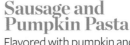
SAUSAGE AND PUMPKIN PASTA

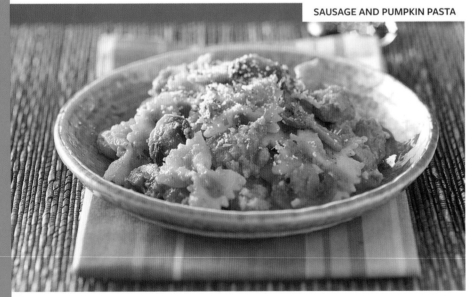

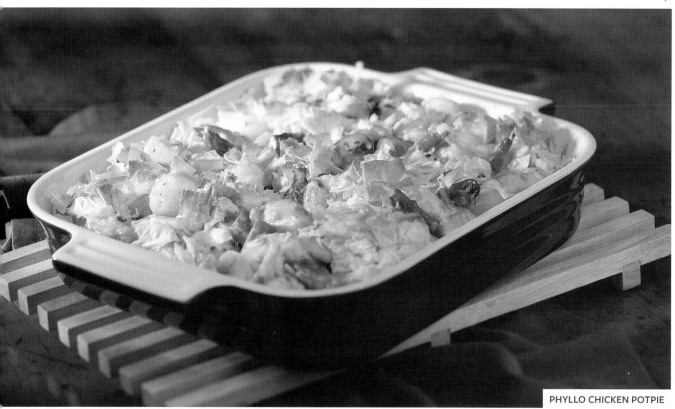

PHYLLO CHICKEN POTPIE

Phyllo Chicken Potpie

Ribbons of buttery phyllo dough provide a crispy topping over pearl onions, mushrooms, asparagus and chicken.

—TASTE OF HOME TEST KITCHEN

PREP: 35 MIN. • **BAKE:** 10 MIN.
MAKES: 6 SERVINGS

- 6 **cups water**
- 2 **cups fresh pearl onions**
- 1½ **pounds boneless skinless chicken breasts, cubed**
- 2 **tablespoons canola oil, divided**
- 2 **medium red potatoes, peeled and chopped**
- 1 **cup sliced fresh mushrooms**
- 1 **can (14½ ounces) reduced-sodium chicken broth**
- ½ **pound fresh asparagus, trimmed and cut into 1-inch pieces**
- 3 **tablespoons sherry or additional reduced-sodium chicken broth**
- 3 **tablespoons cornstarch**
- ½ **cup fat-free milk**
- 1½ **teaspoons minced fresh thyme**
- ½ **teaspoon salt**
- ¼ **teaspoon pepper**
- 10 **sheets phyllo dough (14 inches x 9 inches)**
  Refrigerated butter-flavored spray

1. In a Dutch oven, bring water to a boil. Add the pearl onions; boil for 3 minutes. Drain and rinse in cold water; peel and set aside.

2. In a large skillet, cook chicken in 1 tablespoon oil over medium no longer pink; remove and keep warm. In the same pan, saute potatoes in remaining oil for 5 minutes. Add onions and mushrooms; saute 3 minutes longer. Add the broth, asparagus and sherry or additional broth. Bring to a boil. Reduce heat; cover and simmer for 5 minutes or until potatoes are tender.

3. Combine cornstarch and milk until smooth; stir into skillet. Bring to a boil; cook and stir for 2 minutes or until thickened. Drain chicken; add to onion mixture. Stir in the thyme, salt and pepper. Transfer to an 8-in. square baking dish coated with cooking spray.

4. Stack all 10 phyllo sheets. Roll up, starting at a long side; cut into ½-in. strips. Place in a large bowl and toss to separate strips. Spritz with butter-flavored spray. Arrange over chicken mixture; spritz again.

5. Bake, uncovered, at 425° for 10-15 minutes or until golden brown.

PER SERVING *1 cup equals 325 cal., 8 g fat (1 g sat. fat), 63 mg chol., 542 mg sodium, 33 g carb., 2 g fiber, 29 g pro.* ***Diabetic Exchanges:*** *3 lean meat, 2 vegetable, 1½ starch, 1 fat.*

Honey-of-a-Meal Chicken

My husband is a big fan of honey mustard, so I like to make a little extra of this recipe and slice it up for sandwiches the next day. I've also shredded the chicken and served it on submarine rolls.

—TRACI WYNNE DENVER, PA

START TO FINISH: 30 MIN.
MAKES: 4 SERVINGS

- 4 bone-in chicken breast halves, skin removed (8 ounces each)
- 2 tablespoons olive oil
- 1 medium onion, finely chopped
- 1 cup chicken broth
- 2 tablespoons spicy brown mustard
- ½ teaspoon pepper
- 2 tablespoons honey

1. In a pressure cooker, brown chicken breasts in oil in batches. Set chicken aside. Saute onion in the drippings until tender. Stir in the broth, mustard and pepper. Return chicken to the pan. Close cover securely according to manufacturer's directions.

2. Bring cooker to full pressure over high heat. Reduce heat to medium-high and cook for 8 minutes. (Pressure regulator should maintain a slow steady rocking motion or release of steam; adjust heat if needed.) Immediately cool according to manufacturer's directions until the pressure is completely reduced. Remove chicken and keep warm.

3. Stir honey into sauce. Bring to a boil. Reduce heat; simmer, uncovered, for 8-10 minutes or until thickened. Serve with the chicken.

PER SERVING *314 cal., 11 g fat (2 g sat. fat), 103 mg chol., 433 mg sodium, 13 g carb., 1 g fiber, 38 g pro.* **Diabetic Exchanges:** *4 lean meat, 1 starch, 1 fat.*

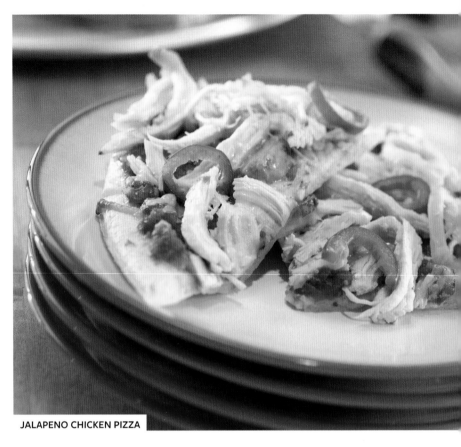

JALAPENO CHICKEN PIZZA

Jalapeno Chicken Pizza

Change up your pizza night! This recipe calls for a prebaked crust, making it quick and easy on busy weeknights.

—LINDA EWANKOWICH RALEIGH, NC

START TO FINISH: 25 MIN.
MAKES: 12 PIECES

- 2 plum tomatoes, quartered
- ½ cup fresh cilantro leaves
- 1 tablespoon tomato paste
- 1 teaspoon chopped chipotle peppers in adobo sauce
- 1 garlic clove, peeled and quartered
- ½ teaspoon salt
- 1 prebaked 12-inch thin pizza crust
- 2 cups shredded cooked chicken breast
- ¾ cup shredded reduced-fat Monterey Jack cheese or Mexican cheese blend
- 2 jalapeno peppers, seeded and sliced into rings

1. Place the first six ingredients in a food processor; cover and process until blended. Place the crust on an ungreased 12-in. pizza pan; spread with tomato mixture. Top with chicken, cheese and jalapenos.

2. Bake at 450° for 10-12 minutes or until heated through and the cheese is melted.

NOTE *Wear disposable gloves when cutting hot peppers; the oils can burn skin. Avoid touching your face.*

PER SERVING *2 pieces equals 262 cal., 8 g fat (2 g sat. fat), 46 mg chol., 613 mg sodium, 26 g carb., 1 g fiber, 23 g pro.* **Diabetic Exchanges:** *3 lean meat, 1½ starch.*

Mashed Potato Sausage Bake

Sausage and savory seasonings like onion and garlic taste great in this casserole.
—**JENNIFER SEEVERS** NORTH BEND, OR

PREP: 35 MIN. • **BAKE:** 10 MIN.
MAKES: 7 SERVINGS

- 5 medium potatoes, peeled and quartered
- ½ cup reduced-fat sour cream
- ¼ cup reduced-sodium chicken broth
- 1 package (14 ounces) smoked turkey kielbasa, sliced
- ½ pound sliced fresh mushrooms
- 1 cup chopped onion
- 1 garlic clove, minced
- ¼ cup shredded reduced-fat cheddar cheese
- 1 teaspoon dried parsley flakes
- 1 teaspoon dried oregano

1. Place potatoes in a large saucepan; cover with water. Bring to a boil. Reduce heat; cover and simmer for 20-25 minutes or until potatoes are very tender; drain.

2. Transfer to a large bowl. Add sour cream and broth; beat on low speed until smooth; set aside. In a large skillet, cook the sausage, mushrooms and onion until vegetables are tender. Add garlic; cook 1 minute longer.

3. Spread half of the potato mixture into a 9-in. x 5-in. loaf pan coated with cooking spray. Top with sausage mixture and remaining potatoes. Sprinkle with the cheese, parsley and oregano.

4. Bake, uncovered, at 350° for 10-15 minutes or until cheese is melted.

PER SERVING *¾ cup equals 255 cal., 6 g fat (3 g sat. fat), 49 mg chol., 706 mg sodium, 34 g carb., 3 g fiber, 17 g pro.* ***Diabetic Exchanges:*** *2 starch, 2 lean meat.*

West African Chicken Stew

I really love African flavors, but you don't encounter them much in this country. Let this combination of native African ingredients, all of which are readily accessible to Americans, take you on a whole new culinary adventure!
—**MICHAEL COHEN** LOS ANGELES, CA

PREP: 20 MIN. • **COOK:** 30 MIN.
MAKES: 8 SERVINGS (2½ QUARTS)

- 1 pound boneless skinless chicken breasts, cut into 1-inch cubes
- ½ teaspoon salt
- ¼ teaspoon pepper
- 3 teaspoons canola oil, divided
- 1 medium onion, thinly sliced
- 6 garlic cloves, minced
- 2 tablespoons minced fresh gingerroot
- 2 cans (15½ ounces each) black-eyed peas, rinsed and drained
- 1 can (28 ounces) crushed tomatoes
- 1 large sweet potato, peeled and cut into 1-inch cubes
- 1 cup reduced-sodium chicken broth
- ¼ cup creamy peanut butter
- 1½ teaspoons minced fresh thyme or ½ teaspoon dried thyme, divided
- ¼ teaspoon cayenne pepper
  Hot cooked brown rice, optional

1. Sprinkle chicken with salt and pepper. In a Dutch oven, cook chicken over medium heat in 2 teaspoons oil for 4-6 minutes or until no longer pink; remove and set aside.

2. In the same pan, saute onion in remaining oil until tender. Add garlic and ginger; cook 1 minute longer.

3. Stir in peas, tomatoes, sweet potato, broth, peanut butter, 1¼ teaspoons thyme and cayenne. Bring to a boil. Reduce heat; cover and simmer for 15-20 minutes or until potato is tender. Add chicken; heat through.

4. Serve with rice if desired. Sprinkle with remaining thyme.

PER SERVING *1¼ cups equals 275 cal., 7 g fat (1 g sat. fat), 31 mg chol., 636 mg sodium, 32 g carb., 6 g fiber, 22 g pro.* ***Diabetic Exchanges:*** *3 lean meat, 2 vegetable, 1 starch, 1 fat.*

WEST AFRICAN CHICKEN STEW

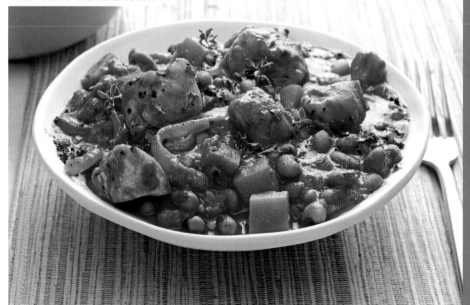

Garden Chicken Cacciatore

When you're expecting company, serve this Italian meal. The slow cooker does all the hard work for you, which frees you up to visit with your guests.

—MARTHA SCHIRMACHER

STERLING HEIGHTS, MI

PREP: 15 MIN. • **COOK:** 8½ HOURS
MAKES: 12 SERVINGS

- 12 boneless skinless chicken thighs (about 3 pounds)
- 2 medium green peppers, chopped
- 1 can (14½ ounces) diced tomatoes with basil, oregano and garlic, undrained
- 1 can (6 ounces) tomato paste
- 1 medium onion, sliced
- ½ cup reduced-sodium chicken broth
- ¼ cup dry red wine or additional reduced-sodium chicken broth
- 3 garlic cloves, minced
- ¾ teaspoon salt
- ⅛ teaspoon pepper
- 2 tablespoons cornstarch
- 2 tablespoons cold water

1. Place chicken in a 4- or 5-qt. slow cooker. In a small bowl, combine the green peppers, tomatoes, tomato paste, onion, broth, wine, garlic, salt and pepper; pour over chicken. Cook, covered, on low 8-10 hours or until chicken is tender.

2. In a small bowl, mix cornstarch and water until smooth; gradually stir into slow cooker. Cook, covered, on high 30 minutes or until sauce is thickened.

PER SERVING *207 cal., 9 g fat (2 g sat. fat), 76 mg chol., 410 mg sodium, 8 g carb., 1 g fiber, 23 g pro.* **Diabetic Exchanges:** *3 lean meat, 1 vegetable, ½ fat.*

GARDEN CHICKEN CACCIATORE

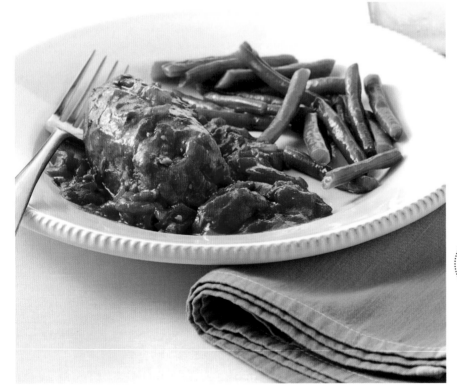

Blueberry-Dijon Chicken

Blueberries and chicken may seem like a strange pairing, but trust me, it's so good! I add a sprinkling of minced fresh basil for the finishing touch.

—SUSAN MARSHALL COLORADO SPRINGS, CO

START TO FINISH: 30 MIN.
MAKES: 4 SERVINGS

- 4 boneless skinless chicken breast halves (6 ounces each)
- ¼ teaspoon salt
- ¼ teaspoon pepper
- 1 tablespoon butter
- ½ cup blueberry preserves
- ⅓ cup raspberry vinegar
- ¼ cup fresh or frozen blueberries
- 3 tablespoons Dijon mustard
  Minced fresh basil or tarragon, optional

1. Sprinkle chicken with salt and pepper. In a large skillet, cook chicken in butter over medium heat for 6-8 minutes on each side or until a thermometer reads 170°. Remove and keep warm.

2. In the same skillet, combine the preserves, vinegar, blueberries and mustard, stirring to loosen browned bits from pan. Bring to a boil; cook and stir until thickened. Serve with chicken. Sprinkle with basil if desired.

PER SERVING *331 cal., 7 g fat (3 g sat. fat), 102 mg chol., 520 mg sodium, 31 g carb., trace fiber, 34 g pro.* **Diabetic Exchanges:** *5 lean meat, 1½ starch, ½ fat.*

top tip
Freeze Berries

Spread berries out on a cookie tray and place the tray in the freezer for about 1½ hours, then transfer the frozen berries to a freezer bag.

—JOHNNIE B. BIRMINGHAM, AL

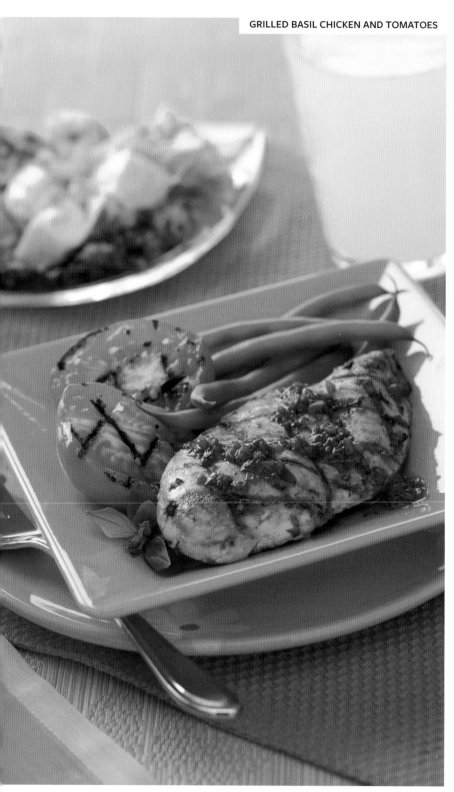

GRILLED BASIL CHICKEN AND TOMATOES

Grilled Basil Chicken and Tomatoes

Relax after work with a cold drink while your savory chicken marinates for an hour, then toss it on the grill.

—LAURA LUNARDI WEST CHESTER, PA

PREP: 15 MIN. + MARINATING
GRILL: 10 MIN.
MAKES: 4 SERVINGS

  8 **plum tomatoes, divided**
  ¾ **cup balsamic vinegar**
  ¼ **cup tightly packed fresh basil leaves**
  2 **tablespoons olive oil**
  1 **garlic clove, minced**
  ½ **teaspoon salt**
  4 **boneless skinless chicken breast halves (4 ounces each)**

1. Cut four tomatoes into quarters and place in a food processor. Add the vinegar, basil, oil, garlic and salt; cover and process until blended.

2. Pour ½ cup dressing into a small bowl; cover and refrigerate until serving. Pour remaining dressing into a large resealable plastic bag; add chicken. Seal bag and turn to coat; refrigerate for up to 1 hour.

3. Drain and discard marinade. Using long-handled tongs, moisten a paper towel with cooking oil and lightly coat the grill rack. Grill chicken, covered, over medium heat or broil 4 in. from the heat for 4-6 minutes on each side or until a thermometer reads 170°.

4. Cut remaining tomatoes in half; grill or broil for 2-3 minutes on each side or until tender. Serve with chicken and reserved dressing.

PER SERVING *174 cal., 5 g fat (1 g sat. fat), 63 mg chol., 179 mg sodium, 7 g carb., 1 g fiber, 24 g pro.* **Diabetic Exchanges:** *3 lean meat, 1 vegetable, ½ fat.*

Makeover Stuffed Chicken Breasts with Mushroom Sauce

This was my great-grandmother's recipe. I have another version made with mushroom soup, which cuts down on prep time, but sometimes you just have to stick with the original!

—**JULIE STACK** PEWAUKEE, WI

PREP: 35 MIN. • **BAKE:** 45 MIN.
MAKES: 4 SERVINGS

- 4 **boneless skinless chicken breast halves (6 ounces each)**
- 1 **small onion, chopped**
- ¼ **cup chopped green pepper**
- ½ **teaspoon canola oil**
- ¾ **cup seasoned bread crumbs**
- ¼ **cup water**
- ½ **teaspoon poultry seasoning**
- ¼ **cup all-purpose flour**
- ¾ **teaspoon paprika**
- ¼ **teaspoon salt**
- ¼ **teaspoon pepper**
  Cooking spray

MUSHROOM SAUCE
- ½ **pound sliced fresh mushrooms**
- ¼ **cup finely chopped onion**
- 2½ **teaspoons canola oil**
- 1 **tablespoon all-purpose flour**
- ½ **cup 2% milk**
- ½ **cup reduced-fat sour cream**
- ¼ **teaspoon salt**
- ⅛ **teaspoon pepper**

1. Flatten chicken to ½-in. thickness. For stuffing, in a small nonstick skillet coated with cooking spray, saute onion and green pepper in oil until tender. Transfer to a small bowl. Stir in the bread crumbs, water and poultry seasoning.

2. Place ¼ cup stuffing over each chicken breast. Roll up from a short side and secure with toothpicks. In a shallow bowl, combine the flour, paprika, salt and pepper. Coat chicken in flour mixture.

3. Place seam side down in an 11-in. x 7-in. baking dish coated with cooking spray. Spritz chicken with cooking spray. Bake, uncovered, at 350° for 45-50 minutes or until a thermometer reads 170°. Discard toothpicks.

4. Meanwhile, in a large skillet, saute mushrooms and onion in oil until tender. Whisk flour and milk; add to

pan. Bring to a boil; cook and stir for 1 minute or until thickened. Remove from the heat; stir in the sour cream, salt and pepper. Serve with chicken.
PER SERVING *401 cal., 13 g fat (3 g sat. fat), 106 mg chol., 627 mg sodium, 27 g carb., 2 g fiber, 43 g pro.* **Diabetic Exchanges:** *5 lean meat, 1 starch, 1 vegetable, 1 fat.*

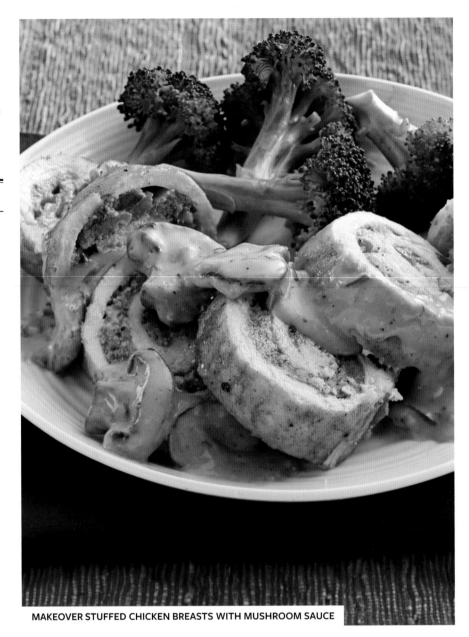

MAKEOVER STUFFED CHICKEN BREASTS WITH MUSHROOM SAUCE

Caribbean Chicken Tenderloins

Give chicken tenderloins a try in this Caribbean-inspired dish. If you're not a big fan of jerk seasoning, the pineapple and brown sugar offset it a bit.

—**LAURA MCALLISTER** MORGANTON, NC

START TO FINISH: 20 MIN.
MAKES: 4 SERVINGS

- 1 **pound chicken tenderloins**
- 2 **teaspoons Caribbean jerk seasoning**
- 3 **teaspoons olive oil, divided**
- 2½ **cups cut fresh asparagus (2-inch pieces)**
- 1 **cup pineapple tidbits, drained**
- 4 **green onions, chopped**
- 2 **teaspoons cornstarch**
- 1 **cup unsweetened pineapple juice**
- 1 **tablespoon spicy brown mustard**
- 2 **cups hot cooked rice**

1. Rub chicken with jerk seasoning. In a large skillet coated with cooking spray, cook chicken in 1 teaspoon oil over medium heat for 3-4 minutes on each side or until juices run clear. Remove and keep warm.

2. In the same skillet, saute asparagus, pineapple and onions in remaining oil for 2-3 minutes or until tender.

3. Combine the cornstarch, pineapple juice and mustard until smooth; gradually stir into the pan. Bring to a boil; cook and stir for 2 minutes or until thickened. Serve with chicken and rice.

PER SERVING *314 cal., 4 g fat (1 g sat. fat), 67 mg chol., 247 mg sodium, 40 g carb., 2 g fiber, 29 g pro.* **Diabetic Exchanges:** *3 lean meat, 2 starch, ½ fruit, ½ fat.*

Chipotle-Lime Chicken Thighs

You can put leftovers from this recipe to good use—the chicken bones can be used to make your own stock or freeze the remaining chipotle peppers and sauce for a smoky Sunday chili.

—**NANCY BROWN** DAHINDA, IL

PREP: 15 MIN. + CHILLING • **GRILL:** 20 MIN.
MAKES: 4 SERVINGS

- 2 **garlic cloves, peeled**
- ¾ **teaspoon salt**
- 1 **tablespoon lime juice**
- 1 **tablespoon minced chipotle pepper in adobo sauce**
- 2 **teaspoons adobo sauce**
- 1 **teaspoon chili powder**
- 4 **bone-in chicken thighs (about 1½ pounds)**

1. Place garlic on a cutting board; sprinkle with salt. Using the flat side of a knife, mash garlic. Continue to mash until it reaches a paste consistency; transfer to a small bowl.

2. Stir in the lime juice, pepper, adobo sauce and chili powder. Gently loosen skin from chicken thighs; rub garlic mixture under the skin. Cover and refrigerate overnight.

3. Moisten a paper towel with cooking oil; using long-handled tongs, lightly coat the grill rack. Grill chicken, covered, over medium-low heat for 20-25 minutes or until a thermometer reads 180°, turning once. Remove and discard skin before serving.

PER SERVING *209 cal., 11 g fat (3 g sat. fat), 87 mg chol., 596 mg sodium, 2 g carb., trace fiber, 25 g pro.* **Diabetic Exchange:** *3 lean meat.*

CHIPOTLE-LIME CHICKEN THIGHS

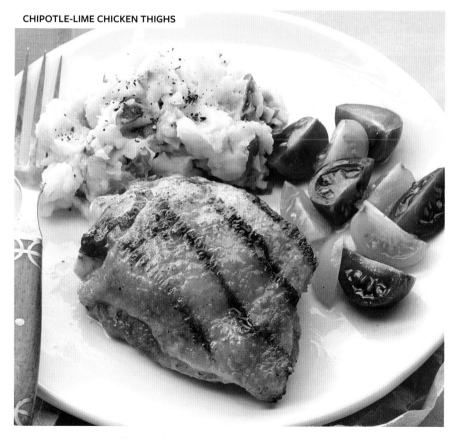

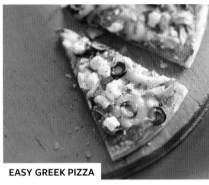

EASY GREEK PIZZA

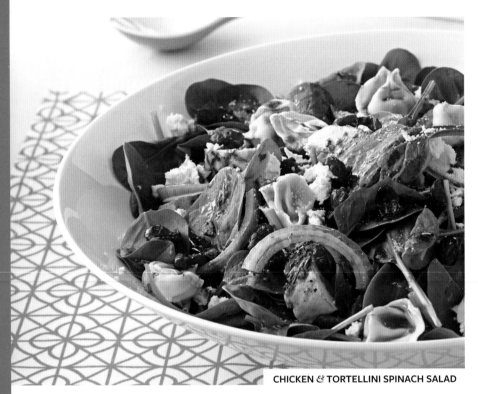

CHICKEN & TORTELLINI SPINACH SALAD

Chicken & Tortellini Spinach Salad

Not only is this attractive salad easy to make, but it is tasty and filling as well.

—MICHELLE ASHTON ST. JOHNS, AZ

PREP: 25 MIN. • **COOK:** 15 MIN.
MAKES: 9 SERVINGS

- 2 packages (9 ounces each) refrigerated cheese tortellini
- 2 packages (6 ounces each) fresh baby spinach
- 1 package (22 ounces) frozen grilled chicken breast strips, cut into 1-inch pieces
- 12 slices red onion, halved
- 1 cup dried cranberries
- 1 cup (4 ounces) crumbled feta cheese

BALSAMIC VINAIGRETTE

- ⅓ cup olive oil
- ⅓ cup balsamic vinegar
- 1 tablespoon tomato paste
- 2 garlic cloves, minced
- 1 teaspoon dried oregano
- ⅛ teaspoon salt
- ⅛ teaspoon pepper
- ¼ cup grated Parmesan cheese

1. In a large saucepan, cook tortellini according to package directions. Meanwhile, in a large bowl, combine the spinach, chicken, onion, cranberries and feta cheese. Drain pasta. Cool for 5 minutes. Add to spinach mixture.
2. For vinaigrette, in a small bowl, whisk the oil, vinegar, tomato paste, garlic, oregano, salt and pepper. Pour over spinach mixture; gently toss to coat. Sprinkle with Parmesan cheese.
PER SERVING *2 cups equals 432 cal., 17 g fat (6 g sat. fat), 74 mg chol., 820 mg sodium, 43 g carb., 4 g fiber, 30 g pro.* **Diabetic Exchanges:** *3 lean meat, 2½ starch, 1½ fat, 1 vegetable.*

Easy Greek Pizza

I created this recipe to use up leftovers from a dinner party. It's even great without the chicken.

—JENNIFER BECK MERIDIAN, ID

START TO FINISH: 30 MIN.
MAKES: 6 SERVINGS

- 1 prebaked 12-inch pizza crust
- ½ cup pizza sauce
- 1 teaspoon lemon-pepper seasoning, divided
- 2 cups shredded cooked chicken breast
- 1½ cups chopped fresh spinach
- 1 small red onion, thinly sliced and separated into rings
- ¼ cup sliced ripe olives
- ¾ cup shredded part-skim mozzarella cheese
- ½ cup crumbled feta cheese

1. Place crust on an ungreased baking sheet; spread with pizza sauce and sprinkle with ½ teaspoon lemon-pepper seasoning. Top with chicken, spinach, onion, olives, cheeses and remaining lemon-pepper seasoning.
2. Bake at 450° for 12-15 minutes or until edges are lightly browned and cheese is melted.
PER SERVING *1 slice equals 321 cal., 9 g fat (4 g sat. fat), 49 mg chol., 719 mg sodium, 32 g carb., 2 g fiber, 26 g pro.* **Diabetic Exchanges:** *3 lean meat, 2 starch, ½ fat.*

Chicken Thighs with Shallots & Spinach

You won't have to worry about making side dishes for supper tonight—this recipe includes a simple spinach side.

—**GENNA JOHANNES** WRIGHTSTOWN, WI

START TO FINISH: 30 MIN.
MAKES: 6 SERVINGS

- 6 **boneless skinless chicken thighs (about 1½ pounds)**
- ½ **teaspoon seasoned salt**
- ½ **teaspoon pepper**
- 1½ **teaspoons olive oil**
- 4 **shallots, thinly sliced**
- ⅓ **cup white wine or reduced-sodium chicken broth**
- 1 **package (10 ounces) fresh spinach**
- ¼ **teaspoon salt**
- ¼ **cup fat-free sour cream**

1. Sprinkle chicken with seasoned salt and pepper. In a large nonstick skillet coated with cooking spray, heat oil over medium heat. Add the chicken; cook 6 minutes on each side or until a thermometer reads 170°. Remove from the pan; keep warm.

2. In the same pan, cook and stir shallots until tender. Add wine; bring to a boil. Cook until wine is reduced by half. Add spinach and salt; cook and stir just until spinach is wilted. Stir in sour cream; serve with chicken.

PER SERVING *1 thigh with ¼ cup spinach mixture equals 225 cal., 10 g fat (2 g sat. fat), 77 mg chol., 338 mg sodium, 8 g carb., 1 g fiber, 24 g pro.* **Diabetic Exchanges:** *3 lean meat, 1½ fat, 1 vegetable.*

Broiled Apricot Chicken

The apricot nectar balances out the bold taste of horseradish in this recipe. You can grill the chicken, too.

—**SUSAN WARREN** NORTH MANCHESTER, IN

START TO FINISH: 30 MIN.
MAKES: 6 SERVINGS

- 1 **cup apricot nectar**
- 3 **tablespoons brown sugar**
- 2 **tablespoons ketchup**
- 2 **teaspoons cornstarch**
- 1 **teaspoon grated orange peel**
- 1 **teaspoon horseradish mustard**
- 6 **boneless skinless chicken breast halves (6 ounces each)**

1. In a small saucepan, combine the first six ingredients. Bring to a boil. Cook and stir for 1 minute or until thickened.

2. Place chicken on a broiler pan coated with cooking spray. Broil 4 in. from the heat for 6-8 minutes on each side or until the chicken juices run clear, basting frequently with the apricot mixture.

PER SERVING *241 cal., 4 g fat (1 g sat. fat), 94 mg chol., 158 mg sodium, 15 g carb., trace fiber, 34 g pro.* **Diabetic Exchanges:** *5 lean meat, 1 starch.*

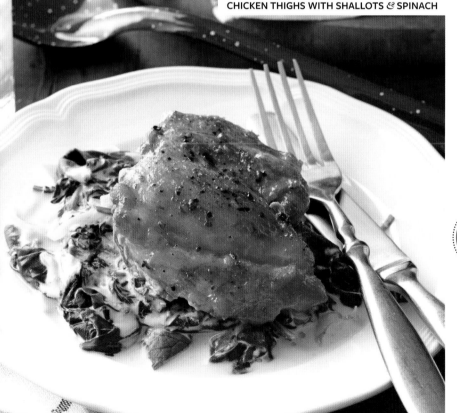

CHICKEN THIGHS WITH SHALLOTS & SPINACH

top tip **Easy Grating**

I freeze an orange the night before I know I'll need it for a recipe. It's much easier to grate that way.

—**JENNIFER B.** SHEBOYGAN, WI

Chicken Breasts with Veggies

This is my own spin on a family-favorite recipe. I think the vegetables are delicious baked right with the chicken because they pick up the marinade flavor.

—**TONY LENTINI** ROGUE RIVER, OR

PREP: 20 MIN. + MARINATING • **BAKE:** 40 MIN.
MAKES: 2 SERVINGS

- 1 **tablespoon olive oil**
- 1 **tablespoon balsamic vinegar**
- 1 **tablespoon Worcestershire sauce**
- 1 **tablespoon reduced-sodium teriyaki sauce**
- 1½ **teaspoons reduced-sodium soy sauce**
- 2 **boneless skinless chicken breast halves (5 ounces each)**
- 1 **small potato, peeled and cut into ½-inch cubes**
- 2 **large fresh mushrooms, sliced**
- 1 **large carrot, sliced**
- 1 **small green pepper, chopped**
- 7 **pitted ripe olives, halved**
- ⅓ **cup chopped onion**
- 1 **tablespoon grated Parmesan cheese**
- ½ **teaspoon Italian seasoning**

1. In a small bowl, combine the first five ingredients. Pour 2 tablespoons marinade into a large resealable plastic bag; add the chicken. Seal bag and turn to coat; refrigerate for up to 4 hours. Cover and refrigerate the remaining marinade.

2. Drain and discard marinade. Place chicken in an 11-in. x 7-in. baking dish coated with cooking spray. Arrange the potato, mushrooms, carrot, green pepper, olives and onion around chicken. Drizzle with reserved marinade. Sprinkle with the cheese and Italian seasoning.

3. Cover and bake at 375° for 40-45 minutes or until a thermometer reads 170°.

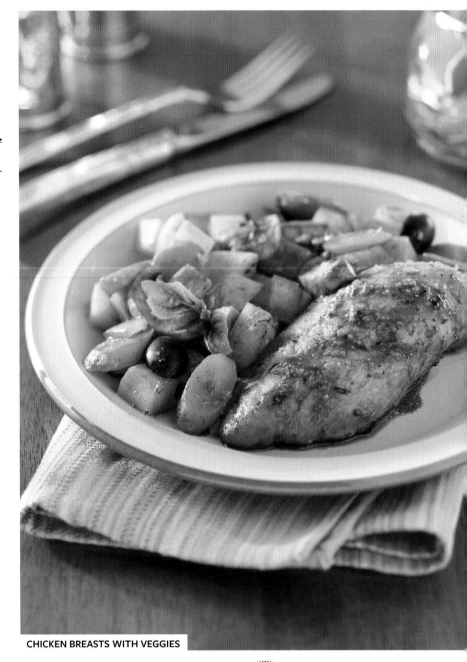

CHICKEN BREASTS WITH VEGGIES

PER SERVING *337 cal., 11 g fat (2 g sat. fat), 81 mg chol., 576 mg sodium, 26 g carb., 4 g fiber, 33 g pro.* **Diabetic Exchanges:** *4 lean meat, 1½ fat, 1 starch, 1 vegetable.*

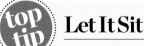

top tip

Let It Sit

Meat tenderizes as it marinates, so follow the recipe's timelines for the best results.

Chicken Sausages with Peppers

Fresh and crispy sweet peppers complement the savory sausage in this family-friendly dish. It requires so little effort to put together!

—**DEBORAH SCHAEFER** DURAND, MI

START TO FINISH: 30 MIN.
MAKES: 4 SERVINGS

- 1 **small onion, halved and sliced**
- 1 **small sweet orange pepper, julienned**
- 1 **small sweet red pepper, julienned**
- 1 **tablespoon olive oil**
- 1 **garlic clove, minced**
- 1 **package (12 ounces) fully cooked apple chicken sausage links or flavor of your choice, cut into 1-inch pieces**

In a large nonstick skillet, saute onion and peppers in oil until crisp-tender. Add garlic; cook 1 minute longer. Stir in sausages; heat through.

PER SERVING *208 cal., 11 g fat (2 g sat. fat), 60 mg chol., 483 mg sodium, 14 g carb., 1 g fiber, 15 g pro.* **Diabetic Exchanges:** *2 lean meat, 1 vegetable, ½ starch, ½ fat.*

CHICKEN SAUSAGES WITH PEPPERS

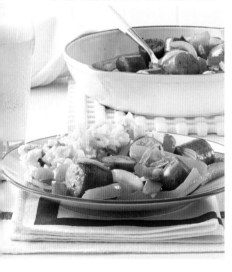

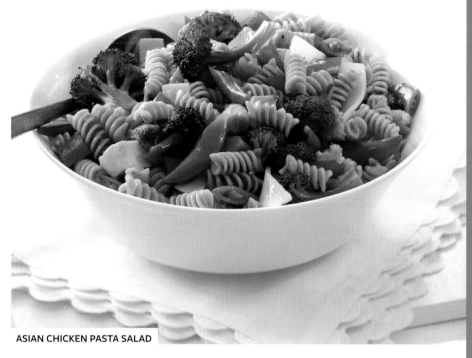

ASIAN CHICKEN PASTA SALAD

Asian Chicken Pasta Salad

Packed with veggies, chicken, whole wheat pasta and just the right amount of heat, this main-dish salad is special and tasty.

—**NICOLE FILIZETTI** JACKSONVILLE, FL

START TO FINISH: 30 MIN.
MAKES: 6 SERVINGS

- 3 **cups uncooked whole wheat spiral pasta**
- 2 **cups cubed cooked chicken breast**
- 2 **cups fresh broccoli florets**
- 1½ **cups fresh sugar snap peas, trimmed and halved**
- 1 **can (8 ounces) bamboo shoots**
- 1 **small sweet red pepper, chopped**
- 3 **tablespoons rice vinegar**
- 3 **tablespoons peanut oil**
- 3 **tablespoons reduced-sodium soy sauce**
- 2 **tablespoons sesame oil**
- 3 **garlic cloves, minced**
- 2 **teaspoons minced fresh gingerroot**
- ½ **teaspoon crushed red pepper flakes**
- ½ **teaspoon pepper**

1. Cook pasta according to package directions. Meanwhile, in a large bowl, combine the chicken, broccoli, peas, bamboo shoots and red pepper.

2. In a small bowl, whisk the remaining ingredients. Pour over chicken mixture; toss to coat. Drain pasta and rinse in cold water; add to salad.

PER SERVING *1⅔ cups equals 321 cal., 14 g fat (2 g sat. fat), 36 mg chol., 344 mg sodium, 29 g carb., 6 g fiber, 21 g pro.* **Diabetic Exchanges:** *2 lean meat, 2 fat, 1½ starch, 1 vegetable.*

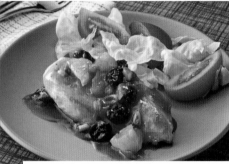

CHICKEN WITH CHERRY PINEAPPLE SALSA

Chicken with Cherry Pineapple Salsa

Cherries and chunks of pineapple turn this chicken into a colorful meal.

—**SALLY MALONEY** DALLAS, GA

START TO FINISH: 25 MIN.
MAKES: 4 SERVINGS

- 4 **boneless skinless chicken breast halves (4 ounces each)**
- ½ **teaspoon garlic salt**
- ¼ **teaspoon ground ginger**
- 2 **teaspoons canola oil**
- 1 **can (8 ounces) unsweetened pineapple chunks**
- ½ **cup sweet-and-sour sauce**
- ¼ **cup dried cherries**
- 2 **green onions, sliced**

1. Sprinkle the chicken with garlic salt and ginger. In a large nonstick skillet coated with cooking spray, brown chicken in oil.
2. Drain pineapple, reserving ¼ cup juice. In a small bowl, combine the sauce, cherries and reserved juice; pour over chicken. Bring to a boil. Reduce heat; cover and simmer for 8-10 minutes or until a thermometer reads 170°, turning chicken once. Stir in pineapple and onions; heat through.
PER SERVING *238 cal., 5 g fat (1 g sat. fat), 63 mg chol., 473 mg sodium, 24 g carb., 1 g fiber, 24 g pro.* **Diabetic Exchanges:** *3 lean meat, ½ starch, ½ fruit, ½ fat.*

CHICKEN WITH BERRY WINE SAUCE

Chicken with Berry Wine Sauce

We like to use merlot in this recipe to bring out the berry flavor.

—**ELIZABETH WRIGHT** RALEIGH, NC

PREP: 35 MIN. • **GRILL:** 10 MIN.
MAKES: 4 SERVINGS

- 1 **cup fresh strawberries, halved**
- 1 **cup fresh raspberries**
- 1 **cup merlot or red grape juice**
- 2 **tablespoons sugar**
- 4 **boneless skinless chicken breast halves (6 ounces each)**
- ½ **teaspoon salt**
- ½ **teaspoon pepper**
  Thinly sliced fresh basil leaves

1. In a small saucepan, combine the strawberries, raspberries, merlot and sugar. Bring to a boil. Reduce heat; simmer, uncovered, for 25-30 minutes or until thickened, stirring occasionally.
2. Meanwhile, moisten a paper towel with cooking oil; using long-handled tongs, lightly coat the grill rack. Sprinkle chicken with salt and pepper. Grill chicken, covered, over medium heat or broil 4 in. from the heat for 4-7 minutes on each side or until a thermometer reads 170°.
3. Serve with the berry sauce; garnish with fresh basil.
PER SERVING *251 cal., 4 g fat (1 g sat. fat), 94 mg chol., 378 mg sodium, 13 g carb., 3 g fiber, 35 g pro.* **Diabetic Exchanges:** *5 lean meat, ½ starch, ½ fruit.*

Apricot-Glazed Turkey Breast

Garlic, ginger and apricot enhance this classic without loading on calories.

—JANET SPRUTE LEWISTON, ID

PREP: 15 MIN. + MARINATING
BAKE: 2 HOURS + STANDING
MAKES: 12 SERVINGS

- 1 **bone-in turkey breast (5 to 6 pounds)**
- 2 **garlic cloves, peeled and thinly sliced**
- 1 **tablespoon sliced fresh gingerroot**
- ½ **cup white wine or reduced-sodium chicken broth**
- ⅓ **cup reduced-sugar apricot preserves**
- 1 **tablespoon spicy brown mustard**
- 2 **teaspoons reduced-sodium soy sauce**

1. With fingers, carefully loosen skin from turkey breast. With a sharp knife, cut ten 2-in.-long slits in meat under the skin; insert a garlic clove slice and a ginger slice into each slit.

2. Place turkey in a large bowl; pour ¼ cup wine under the skin. Secure skin to underside of breast with toothpicks. Pour remaining wine over turkey. Cover and refrigerate for 6 hours or overnight.

3. In a small bowl, combine the preserves, mustard and soy sauce; set aside. Drain and discard marinade; place turkey on a rack in a foil-lined roasting pan.

4. Bake at 325° for 2 to 2½ hours or until a thermometer reads 170°, basting with apricot mixture every 30 minutes (cover loosely with foil if turkey browns too quickly). Cover and let stand for 15 minutes before carving.

PER SERVING *5 ounces cooked turkey equals 276 cal., 10 g fat (3 g sat. fat), 102 mg chol., 137 mg sodium, 3 g carb., trace fiber, 40 g pro.* **Diabetic Exchange:** *5 medium-fat meat.*

APRICOT-GLAZED TURKEY BREAST

Italian Restaurant Chicken

While the chicken and sauce cook, I make pasta to serve alongside. Your family will definitely be impressed with this entree.

—PATRICIA NIEH PORTOLA VALLEY, CA

PREP: 25 MIN. • **BAKE:** 50 MIN.
MAKES: 6 SERVINGS

- 1 **broiler/fryer chicken (3 pounds), cut up and skin removed**
- ½ **teaspoon salt**
- ¼ **teaspoon pepper**
- 2 **tablespoons olive oil**
- 1 **small onion, finely chopped**
- ¼ **cup finely chopped celery**
- ¼ **cup finely chopped carrot**
- 3 **garlic cloves, minced**
- ½ **cup dry red wine or reduced-sodium chicken broth**
- 1 **can (28 ounces) crushed tomatoes**
- 1 **bay leaf**
- 1 **teaspoon minced fresh rosemary or ¼ teaspoon dried rosemary, crushed**
- ¼ **cup minced fresh basil**

1. Preheat oven to 325°. Sprinkle chicken with salt and pepper. In an ovenproof Dutch oven, brown the chicken in oil in batches. Remove and keep warm.

2. In the same pan, saute onion, celery, carrot and garlic in pan drippings until tender. Add wine, stirring to loosen browned bits from pan. Stir in the tomatoes, bay leaf, rosemary and chicken; bring to a boil.

3. Cover and bake 50-60 minutes or until juices run clear. Discard bay leaf; sprinkle with basil.

PER SERVING *3 ounces cooked chicken with ⅔ cup sauce equals 254 cal., 11 g fat (2 g sat. fat), 73 mg chol., 442 mg sodium, 12 g carb., 3 g fiber, 27 g pro.* **Diabetic Exchanges:** *3 lean meat, 2 vegetable, 1 fat.*

Chicken Enchilada Casserole

If you like your enchiladas with a little extra "oomph," sprinkle seeded fresh chopped jalapenos and cilantro on top.

—**AMY JOHNSON** NEW BRAUNFELS, TX

PREP: 30 MIN. • **BAKE:** 30 MIN.
MAKES: 6 SERVINGS

- 1 **large onion, chopped**
- 1 **medium green pepper, chopped**
- 1 **teaspoon butter**
- 3 **cups shredded cooked chicken breast**
- 2 **cans (4 ounces each) chopped green chilies**
- ¼ **cup all-purpose flour**
- 1½ **to 2 teaspoons ground coriander**
- 2½ **cups reduced-sodium chicken broth**
- 1 **cup (8 ounces) reduced-fat sour cream**
- 1 **cup (4 ounces) reduced-fat Monterey Jack or reduced-fat Mexican cheese blend, divided**
- 12 **corn tortillas (6 inches), warmed**

1. In a small skillet, saute onion and green pepper in butter until tender. In a large bowl, combine the chicken, green chilies and onion mixture.

2. In a small saucepan, combine flour and coriander. Add broth; stir until smooth. Cook and stir over medium heat until mixture comes to a boil. Cook and stir 1-2 minutes longer or until thickened. Remove from the heat; stir in sour cream and ½ cup cheese. Stir ¾ cup sauce into chicken mixture.

3. Place ⅓ cup chicken mixture down the center of each tortilla. Roll up and place seam side down in a 13-in. x 9-in. baking dish coated with cooking spray. Pour remaining sauce over top; sprinkle with remaining cheese. Bake, uncovered, at 350° for 30-35 minutes or until heated through.

PER SERVING *2 enchiladas equals 383 cal., 12 g fat (6 g sat. fat), 82 mg chol., 710 mg sodium, 37 g carb., 5 g fiber, 33 g pro.* **Diabetic Exchanges:** *4 lean meat, 2 starch, 1 fat.*

CHICKEN ENCHILADA CASSEROLE

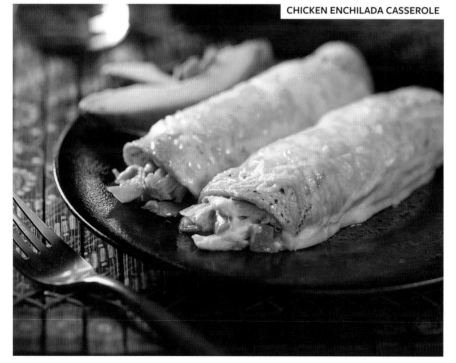

Turkey Spaghetti Sauce

Top your spaghetti (or other pasta) with this special sauce. It's lower in sodium than jarred meat sauce.

—**JENNIFER KOLB** OVERLAND PARK, KS

PREP: 25 MIN. • **COOK:** 40 MIN.
MAKES: 7½ CUPS

- 1 **pound Italian turkey sausage links, casings removed**
- ½ **pound extra-lean ground turkey**
- 1¾ **cups sliced fresh mushrooms**
- 1 **medium green pepper, chopped**
- 1 **medium onion, chopped**
- 1 **can (29 ounces) tomato puree**
- 1 **can (14½ ounces) diced tomatoes, undrained**
- 1 **can (6 ounces) tomato paste**
- 2 **bay leaves**
- 1 **tablespoon dried oregano**
- 1 **teaspoon garlic powder**
- 1 **teaspoon dried basil**
- ½ **teaspoon salt**
- ¼ **teaspoon pepper**
  Hot cooked multigrain spaghetti

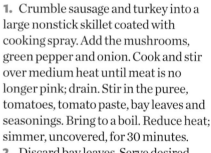

1. Crumble sausage and turkey into a large nonstick skillet coated with cooking spray. Add the mushrooms, green pepper and onion. Cook and stir over medium heat until meat is no longer pink; drain. Stir in the puree, tomatoes, tomato paste, bay leaves and seasonings. Bring to a boil. Reduce heat; simmer, uncovered, for 30 minutes.

2. Discard bay leaves. Serve desired amount with spaghetti. Cool remaining sauce; transfer to freezer containers. Freeze for up to 3 months.

TO USE FROZEN SAUCE *Thaw in the refrigerator overnight. Place in a saucepan and heat through.*

PER SERVING *½ cup (calculated without spaghetti) equals 103 cal., 3 g fat (1 g sat. fat), 24 mg chol., 325 mg sodium, 9 g carb., 2 g fiber, 10 g pro.* **Diabetic Exchanges:** *2 vegetable, 1 lean meat.*

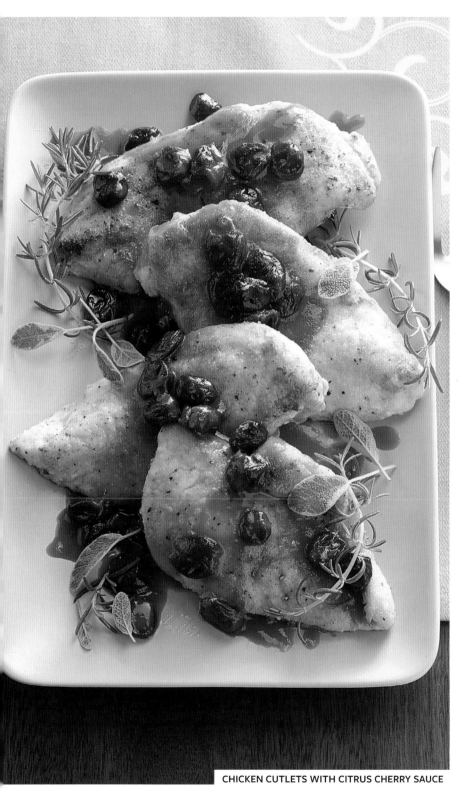

CHICKEN CUTLETS WITH CITRUS CHERRY SAUCE

Chicken Cutlets with Citrus Cherry Sauce

You'll love the tangy sweet-tart flavor this recipe offers. It's just as good made with pork cutlets and dried cranberries in place of the chicken and cherries.

—**CHARLENE CHAMBERS** ORMOND BEACH, FL

START TO FINISH: 30 MIN.
MAKES: 4 SERVINGS

4	boneless skinless chicken breast halves (6 ounces each)
½	teaspoon salt
¼	teaspoon pepper
¼	cup all-purpose flour
½	cup ruby red grapefruit juice
½	cup orange juice
⅓	cup dried cherries
2	teaspoons Dijon mustard
1	tablespoon butter
1	tablespoon canola oil

1. Flatten chicken breasts to ½-in. thickness; sprinkle with salt and pepper. Place flour in a large resealable plastic bag. Add chicken, a few pieces at a time, and shake to coat; set aside.

2. In a small saucepan, combine the juices, cherries and mustard. Bring to a boil; cook until the liquid is reduced to ½ cup.

3. In a large skillet over medium heat, cook chicken in butter and oil for 5-7 minutes on each side or until juices run clear. Serve with sauce.

PER SERVING *316 cal., 10 g fat (3 g sat. fat), 102 mg chol., 458 mg sodium, 18 g carb., trace fiber, 35 g pro.* **Diabetic Exchanges:** *5 lean meat, 1 starch, 1 fat.*

seafood & meatless

It's time to **dig into goodness.** You can still enjoy a filling, delicious meal while sticking to your diet. Dare to go meatless or discover a new **catch-of-the-day recipe** that's sure to wow your crowd.

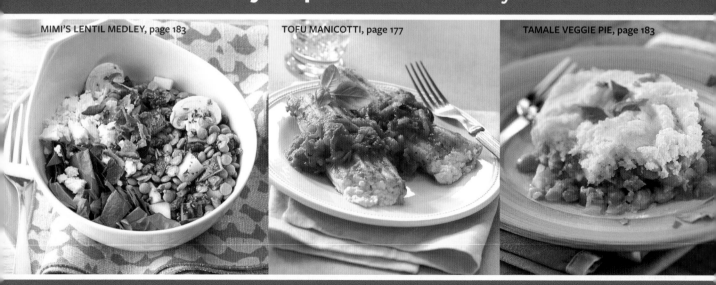

MIMI'S LENTIL MEDLEY, page 183

TOFU MANICOTTI, page 177

TAMALE VEGGIE PIE, page 183

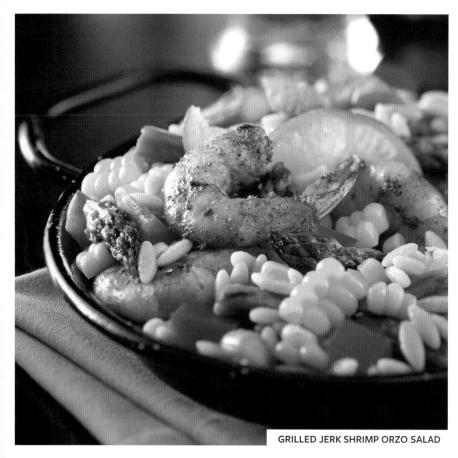

GRILLED JERK SHRIMP ORZO SALAD

Grilled Jerk Shrimp Orzo Salad

It doesn't matter what the temperature is outside—you'll feel like you're in the Caribbean when you take your first bite of this salad!

—**EILEEN BUDNYK** PALM BEACH GARDENS, FL

PREP: 25 MIN. • **GRILL:** 25 MIN.
MAKES: 2 SERVINGS

- 1 **large ear sweet corn in husk**
- 1 **teaspoon olive oil**
- ⅓ **cup uncooked whole wheat orzo pasta**
- 6 **fresh asparagus spears, trimmed**
- ½ **pound uncooked medium shrimp, peeled and deveined**
- 1 **tablespoon Caribbean jerk seasoning**
- 1 **small sweet red pepper, chopped**

DRESSING

- 2 **tablespoons white vinegar**
- 1 **tablespoon water**
- 1 **tablespoon lime juice**
- 1 **tablespoon olive oil**
- ⅛ **teaspoon salt**
- ⅛ **teaspoon pepper**

1. Carefully peel back corn husk to within 1 in. of bottom; remove silk. Brush corn with oil. Rewrap corn in husk and secure with kitchen string. Grill corn, covered, over medium heat for 25-30 minutes or until tender, turning often.

2. Meanwhile, cook orzo according to package directions. Drain and rinse in cold water; set aside.

3. Thread asparagus spears onto two parallel metal or soaked wooden skewers. Rub shrimp with jerk seasoning; thread onto two skewers. Grill asparagus and shrimp, covered, over medium heat for 5-8 minutes or until asparagus is crisp-tender and shrimp turn pink, turning once.

4. Cut corn from cob; place in a large bowl. Cut asparagus into 1-in. pieces; add to bowl. Add the shrimp, orzo and pepper. In a small bowl, whisk the dressing ingredients. Pour over salad; toss to coat.

PER SERVING *352 cal., 12 g fat (2 g sat. fat), 138 mg chol., 719 mg sodium, 38 g carb., 8 g fiber, 26 g pro.* **Diabetic Exchanges:** *3 lean meat, 2 starch, 1 vegetable, 1 fat.*

Greek Pizza

Every year my sisters and I have a Sister's Day, which includes a special lunch, and this pizza usually makes an appearance. Who knew pizza could be good for you?

—**DEBORAH PREVOST** BARNET, VT

START TO FINISH: 20 MIN.
MAKES: 12 PIECES

- 1 **prebaked 12-inch thin whole wheat pizza crust**
- 3 **tablespoons prepared pesto**
- 2 **medium tomatoes, thinly sliced**
- ¾ **cup water-packed artichoke hearts, rinsed, drained and chopped**
- ½ **cup crumbled reduced-fat feta cheese**
- ¼ **cup sliced ripe olives**

1. Place the crust on an ungreased 12-in. pizza pan; spread with pesto. Top with the tomatoes, artichokes, cheese and olives.

2. Bake at 450° for 10-12 minutes or until heated through.

PER SERVING *2 pieces equals 206 cal., 8 g fat (3 g sat. fat), 6 mg chol., 547 mg sodium, 27 g carb., 4 g fiber, 10 g pro.* **Diabetic Exchanges:** *2 starch, 1½ fat.*

Halibut Steaks with Papaya Mint Salsa

Zesty salsa and smoky-flavored fish together make this dish a stunner!

—**SONYA LABBE** WEST HOLLYWOOD, CA

START TO FINISH: 20 MIN.
MAKES: 4 SERVINGS

1 medium papaya, peeled, seeded and chopped
¼ cup chopped red onion
¼ cup fresh mint leaves
1 teaspoon finely chopped chipotle pepper in adobo sauce
1 tablespoon olive oil
1 tablespoon honey
4 halibut steaks (6 ounces each)
1 tablespoon olive oil

1. In a small bowl, combine the papaya, onion, mint, chipotle pepper, oil and honey. Cover and refrigerate the salsa until serving.
2. In a large skillet, cook halibut in oil for 4-6 minutes on each side or until fish flakes easily with a fork. Serve with the salsa.
PER SERVING *300 cal., 11 g fat (2 g sat. fat), 54 mg chol., 105 mg sodium, 13 g carb., 2 g fiber, 36 g pro.* **Diabetic Exchanges:** *5 lean meat, 1 starch, 1 fat.*

HALIBUT STEAKS WITH PAPAYA MINT SALSA

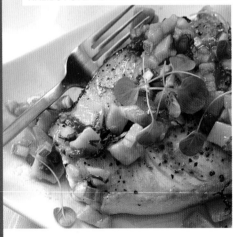

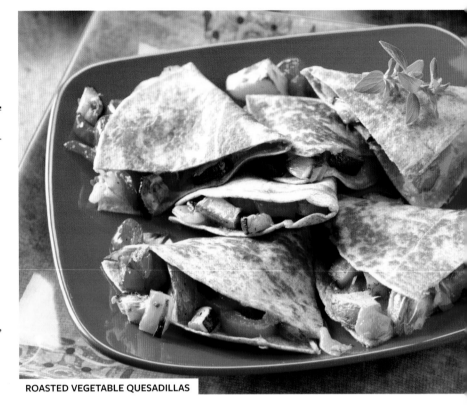

ROASTED VEGETABLE QUESADILLAS

Roasted Vegetable Quesadillas

You can change up the vegetables in this delightful recipe and use mushrooms, eggplant, asparagus and broccoli. Just remember to roast your vegetables before making the quesadillas. Find out what tastes best to you!

—**KATHY CARLAN** CANTON, GA

PREP: 40 MIN. • **COOK:** 5 MIN./BATCH
MAKES: 8 SERVINGS

2 medium red potatoes, quartered and sliced
1 medium zucchini, quartered and sliced
1 medium sweet red pepper, sliced
1 small onion, chopped
2 tablespoons olive oil
1 garlic clove, minced
½ teaspoon salt
½ teaspoon dried oregano
¼ teaspoon pepper
1 cup (4 ounces) shredded part-skim mozzarella cheese
1 cup (4 ounces) shredded reduced-fat cheddar cheese
8 whole wheat tortillas (8 inches)

1. In a large bowl, combine the first nine ingredients. Transfer to a 15-in. x 10-in. x 1-in. baking pan. Bake at 425° for 24-28 minutes or until the potatoes are tender.
2. In a small bowl, combine cheeses. Place tortillas on a griddle coated with cooking spray. Spread ⅓ cup vegetable mixture over half of each tortilla. Sprinkle with ¼ cup cheese. Fold over and cook over low heat for 1-2 minutes on each side or until cheese is melted.
PER SERVING *279 cal., 12 g fat (4 g sat. fat), 18 mg chol., 479 mg sodium, 30 g carb., 3 g fiber, 12 g pro.* **Diabetic Exchanges:** *2 starch, 1½ fat, 1 lean meat.*

Tofu Manicotti

To create a light main course, I took the best elements from a few favorite recipes, including my mom's lasagna. No one suspects that the creamy filling is actually made with tofu.

—CAROLYN DIANA SCOTTSDALE, AZ

PREP: 25 MIN. • **BAKE:** 50 MIN.
MAKES: 5 SERVINGS

- 2 cups meatless spaghetti sauce
- 1 can (14½ ounces) diced tomatoes, undrained
- ⅓ cup finely shredded zucchini
- ¼ cup finely shredded carrot
- ½ teaspoon Italian seasoning
- 1 package (12.3 ounces) silken firm tofu
- 1 cup (8 ounces) 1% cottage cheese
- 1 cup (4 ounces) shredded part-skim mozzarella cheese
- 1 tablespoon grated Parmesan cheese
- 10 uncooked manicotti shells

1. Combine spaghetti sauce, tomatoes, zucchini, carrot and Italian seasoning; spread ¾ cup into a 13-in. x 9-in. baking dish coated with cooking spray.
2. Combine the tofu and cheeses; stuff into uncooked manicotti shells. Place over spaghetti sauce; top with remaining sauce.
3. Cover and bake at 375° for 50-55 minutes or until noodles are tender. Let stand for 5 minutes before serving.
PER SERVING *319 cal., 7 g fat (3 g sat. fat), 16 mg chol., 885 mg sodium, 42 g carb., 4 g fiber, 23 g pro.* **Diabetic Exchanges:** *3 starch, 2 lean meat.*

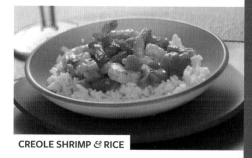

CREOLE SHRIMP & RICE

Creole Shrimp & Rice

Running out of time to make dinner? Turn to this simple weekday supper with lots of Creole flavor.

—ELSIE EPP NEWTON, KS

PREP: 25 MIN. • **COOK:** 20 MIN.
MAKES: 4 SERVINGS

- 1 celery rib, chopped
- 1 small onion, chopped
- 1 small green pepper, chopped
- 1 tablespoon canola oil
- 1 garlic clove, minced
- 1 can (14½ ounces) diced tomatoes, undrained
- 2 tablespoons savory herb with garlic soup mix
- 1 teaspoon Worcestershire sauce
- 1 bay leaf
- ⅛ teaspoon cayenne pepper
- 1 pound cooked medium shrimp, peeled and deveined
- 2 cups hot cooked rice

1. In a large skillet, saute the celery, onion and green pepper in oil until tender. Add garlic; cook 1 minute longer. Add the tomatoes, soup mix, Worcestershire sauce, bay leaf and cayenne. Bring to a boil. Reduce heat; cover and simmer for 15 minutes.
2. Add shrimp; heat through. Discard bay leaf. Serve with rice.
PER SERVING *304 cal., 6 g fat (1 g sat. fat), 172 mg chol., 622 mg sodium, 34 g carb., 3 g fiber, 27 g pro.* **Diabetic Exchanges:** *3 lean meat, 2 vegetable, 1½ starch.*

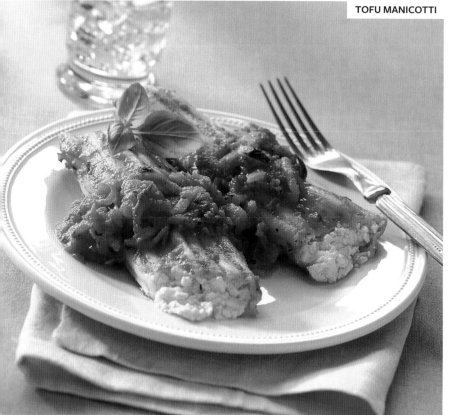

TOFU MANICOTTI

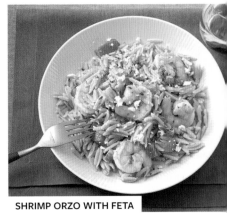

SHRIMP ORZO WITH FETA

Shrimp Orzo with Feta

Shrimp is good for you, and garlic and a splash of lemon add freshness to this seafood and pasta dish.

—**SARAH HUMMEL** MOON TOWNSHIP, PA

START TO FINISH: 25 MIN.
MAKES: 4 SERVINGS

- 1¼ cups uncooked whole wheat orzo pasta
- 2 garlic cloves, minced
- 2 tablespoons olive oil
- 2 medium tomatoes, chopped
- 2 tablespoons lemon juice
- 1¼ pounds uncooked large shrimp, peeled and deveined
- 2 tablespoons minced fresh cilantro
- ¼ teaspoon pepper
- ½ cup crumbled feta cheese

1. Cook orzo according to package directions. Meanwhile, in a large skillet, saute garlic in oil for 1 minute. Add tomatoes and lemon juice. Bring to a boil. Reduce heat; stir in shrimp. Simmer, uncovered, for 4-5 minutes or until shrimp turn pink.
2. Drain orzo. Add the orzo, cilantro and pepper to shrimp mixture; heat through. Sprinkle with feta cheese.
PER SERVING *406 cal., 12 g fat (3 g sat. fat), 180 mg chol., 307 mg sodium, 40 g carb., 9 g fiber, 33 g pro.* **Diabetic Exchanges:** *4 lean meat, 2 starch, 1 fat.*

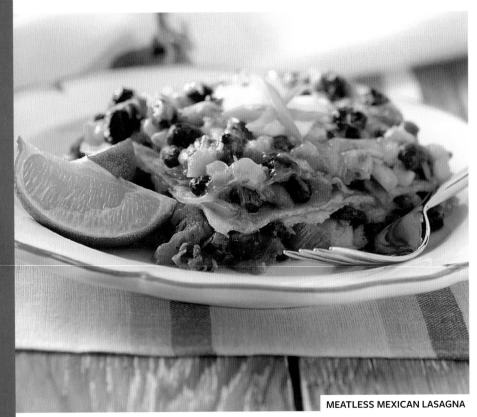

MEATLESS MEXICAN LASAGNA

Meatless Mexican Lasagna

Have fun assembling this quick twist on lasagna tonight. Instead of traditional lasagna noodles, layer corn tortillas between Mexican-style cheese and a Southwestern-style corn filling for a satisfying fiesta of a meal.

—**JEAN ECOS** HARTLAND, WI

PREP: 20 MIN. • **BAKE:** 15 MIN.
MAKES: 6 SERVINGS

- 2 cups frozen corn, thawed
- 1 can (15 ounces) black beans, rinsed and drained
- 1 can (14½ ounces) diced tomatoes with basil, oregano and garlic, undrained
- 1 can (4 ounces) chopped green chilies
- 3 green onions, sliced
- 2 teaspoons dried oregano
- 2 teaspoons ground cumin
- 4 corn tortillas (6 inches)
- 1½ cups (6 ounces) shredded Mexican cheese blend
- 6 tablespoons plain yogurt

1. In a large bowl, combine the first seven ingredients. Place two tortillas in an 11-in. x 7-in. baking dish coated with cooking spray. Spread with half of the corn mixture; sprinkle with half of the cheese. Repeat layers.
2. Bake, uncovered, at 400° for 15-20 minutes or until heated through. Let stand for 5 minutes. Garnish each serving with a dollop of yogurt.
PER SERVING *1 piece equals 291 cal., 11 g fat (6 g sat. fat), 25 mg chol., 781 mg sodium, 38 g carb., 6 g fiber, 14 g pro.* **Diabetic Exchanges:** *2 starch, 1 lean meat, 1 vegetable, 1 fat.*

Pan-Fried Scallops with White Wine Reduction

Don't let this recipe's fancy title scare you away! This special-occasion entree isn't at all difficult to prepare.

—KATHERINE ROBINSON
GLENWOOD SPRINGS, CO

START TO FINISH: 30 MIN.
MAKES: 8 SERVINGS

- 2 **pounds sea scallops**
- 1 **teaspoon salt**
- ¼ **teaspoon pepper**
- 2 **tablespoons olive oil**

WHITE WINE REDUCTION
- ½ **cup white wine or chicken broth**
- ⅓ **cup orange juice**
- ¼ **cup finely chopped onion**
- 1 **teaspoon dried oregano**
- 1 **teaspoon Dijon mustard**
- 1 **garlic clove, minced**
- 3 **tablespoons cold butter, cubed**

1. Sprinkle scallops with salt and pepper. In a large skillet, saute scallops in oil until firm and opaque. Remove and keep warm.

2. Add wine to the skillet, stirring to loosen browned bits from pan. Stir in the orange juice, onion, oregano, mustard and garlic. Bring to a boil; cook and stir for 2-3 minutes or until reduced by half. Remove from the heat; stir in butter until melted. Serve with scallops.

PER SERVING *4 scallops with 2 tablespoons sauce equals 181 cal., 9 g fat (3 g sat. fat), 49 mg chol., 524 mg sodium, 5 g carb., trace fiber, 19 g pro.* **Diabetic Exchanges:** *3 lean meat, 2 fat.*

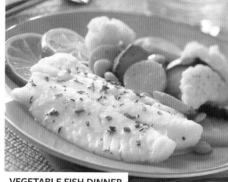

VEGETABLE FISH DINNER

Vegetable Fish Dinner

I use the microwave to cook this because it keeps the fish from drying out. It's also a healthier alternative to frying the fillets.

—PAULA MARCHESI LENHARTSVILLE, PA

START TO FINISH: 15 MIN.
MAKES: 2 SERVINGS

- 2 **orange roughy fillets (6 ounces each)**
- 2 **tablespoons minced chives**
- 2 **teaspoons minced fresh thyme**
- 1 **medium lime, thinly sliced**
- 3 **cups frozen Italian vegetables, thawed**
- 2 **teaspoons butter, melted**
- ¼ **teaspoon salt**
- ⅛ **teaspoon pepper**

1. Place fish fillets in an 8-in. square microwave-safe dish. Sprinkle with chives and thyme. Top with lime and vegetables. Drizzle with butter; sprinkle with salt and pepper.

2. Cover and microwave on high for 5-7 minutes or until fish flakes easily with a fork and the vegetables are heated through.

NOTE *This recipe was tested in a 1,100-watt microwave.*

PER SERVING *247 cal., 5 g fat (2 g sat. fat), 112 mg chol., 517 mg sodium, 16 g carb., 6 g fiber, 31 g pro.* **Diabetic Exchanges:** *5 lean meat, 2 vegetable, 1 fat.*

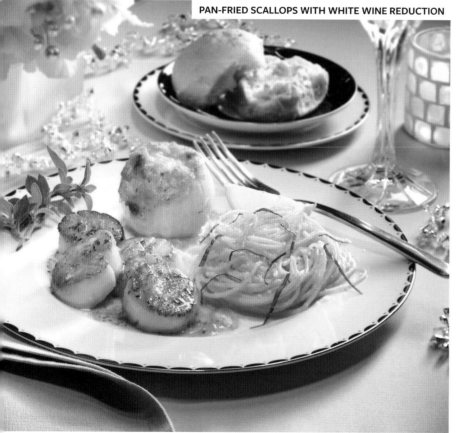

PAN-FRIED SCALLOPS WITH WHITE WINE REDUCTION

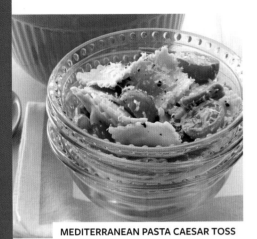

MEDITERRANEAN PASTA CAESAR TOSS

Mediterranean Pasta Caesar Toss

Get creative using convenience items for a fresh take on ravioli. Try this lightened-up pasta toss for an alfresco dinner, or double it for a family picnic.

—**LIBBY WALP** CHICAGO, IL

START TO FINISH: 30 MIN.
MAKES: 4 SERVINGS

- 1 **package (9 ounces) refrigerated cheese ravioli**
- 1 **cup frozen cut green beans, thawed**
- 1 **cup cherry tomatoes, halved**
- ¾ **teaspoon coarsely ground pepper**
- ⅓ **cup reduced-fat creamy Caesar salad dressing**
- 3 **tablespoons shredded Parmesan cheese**

1. In a large saucepan, cook ravioli according to package directions, adding beans during the last 3 minutes of cooking. Drain.
2. In a serving bowl, combine the ravioli mixture, tomatoes and pepper. Add dressing; toss to coat. Sprinkle with cheese.
PER SERVING *264 cal., 10 g fat (4 g sat. fat), 28 mg chol., 649 mg sodium, 31 g carb., 3 g fiber, 12 g pro.* **Diabetic Exchanges:** *1½ starch, 1 lean meat, 1 vegetable, 1 fat.*

Salmon with Lemon-Dill Butter

Fast and healthy, this recipe has it all. I recommend rounding out the meal with steamed sugar snap peas.

—**JENNIE RICHARDS** RIVERTON, UT

START TO FINISH: 15 MIN.
MAKES: 2 SERVINGS

- 2 **salmon fillets (4 ounces each)**
- 5 **teaspoons reduced-fat butter, melted**
- ¾ **teaspoon lemon juice**
- ½ **teaspoon grated lemon peel**
- ½ **teaspoon snipped fresh dill**

Place salmon skin side down on a broiler pan. Combine the butter, lemon juice, lemon peel and dill. Brush one-third of mixture over salmon. Broil 3-4 in. from the heat for 7-9 minutes or until fish flakes easily with a fork, basting occasionally with remaining butter mixture.

PER SERVING *219 cal., 15 g fat (5 g sat. fat), 69 mg chol., 136 mg sodium, 1 g carb., trace fiber, 19 g pro.* **Diabetic Exchanges:** *3 lean meat, 1½ fat.*
SESAME-ORANGE SALMON *Follow method as directed but combine the butter with 1½ tsp. reduced-sodium soy sauce, ¾ tsp. grated orange peel and ½ tsp. sesame seeds.* **Per Serving** *1 fillet equals 224 cal., 16 g fat (5 g sat. fat), 69 mg chol., 288 mg sodium, 1 g carb., trace fiber, 19 g pro.* **Diabetic Exchanges:** *3 lean meat, 1½ fat.*
SALMON WITH GARLIC ROSEMARY BUTTER *Follow method as directed but combine the butter with ¾ tsp. honey, 1 minced garlic clove and ¼ tsp. crushed dried rosemary.* **Per Serving** *1 fillet equals 229 cal., 15 g fat (5 g sat. fat), 69 mg chol., 136 mg sodium, 4 g carb., trace fiber, 19 g pro.* **Diabetic Exchanges:** *3 lean meat, 1½ fat.*
NOTE *This recipe was tested with Land O'Lakes light stick butter.*

SALMON WITH LEMON-DILL BUTTER

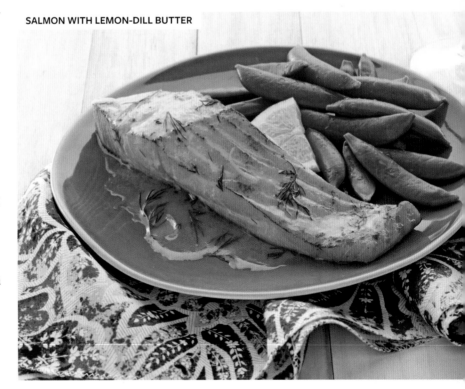

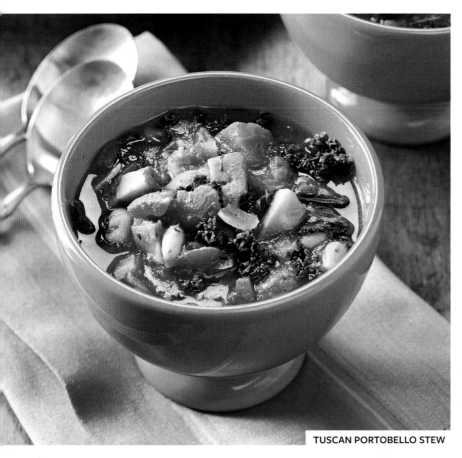

TUSCAN PORTOBELLO STEW

Baked Flounder

Since my husband is on a low-calorie diet, I fix this fish entree often. The flounder is baked on a bed of mushrooms and green onions, then topped with bread crumbs and reduced-fat cheese.

—**BRENDA TAYLOR** BENTON, KY

START TO FINISH: 20 MIN.
MAKES: 6 SERVINGS

- ⅔ **cup sliced green onions**
- ½ **cup sliced fresh mushrooms**
- 2 **pounds flounder or sole fillets**
- 1 **teaspoon dried marjoram**
- ½ **teaspoon salt**
- ⅛ **teaspoon pepper**
- 2 **tablespoons dry white wine or chicken broth**
- 2 **teaspoons lemon juice**
- ¼ **cup shredded reduced-fat Mexican cheese blend**
- ¼ **cup soft whole wheat bread crumbs**
- 2 **tablespoons butter, melted**

1. Sprinkle the green onions and mushrooms into a 13-in. x 9-in. baking dish coated with cooking spray. Arrange the fish over vegetables, overlapping the thickest end of fillets over the thin ends. Sprinkle with the marjoram, salt and pepper.

2. Pour wine and lemon juice over fish. Cover with cheese and bread crumbs; drizzle with butter. Bake, uncovered, at 400° for 10-12 minutes or until fish flakes easily with a fork.

PER SERVING *1 fillet equals 212 cal., 7 g fat (4 g sat. fat), 86 mg chol., 438 mg sodium, 5 g carb., 1 g fiber, 31 g pro.* ***Diabetic Exchanges:*** *4 lean meat, 1 fat.*

Tuscan Portobello Stew

Make this delicious stew all in one skillet— it's less cleanup for you later!

—**JANE SIEMON** VIROQUA, WI

PREP: 20 MIN. • **COOK:** 20 MIN.
MAKES: 4 SERVINGS

- 2 **large portobello mushrooms, coarsely chopped**
- 1 **medium onion, chopped**
- 3 **garlic cloves, minced**
- 2 **tablespoons olive oil**
- ½ **cup white wine or vegetable broth**
- 1 **can (28 ounces) diced tomatoes, undrained**
- 2 **cups chopped fresh kale**
- 1 **bay leaf**
- 1 **teaspoon dried thyme**
- ½ **teaspoon dried basil**
- ½ **teaspoon dried rosemary, crushed**
- ¼ **teaspoon salt**
- ¼ **teaspoon pepper**
- 2 **cans (15 ounces each) white kidney or cannellini beans, rinsed and drained**

1. In a large skillet, saute mushrooms, onion and garlic in oil until tender. Add the wine. Bring to a boil; cook until liquid is reduced by half. Stir in the tomatoes, kale and seasonings. Bring to a boil. Reduce heat; cover and simmer for 8-10 minutes.

2. Add beans; heat through. Discard the bay leaf.

PER SERVING *309 cal., 8 g fat (1 g sat. fat), 0 chol., 672 mg sodium, 46 g carb., 13 g fiber, 12 g pro.* ***Diabetic Exchanges:*** *2 starch, 2 vegetable, 1½ fat, 1 lean meat.*

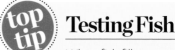

top tip

Testing Fish

When fish fillets are opaque and flake easily into sections with a fork, they're ready.

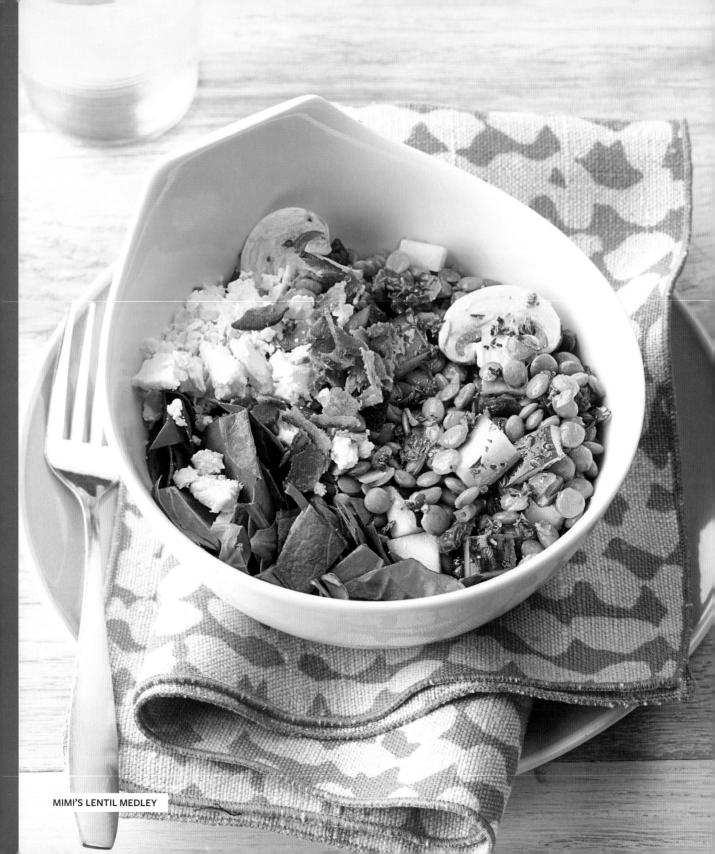

MIMI'S LENTIL MEDLEY

Mimi's Lentil Medley

I put this together one summer evening by using just what I had on hand. It earned my husband Ken's top rating—he said, "You can make this again soon."

—MARY ANN HAZEN ROCHESTER HILLS, MI

PREP: 10 MIN. • **COOK:** 30 MIN.
MAKES: 8 SERVINGS

- 1 cup dried lentils, rinsed
- 2 cups water
- 2 cups sliced fresh mushrooms
- 1 medium cucumber, cubed
- 1 medium zucchini, cubed
- 1 small red onion, chopped
- ½ cup chopped sun-dried tomatoes (not packed in oil)
- ½ cup rice vinegar
- ¼ cup minced fresh mint
- 3 tablespoons olive oil
- 2 teaspoons honey
- 1 teaspoon dried basil
- 1 teaspoon dried oregano
- 4 cups fresh baby spinach, chopped
- 1 cup (4 ounces) crumbled feta cheese
- 4 bacon strips, cooked and crumbled

1. In a small saucepan, bring lentils and water to a boil. Reduce heat; cover and simmer for 20-25 minutes or until tender. Drain and rinse in cold water.
2. Transfer to a large bowl. Add the mushrooms, cucumber, zucchini, onion and tomatoes. In a small bowl, whisk the vinegar, mint, oil, honey, basil and oregano. Drizzle over lentil mixture; toss to coat. Add the spinach, cheese and bacon; toss to combine.

PER SERVING *1¼ cups equals 226 cal., 9 g fat (3 g sat. fat), 11 mg chol., 299 mg sodium, 25 g carb., 10 g fiber, 12 g pro. **Diabetic Exchanges:** 2 fat, 1 starch, 1 vegetable.*

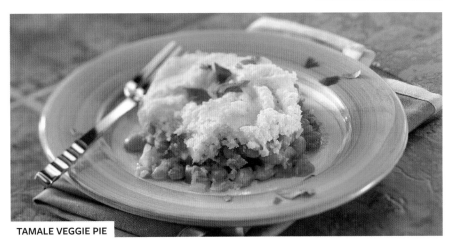
TAMALE VEGGIE PIE

Tamale Veggie Pie

Beans and veggies make up the filling, while a tender corn bread completes this pie. It's great served with a small garden salad.

—DEB PERRY BLUFFTON, IN

PREP: 25 MIN. • **BAKE:** 20 MIN.
MAKES: 6 SERVINGS

- 1 cup chopped onion
- 1 teaspoon canola oil
- 1 garlic clove, minced
- 1 can (14½ ounces) Mexican diced tomatoes
- 1 can (15 ounces) pinto beans, rinsed and drained
- 1 cup (4 ounces) shredded reduced-fat cheddar cheese
- 1 can (4 ounces) chopped green chilies
- 1 jalapeno pepper, seeded and chopped
- ¾ teaspoon ground cumin
- ¾ teaspoon chili powder

TOPPING

- ½ cup plus 1 tablespoon all-purpose flour
- ½ cup yellow cornmeal
- ½ teaspoon baking powder
- ¼ teaspoon baking soda
- ¼ teaspoon salt
- 1 egg
- ½ cup plain yogurt
- 2 teaspoons butter, melted

1. In a small nonstick skillet coated with cooking spray, cook onion in oil until tender. Add garlic; cook 1 minute longer. Transfer to a large bowl. Drain tomatoes, reserving 2 tablespoons juice; add tomatoes and juice to the onion mixture.
2. Stir in the beans, cheese, chilies, jalapeno, cumin and chili powder. Transfer to an 8-in. square baking dish coated with cooking spray.
3. For topping, in a small bowl, combine the flour, cornmeal, baking powder, baking soda and salt. Whisk together the egg, yogurt and butter; stir into dry ingredients just until moistened. Spoon over filling; gently spread to cover top.
4. Bake, uncovered, at 375° for 20-25 minutes or until filling is bubbly and a toothpick inserted into topping comes out clean.

NOTE *Wear disposable gloves when cutting hot peppers; the oils can burn skin. Avoid touching your face.*
PER SERVING *1 piece equals 280 cal., 8 g fat (4 g sat. fat), 55 mg chol., 746 mg sodium, 39 g carb., 6 g fiber, 13 g pro. **Diabetic Exchanges:** 2 starch, 1 lean meat, 1 vegetable, 1 fat.*

Curried Tofu with Rice

Replace meat with tofu in this hearty dish. It's packed with curry and cilantro, too, so you won't even miss the meat.

—CRYSTAL JO BRUNS ILIFF, CO

PREP: 15 MIN. • **COOK:** 20 MIN.
MAKES: 4 SERVINGS

- 1 **package (12.3 ounces) extra-firm tofu, drained and cubed**
- 1 **teaspoon seasoned salt**
- 1 **tablespoon canola oil**
- 1 **small onion, chopped**
- 3 **garlic cloves, minced**
- ½ **cup light coconut milk**
- ¼ **cup minced fresh cilantro**
- 1 **teaspoon curry powder**
- ¼ **teaspoon salt**
- ¼ **teaspoon pepper**
- 2 **cups cooked brown rice**

1. Sprinkle tofu with seasoned salt. In a large nonstick skillet coated with cooking spray, saute the tofu in oil until lightly browned. Remove and keep warm.

2. In the same skillet, saute onion and garlic for 1-2 minutes or until crisp-tender. Stir in the coconut milk, cilantro, curry, salt and pepper. Bring to a boil. Reduce heat; simmer, uncovered, for 4-5 minutes or until sauce is slightly thickened. Stir in tofu; heat through. Serve with rice.

PER SERVING *240 cal., 11 g fat (3 g sat. fat), 0 chol., 540 mg sodium, 27 g carb., 3 g fiber, 10 g pro.* **Diabetic Exchanges:** *1½ starch, 1 medium-fat meat, 1 fat.*

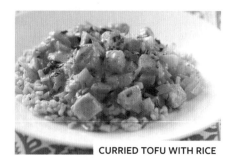

CURRIED TOFU WITH RICE

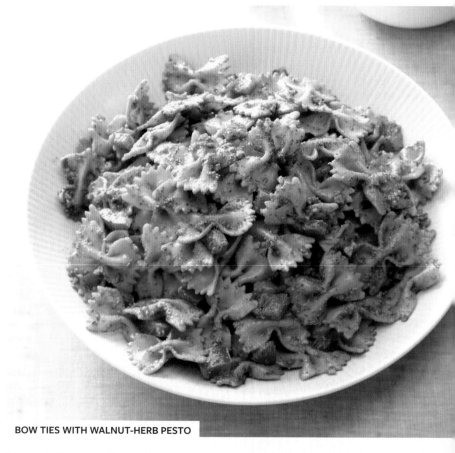

BOW TIES WITH WALNUT-HERB PESTO

Bow Ties with Walnut-Herb Pesto

I can't resist having pasta at least once a week, but I don't want or need all the fat and extra calories. So I created this dish, and now I can sometimes even have second helpings!

—DIANE NEMITZ LUDINGTON, MI

START TO FINISH: 20 MIN.
MAKES: 6 SERVINGS

- 4 **cups uncooked whole wheat bow tie pasta**
- 1 **cup fresh arugula**
- ½ **cup packed fresh parsley sprigs**
- ½ **cup loosely packed basil leaves**
- ¼ **cup grated Parmesan cheese**
- ½ **teaspoon salt**
- ⅛ **teaspoon crushed red pepper flakes**
- ¼ **cup chopped walnuts**
- ⅓ **cup olive oil**
- 1 **plum tomato, seeded and chopped**

1. Cook pasta according to package directions.

2. Meanwhile, place the arugula, parsley, basil, cheese, salt and pepper flakes in a food processor; cover and pulse until chopped. Add walnuts; cover and process until blended. While processing, gradually add the oil in a steady stream.

3. Drain the pasta, reserving 3 tablespoons cooking water. In a large bowl, toss pasta with pesto, tomato and reserved water.

PER SERVING *1 cup equals 323 cal., 17 g fat (3 g sat. fat), 3 mg chol., 252 mg sodium, 34 g carb., 6 g fiber, 10 g pro.* **Diabetic Exchanges:** *2½ fat, 2 starch.*

Feta Shrimp Skillet

A Mediterranean blend of feta, wine, garlic and oregano seasons this bold, beautiful dish. Soak up the sauce with a slice of thick, crusty bread.

—**SONALI RUDER** NEW YORK, NY

START TO FINISH: 30 MIN.
MAKES: 4 SERVINGS

- 1 tablespoon olive oil
- 1 medium onion, finely chopped
- 3 garlic cloves, minced
- 1 teaspoon dried oregano
- ½ teaspoon pepper
- ¼ teaspoon salt
- 2 cans (14½ ounces each) diced tomatoes, undrained
- ¼ cup white wine, optional
- 1 pound uncooked medium shrimp, peeled and deveined
- 2 tablespoons minced fresh parsley
- ¾ cup crumbled feta cheese

1. In a large nonstick skillet, heat oil over medium-high heat. Add onion; cook and stir 4-6 minutes or until tender. Add garlic and seasonings; cook 1 minute longer. Stir in tomatoes and, if desired, wine. Bring to a boil. Reduce heat; simmer, uncovered, 5-7 minutes or until sauce is slightly thickened.
2. Add shrimp and parsley; cook 5-6 minutes or until shrimp turn pink, stirring occasionally. Remove from heat; sprinkle with cheese. Let stand, covered, until cheese is softened.
PER SERVING *240 cal., 8 g fat (3 g sat. fat), 149 mg chol., 748 mg sodium, 16 g carb., 5 g fiber, 25 g pro.* **Diabetic Exchanges:** *3 lean meat, 1 starch, 1 fat.*

Baked Cod with Mushrooms

I created this recipe when I was on a low-carb diet. Use a bit less jalapeno if you're not a big fan of its heat.

—**KIM THOMAS** MONAHANS, TX

START TO FINISH: 30 MIN.
MAKES: 2 SERVINGS

- 5 small fresh mushrooms, sliced
- 1 jalapeno pepper, seeded and finely chopped
- 2 tablespoons chopped onion
- 3 teaspoons butter, divided
- 2 cod fillets (4 ounces each)
- ½ teaspoon lemon-pepper seasoning
- ½ teaspoon steak seasoning
- 1 tablespoon dry bread crumbs
- ¼ cup shredded reduced-fat cheddar cheese

1. In a large skillet, saute the mushrooms, jalapeno and onion in 2 teaspoons butter until tender. Place fillets in an ungreased 8-in. square baking dish. Sprinkle with lemon-pepper, steak seasoning and bread crumbs. Top with mushroom mixture. Divide remaining butter and place on each fillet.
2. Cover and bake at 400° for 10 minutes. Uncover; sprinkle with cheese. Bake 5-8 minutes longer or until fish flakes easily with a fork.
NOTES *This recipe was tested with McCormick's Montreal Steak Seasoning. Look for it in the spice aisle. Wear disposable gloves when cutting hot peppers; the oils can burn skin. Avoid touching your face.*
PER SERVING *199 cal., 10 g fat (6 g sat. fat), 68 mg chol., 503 mg sodium, 5 g carb., 1 g fiber, 23 g pro.* **Diabetic Exchanges:** *3 lean meat, 2 fat.*

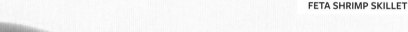

FETA SHRIMP SKILLET

Curried Halibut Skillet

I've been experimenting with coconut in main dishes recently. This was definitely a successful attempt.

—**KAREN KUEBLER** DALLAS, TX

START TO FINISH: 25 MIN.
MAKES: 4 SERVINGS

- 4 **halibut fillets (4 ounces each)**
- ½ **teaspoon salt**
- 4 **teaspoons curry powder**
- 2 **tablespoons olive oil, divided**
- 1 **large sweet onion, chopped**
- 1 **can (14½ ounces) diced tomatoes, undrained**
- 2 **tablespoons lime juice**
- 1½ **teaspoons grated lime peel**
- 1 **teaspoon minced fresh gingerroot**
- ¼ **cup flaked coconut, toasted**
- ¼ **cup minced fresh cilantro**

1. Sprinkle fillets with salt; coat with curry. In a large nonstick skillet coated with cooking spray, brown fillets in 1 tablespoon oil; remove and set aside.

2. In the same pan, saute onion in remaining oil for 1 minute. Stir in the tomatoes, lime juice, lime peel and ginger. Bring to a boil. Return fillets to the pan; cover and simmer for 10-12 minutes or until fish flakes easily with a fork. Serve with tomato mixture; sprinkle with coconut and cilantro.

PER SERVING *270 cal., 12 g fat (3 g sat. fat), 36 mg chol., 510 mg sodium, 16 g carb., 3 g fiber, 26 g pro.* **Diabetic Exchanges:** *3 lean meat, 2 vegetable, 1½ fat.*

top tip

The Best Fish

When buying fresh fish, search for fillets that don't smell too strongly or look discolored. Store fresh fish in the refrigerator for no more than two days.

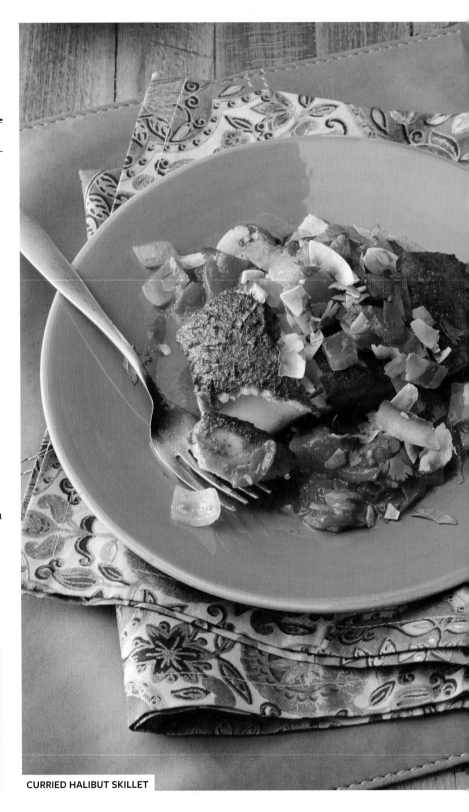

CURRIED HALIBUT SKILLET

Slow-Cooked Stuffed Peppers

Fix stuffed peppers without worrying about parboiling! Packed with Southwest flavor, these also come with 8 grams of fiber per serving. You can't go wrong with this meal!

—**MICHELLE GURNSEY** LINCOLN, NE

PREP: 15 MIN. • **COOK:** 3 HOURS
MAKES: 4 SERVINGS

- 4 medium sweet red peppers
- 1 can (15 ounces) black beans, rinsed and drained
- 1 cup (4 ounces) shredded pepper jack cheese
- ¾ cup salsa
- 1 small onion, chopped
- ½ cup frozen corn
- ⅓ cup uncooked converted long grain rice
- 1¼ teaspoons chili powder
- ½ teaspoon ground cumin
    Reduced-fat sour cream, optional

1. Cut and discard tops from peppers; remove seeds. In a large bowl, mix beans, cheese, salsa, onion, corn, rice, chili powder and cumin; spoon into peppers. Place in a 5-qt. slow cooker coated with cooking spray.

2. Cook, covered, on low 3-4 hours or until peppers are tender and filling is heated through. If desired, serve with sour cream.

PER SERVING *317 cal., 10 g fat (5 g sat. fat), 30 mg chol., 565 mg sodium, 43 g carb., 8 g fiber, 15 g pro.* **Diabetic Exchanges:** *2 starch, 2 lean meat, 2 vegetable, 1 fat.*

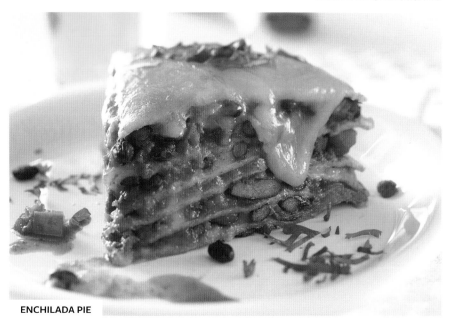

ENCHILADA PIE

Enchilada Pie

Layer it up! This meatless pie will have you satisfied in no time.

—**JACQUELINE CORREA** LANDING, NJ

PREP: 40 MIN. • **COOK:** 4 HOURS
MAKES: 8 SERVINGS

- 1 package (12 ounces) frozen vegetarian meat crumbles
- 1 cup chopped onion
- ½ cup chopped green pepper
- 2 teaspoons canola oil
- 1 can (16 ounces) kidney beans, rinsed and drained
- 1 can (15 ounces) black beans, rinsed and drained
- 1 can (10 ounces) diced tomatoes and green chilies, undrained
- ½ cup water
- 1½ teaspoons chili powder
- ½ teaspoon ground cumin
- ¼ teaspoon pepper
- 6 whole wheat tortillas (8 inches)
- 2 cups (8 ounces) shredded reduced-fat cheddar cheese

1. Cut three 25-in. x 3-in. strips of heavy-duty foil; crisscross so they resemble spokes of a wheel. Place strips on the bottom and up the sides of a 5-qt. slow cooker. Coat the strips with cooking spray.

2. In a large saucepan, cook the meat crumbles, onion and green pepper in oil until vegetables are tender. Stir in both cans of beans, tomatoes, water, chili powder, cumin and pepper. Bring to a boil. Reduce heat; simmer, uncovered, for 10 minutes.

3. In the prepared slow cooker, layer one tortilla, about a cup of bean mixture and ⅓ cup cheese. Repeat layers five times. Cover and cook on low for 4-5 hours or until heated through and cheese is melted.

4. Using foil strips as handles, remove the pie to a platter.

NOTE *Vegetarian meat crumbles are a nutritious protein source made from soy. Look for them in the natural foods freezer section.*

PER SERVING *1 piece equals 367 cal., 11 g fat (4 g sat. fat), 20 mg chol., 818 mg sodium, 41 g carb., 9 g fiber, 25 g pro.* **Diabetic Exchanges:** *3 starch, 2 lean meat, 1 fat.*

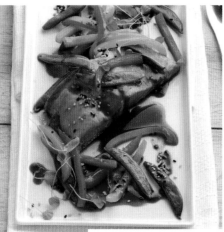

GRILLED SALMON PACKETS

Grilled Salmon Packets

I generally don't like plain salmon, but this offers a stir-fry taste without all the fuss. I love it!

—**MIKE MILLER** CRESTON, IA

START TO FINISH: 25 MIN.
MAKES: 4 SERVINGS

- 4 salmon fillets (6 ounces each)
- 3 cups fresh sugar snap peas
- 1 small sweet red pepper, cut into strips
- 1 small sweet yellow pepper, cut into strips
- ¼ cup reduced-fat Asian toasted sesame salad dressing

1. Place each salmon fillet on a double thickness of heavy-duty foil (about 12 in. square). Combine sugar snap peas and peppers; spoon over salmon. Drizzle with salad dressing. Fold foil around mixture and seal tightly.
2. Grill, covered, over medium heat for 15-20 minutes or until fish flakes easily with a fork. Open foil carefully to allow steam to escape.
PER SERVING *350 cal., 17 g fat (3 g sat. fat), 85 mg chol., 237 mg sodium, 14 g carb., 4 g fiber, 34 g pro.* **Diabetic Exchanges:** *4 lean meat, 2 vegetable, 2 fat.*

Snapper with Zucchini & Mushrooms

Get your veggies in for the day while savoring some red snapper. Colorful tomatoes, mushrooms and zucchini make a surprising topping for the fish. You can serve these veggies with pork, too.

—**LISA GLOGOW** ALISO VIEJO, CA

PREP: 25 MIN. • **COOK:** 10 MIN.
MAKES: 4 SERVINGS

- 3 cups diced zucchini
- 2 cups halved fresh mushrooms
- ¾ cup chopped sweet onion
- 2 tablespoons olive oil, divided
- 3 garlic cloves, minced
- 1 can (14½ ounces) diced tomatoes, undrained
- 2 teaspoons minced fresh basil or ½ teaspoon dried basil
- 2 teaspoons minced fresh oregano or ½ teaspoon dried oregano
- ¼ teaspoon salt
- ¼ teaspoon pepper
- ¼ teaspoon crushed red pepper flakes, optional
- 4 red snapper or orange roughy fillets (6 ounces each)

1. In a large nonstick skillet coated with cooking spray, saute the zucchini, mushrooms and onion in 1 tablespoon oil until crisp-tender. Add garlic; cook 1 minute longer. Stir in the tomatoes, basil, oregano, salt, pepper and pepper flakes if desired. Bring to a boil. Reduce heat; cover and simmer for 12-15 minutes or until vegetables are tender.
2. Meanwhile, in another large nonstick skillet coated with cooking spray, cook fillets in remaining oil over medium heat for 4-6 minutes on each side or until fish flakes easily with a fork. Serve with vegetable mixture.
PER SERVING *253 cal., 8 g fat (1 g sat. fat), 102 mg chol., 414 mg sodium, 14 g carb., 4 g fiber, 32 g pro.* **Diabetic Exchanges:** *4 lean meat, 2 vegetable, 1½ fat.*

SNAPPER WITH ZUCCHINI & MUSHROOMS

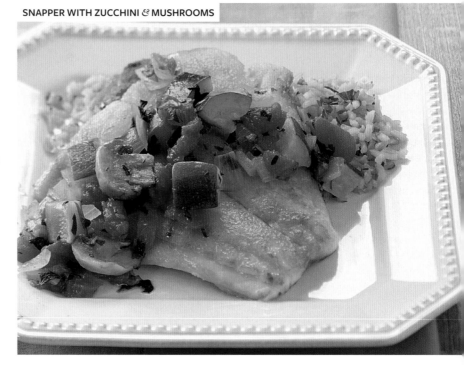

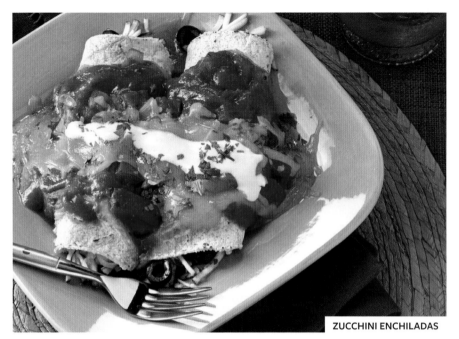

ZUCCHINI ENCHILADAS

Zucchini Enchiladas

When my garden is bursting with zucchini, I rely on this recipe to make the most of it.

—ANGELA LEINENBACH MECHANICSVILLE, VA

PREP: 1½ HOURS • **BAKE:** 30 MIN.
MAKES: 12 SERVINGS

- 1 **medium sweet yellow pepper, chopped**
- 1 **medium green pepper, chopped**
- 1 **large sweet onion, chopped**
- 2 **tablespoons olive oil**
- 2 **garlic cloves, minced**
- 2 **cans (15 ounces each) tomato sauce**
- 2 **cans (14½ ounces each) no-salt-added diced tomatoes, undrained**
- 2 **tablespoons chili powder**
- 2 **teaspoons sugar**
- 2 **teaspoons dried marjoram**
- 1 **teaspoon dried basil**
- 1 **teaspoon ground cumin**
- ¼ **teaspoon salt**
- ¼ **teaspoon cayenne pepper**
- 1 **bay leaf**
- 3 **pounds zucchini, shredded (about 8 cups)**
- 24 **corn tortillas (6 inches), warmed**
- 4 **cups (16 ounces) shredded reduced-fat cheddar cheese**
- 2 **cans (2¼ ounces each) sliced ripe olives, drained**
- ½ **cup minced fresh cilantro Reduced-fat sour cream, optional**

1. In a large saucepan, saute peppers and onion in oil until tender. Add garlic; cook 1 minute longer. Stir in the tomato sauce, tomatoes, chili powder, sugar, marjoram, basil, cumin, salt, cayenne and bay leaf. Bring to a boil. Reduce heat; simmer, uncovered, for 30-35 minutes or until slightly thickened. Discard bay leaf.

2. Place ⅓ cup zucchini down the center of each tortilla; top with 2 tablespoons cheese and 1 tablespoon olives. Roll up and place seam side down in two 13-in. x 9-in. baking dishes coated with cooking spray. Pour sauce over the top; sprinkle with remaining cheese.

3. Bake, uncovered, at 350° for 30-35 minutes or until heated through. Sprinkle with cilantro. Serve with sour cream if desired.

PER SERVING *2 enchiladas (calculated without sour cream) equals 326 cal., 13 g fat (6 g sat. fat), 27 mg chol., 846 mg sodium, 42 g carb., 7 g fiber, 16 g pro.* **Diabetic Exchanges:** *2 starch, 2 medium-fat meat, 2 vegetable, ½ fat.*

Shrimp Quesadillas

Switch up your normal quesadilla ingredients with this recipe.

—TIFFANY BRYSON SAN ANTONIO, TX

START TO FINISH: 30 MIN.
MAKES: 2 SERVINGS

- ¼ **cup chopped onion**
- 1 **tablespoon finely chopped jalapeno pepper**
- ½ **pound uncooked shrimp, peeled, deveined and chopped**
- ¼ **teaspoon ground cumin**
- ⅛ **teaspoon pepper**
- ¼ **cup chopped tomato**
- 4 **flour tortillas (6 inches)**
- ⅓ **cup shredded reduced-fat Mexican cheese blend**

1. In a large nonstick skillet coated with cooking spray, cook and stir onion and jalapeno until tender. Add the shrimp, cumin and pepper; cook and stir until shrimp turn pink. Transfer to a small bowl; stir in tomato.

2. Coat the same skillet with cooking spray; add one tortilla. Top with half the cheese, half the shrimp mixture and one tortilla. Cook over medium heat for 2-3 minutes on each side or until lightly browned; remove. Repeat with remaining tortillas, cheese and shrimp mixture, spraying pan as needed. Cut into wedges.

NOTE *Wear disposable gloves when cutting hot peppers; the oils can burn skin. Avoid touching your face.*

PER SERVING *333 cal., 11 g fat (2 g sat. fat), 181 mg chol., 777 mg sodium, 30 g carb., 1 g fiber, 30 g pro.* **Diabetic Exchanges:** *3 lean meat, 2 starch.*

Shrimp 'n' Noodle Bowls

It'll look like you got takeout, but surprise! This dish comes right out of your kitchen. Precooked shrimp, bagged slaw and bottled dressing reduce the prep time.

—MARY BERGFELD EUGENE, OR

START TO FINISH: 25 MIN.
MAKES: 6 SERVINGS

- 8 **ounces uncooked angel hair pasta**
- 1 **pound cooked small shrimp**
- 2 **cups broccoli coleslaw mix**
- 6 **green onions, thinly sliced**
- ½ **cup minced fresh cilantro**
- ⅔ **cup reduced-fat sesame ginger salad dressing**

Cook pasta according to package directions; drain and rinse in cold water. Transfer to a large bowl. Add the shrimp, coleslaw mix, onions and cilantro. Drizzle with dressing; toss to coat. Cover and refrigerate until serving.

PER SERVING *1⅓ cups equals 260 cal., 3 g fat (trace sat. fat), 147 mg chol., 523 mg sodium, 36 g carb., 2 g fiber, 22 g pro.* **Diabetic Exchanges:** *2 starch, 2 lean meat, 1 vegetable.*

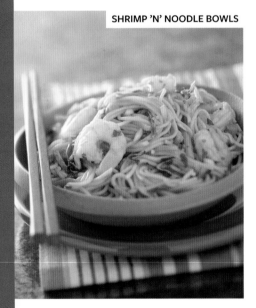

SHRIMP 'N' NOODLE BOWLS

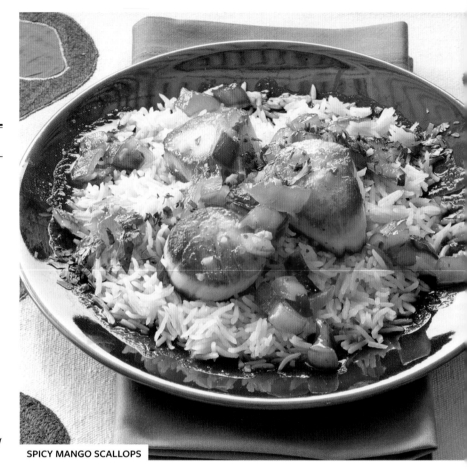

SPICY MANGO SCALLOPS

Spicy Mango Scallops

Warm up your whole family with this spicy-sweet dish! Be sure to buy the larger sea scallops; the cooking times would be off if you used the smaller bay scallops.

—NICOLE FILIZETTI JACKSONVILLE, FL

START TO FINISH: 30 MIN.
MAKES: 4 SERVINGS

- 12 **sea scallops (1½ pounds)**
- 1 **tablespoon peanut oil**
- 1 **medium red onion, chopped**
- 1 **garlic clove, minced**
- ¼ **to ½ teaspoon crushed red pepper flakes**
- ½ **cup unsweetened pineapple juice**
- ¼ **cup mango chutney**
- 2 **cups hot cooked basmati rice**
  Minced fresh cilantro

1. In a large skillet, saute scallops in oil for 1½ to 2 minutes on each side or until firm and opaque. Remove and keep warm.

2. In the same skillet, saute onion until tender. Add garlic and pepper flakes; cook 1 minute longer. Stir in pineapple juice. Bring to a boil; cook until liquid is reduced by half. Remove from the heat. Add chutney and scallops; stir to coat. Serve with rice; drizzle with sauce. Sprinkle with cilantro.

PER SERVING *371 cal., 5 g fat (1 g sat. fat), 56 mg chol., 447 mg sodium, 47 g carb., 1 g fiber, 31 g pro.* **Diabetic Exchanges:** *4 lean meat, 3 starch, ½ fat.*

Taco Salad with a Twist

Beans, veggies and a mouthwatering Southwest flavor give you a taco salad you'll want to serve again and again.

—HEATHER CARROLL

COLORADO SPRINGS, CO

START TO FINISH: 25 MIN.
MAKES: 4 SERVINGS

- 1 **package (5 ounces) spring mix salad greens**
- 1 **large tomato, seeded and chopped**
- 1 **large red onion, chopped**
- 1 **medium ripe avocado, peeled and chopped**
- 1 **cup canned black beans, rinsed and drained**
- 4 **green onions, chopped**
- ½ **cup shredded reduced-fat cheddar cheese**
- ½ **cup minced fresh cilantro**

DRESSING

- ½ **cup salsa verde**
- ½ **cup fat-free plain Greek yogurt**
- 2 **tablespoons minced fresh cilantro**
- 1 **tablespoon thinly sliced green onion**
- 1 **tablespoon lemon juice**
- 1 **tablespoon white wine vinegar**
- 1 **tablespoon olive oil**
- 1½ **teaspoons honey**
- ⅛ **teaspoon pepper**

In a large bowl, combine the first eight ingredients. In a small bowl, whisk the remaining ingredients. Pour over the salad mixture; toss to coat. Serve immediately.

PER SERVING *277 cal., 14 g fat (3 g sat. fat), 10 mg chol., 439 mg sodium, 29 g carb., 10 g fiber, 14 g pro.* **Diabetic Exchanges:** *2 lean meat, 2 vegetable, 1½ fat, 1 starch.*

Lactose-Free Spinach Lasagna

If you think you don't like tofu, you simply must give it a try in this lasagna.

—PEGGY KERN RIVERSIDE, CA

PREP: 45 MIN. • **BAKE:** 35 MIN. + STANDING
MAKES: 12 SERVINGS

- 1¾ **cups sliced fresh mushrooms**
- ¼ **cup chopped onion**
- 1 **tablespoon olive oil**
- 1 **package (10 ounces) frozen chopped spinach, thawed and squeezed dry**
- 2 **garlic cloves, minced**
- 2 **cans (14½ ounces each) diced tomatoes, undrained**
- 1 **can (8 ounces) tomato sauce**
- 1 **can (6 ounces) tomato paste**
- 2 **tablespoons minced fresh basil or 2 teaspoons dried basil**
- 1 **teaspoon dried marjoram**
- 9 **uncooked lasagna noodles**
- 1 **package (14 ounces) firm tofu, drained and cubed**
- 2 **eggs, lightly beaten**
- 2 **tablespoons dried parsley flakes**
- ½ **teaspoon salt**
- ¼ **teaspoon pepper**
- 1½ **cups (6 ounces) shredded mozzarella-flavored soy cheese**
- 1 **cup (4 ounces) shredded cheddar-flavored soy cheese**

1. In a large nonstick skillet coated with cooking spray, saute mushrooms and onion in oil until tender. Add spinach and garlic; cook 2 minutes longer. Stir in the tomatoes, tomato sauce, tomato paste, basil and marjoram. Bring to a boil. Reduce heat; cover and simmer for 15 minutes, stirring occasionally.

2. Meanwhile, cook lasagna noodles according to package directions; drain.

3. In a small bowl, combine the tofu, eggs, parsley, salt and pepper. Place three noodles in the bottom of a 13-in. x 9-in. baking dish coated with cooking spray. Layer with half of the tofu mixture, 1½ cups spinach mixture, ½ cup mozzarella-flavored soy cheese and ⅓ cup cheddar-flavored soy cheese. Repeat layers. Top with remaining the noodles and spinach mixture; sprinkle with the remaining cheeses.

4. Cover and bake at 375° for 35-40 minutes or until heated through. Let stand for 10 minutes before cutting.

PER SERVING *1 piece equals 216 cal., 7 g fat (1 g sat. fat), 35 mg chol., 531 mg sodium, 24 g carb., 3 g fiber, 14 g pro.* **Diabetic Exchanges:** *2 vegetable, 1 medium-fat meat, 1 starch.*

LACTOSE-FREE SPINACH LASAGNA

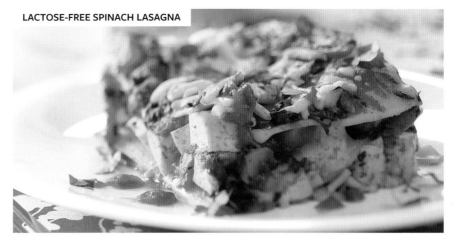

Egg Foo Yong

Forget ordering Chinese food—make it yourself! Throw together this easy version of an Asian classic in a half-hour.

—SHERRI MELOTIK OAK CREEK, WI

START TO FINISH: 30 MIN.
MAKES: 4 SERVINGS

- 1 can (14 ounces) chop suey vegetables, drained
- ½ pound peeled and deveined cooked small shrimp, coarsely chopped
- 4 green onions, thinly sliced
- 4 eggs, beaten
- 2 tablespoons canola oil

GREEN PEA SAUCE

- 2 tablespoons cornstarch
- 1 teaspoon chicken bouillon granules
- 2 cups water
- 1½ teaspoons reduced-sodium soy sauce
- ½ cup frozen peas, thawed

1. In a large bowl, combine the chop suey vegetables, shrimp and green onions. Stir in eggs. In a large nonstick skillet, heat 1 teaspoon oil. Drop the vegetable mixture by ¼ cupfuls into the skillet. Cook in batches until browned on both sides, using remaining oil as needed.

2. In a small saucepan, combine cornstarch and bouillon. Gradually stir in water and soy sauce. Bring to a boil; cook and stir for 2 minutes or until thickened. Stir in peas; heat through. Serve with egg foo yong.

PER SERVING *242 cal., 13 g fat (2 g sat. fat), 298 mg chol., 497 mg sodium, 10 g carb., 2 g fiber, 20 g pro.* **Diabetic Exchanges:** *3 lean meat, 1½ fat, ½ starch.*

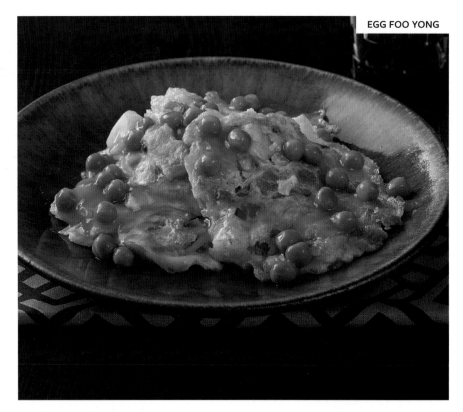

EGG FOO YONG

Crusty Red Snapper

Baking this fish on top of the veggies saves you so much time! The fillets will come out very moist, too.

—KELLY REMINGTON ARCATA, CA

PREP: 25 MIN. • **BAKE:** 20 MIN.
MAKES: 6 SERVINGS

- 2 medium tomatoes, chopped
- 1 each medium green, sweet yellow and red pepper, chopped
- 1 cup chopped leeks (white portion only)
- ½ cup chopped celery leaves
- 2 garlic cloves, minced
- 6 red snapper fillets (4 ounces each)

TOPPING

- ½ cup panko (Japanese) bread crumbs
- ½ cup coarsely crushed baked Parmesan and Tuscan herb potato chips
- ¼ cup grated Parmesan cheese
- ½ teaspoon salt
- ½ teaspoon paprika
- ¼ teaspoon cayenne pepper
- ¼ teaspoon pepper
- 2 tablespoons butter, melted

1. In a 15x10x1-in. baking pan coated with cooking spray, combine the tomatoes, peppers, leeks, celery leaves and garlic; arrange fillets over the vegetable mixture.

2. In a small bowl, combine the bread crumbs, chips, cheese, salt, paprika, cayenne and pepper; stir in butter. Sprinkle over fillets. Bake, uncovered, at 425° for 18-22 minutes or until fish flakes easily with a fork.

PER SERVING *237 cal., 7 g fat (3 g sat. fat), 53 mg chol., 396 mg sodium, 16 g carb., 3 g fiber, 26 g pro.* **Diabetic Exchanges:** *3 lean meat, 1 vegetable, 1 fat, ½ starch.*

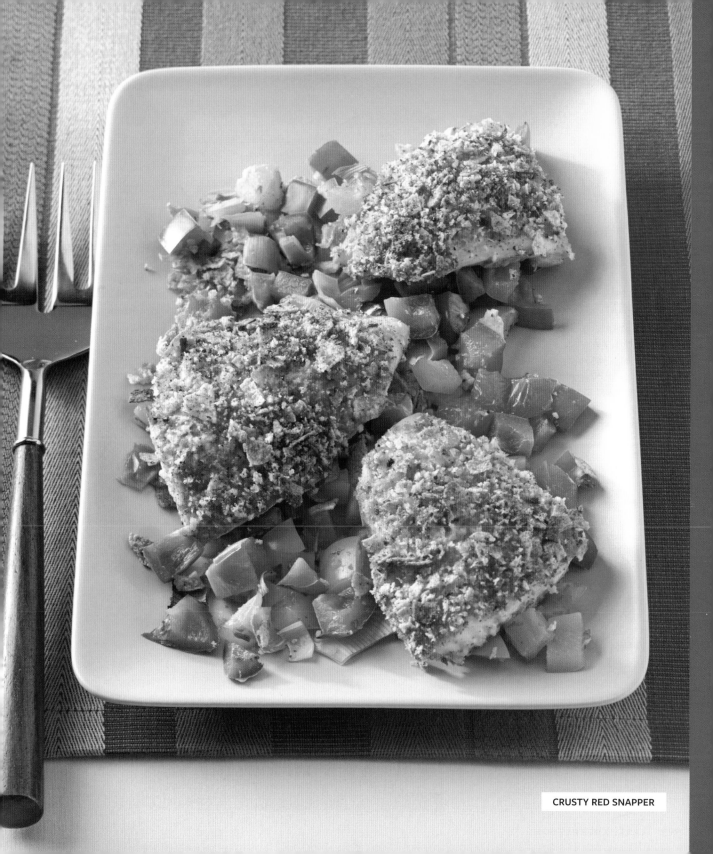

CRUSTY RED SNAPPER

Mediterranean Shrimp and Linguine

This dish is lower in fat but looks like it came from an Italian restaurant. You can make it ahead and reheat later for convenience.

—**NANCY DEANS** ACTON, ME

START TO FINISH: 30 MIN.
MAKES: 6 SERVINGS

- 9 **ounces uncooked linguine**
- 2 **tablespoons olive oil**
- 1 **cup sliced fresh mushrooms**
- 1 **pound uncooked medium shrimp, peeled and deveined**
- 3 **medium tomatoes, chopped**
- 1 **can (14 ounces) water-packed artichoke hearts, rinsed, drained and halved**
- 1 **can (6 ounces) pitted ripe olives, drained and halved**
- 2 **garlic cloves, minced**
- 1 **teaspoon dried oregano**
- ½ **teaspoon salt**
- ½ **teaspoon dried basil**
- ⅛ **teaspoon pepper**

1. Cook linguine according to package directions. Meanwhile, in a large skillet, heat oil over medium-high heat. Add mushrooms; cook and stir 4 minutes. Add remaining ingredients; cook and stir 5 minutes or until heated through and shrimp turn pink.

2. Drain linguine; serve with shrimp mixture.

PER SERVING *1 cup shrimp mixture with ¾ cup linguine equals 328 cal., 9 g fat (1 g sat. fat), 112 mg chol., 748 mg sodium, 41 g carb., 3 g fiber, 21 g pro. **Diabetic Exchanges:** 2 starch, 2 lean meat, 1½ fat, 1 vegetable.*

MEDITERRANEAN SHRIMP AND LINGUINE

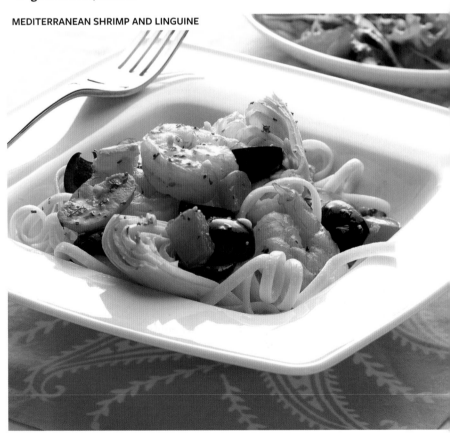

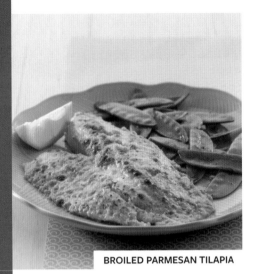

BROILED PARMESAN TILAPIA

Broiled Parmesan Tilapia

Even picky eaters will find a way to love fish when you plate up this toasty, cheesy dish. I serve it with mashed cauliflower and a green salad for a low-carb meal that everyone can enjoy.

—**TRISHA KRUSE** EAGLE, ID

START TO FINISH: 20 MIN.
MAKES: 6 SERVINGS

- 6 **tilapia fillets (6 ounces each)**
- ¼ **cup grated Parmesan cheese**
- ¼ **cup reduced-fat mayonnaise**
- 2 **tablespoons lemon juice**
- 1 **tablespoon butter, softened**
- 1 **garlic clove, minced**
- 1 **teaspoon minced fresh basil or ¼ teaspoon dried basil**
- ½ **teaspoon seafood seasoning**

1. Place fillets on a broiler pan coated with cooking spray. In a small bowl, combine the remaining ingredients; spread over fillets.

2. Broil 3-4 in. from the heat for 10-12 minutes or until the fish flakes easily with a fork.

PER SERVING *207 cal., 8 g fat (3 g sat. fat), 94 mg chol., 260 mg sodium, 2 g carb., trace fiber, 33 g pro. **Diabetic Exchanges:** 5 lean meat, 1 fat.*

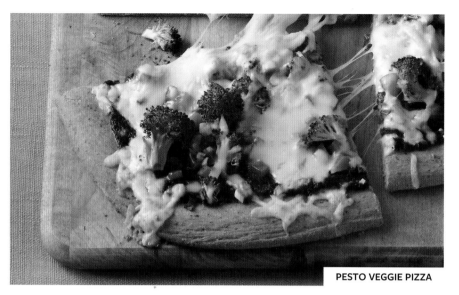

PESTO VEGGIE PIZZA

Soy-Glazed Scallops

A great source of vitamin B12 and heart-healthy minerals such as magnesium, scallops are a worthy dinner option. Here, a no-fuss marinade adds a lovely burst of flavor to the scallops.

—**APRIL KORANDO** AVA, IL

PREP: 25 MIN. + MARINATING • **BROIL:** 5 MIN.
MAKES: 4 SERVINGS

- ¼ **cup lemon juice**
- 2 **tablespoons canola oil**
- 2 **tablespoons reduced-sodium soy sauce**
- 2 **tablespoons honey**
- 2 **garlic cloves, minced**
- ½ **teaspoon ground ginger**
- 12 **sea scallops (about 1½ pounds)**

1. In a small bowl, combine the first six ingredients. Pour ⅓ cup marinade into a large resealable plastic bag. Add the scallops; seal bag and turn to coat. Refrigerate for 20 minutes.

2. Place remaining marinade in a small saucepan. Bring to a boil. Reduce heat; simmer, uncovered, for 8-10 minutes or until slightly thickened.

3. Drain and discard marinade. Thread scallops onto four metal or soaked wooden skewers.

4. Broil 4 in. from the heat for 2-4 minutes on each side or until scallops are firm and opaque, basting occasionally with the remaining marinade.

PER SERVING *250 cal., 8 g fat (1 g sat. fat), 54 mg chol., 567 mg sodium, 15 g carb., trace fiber, 28 g pro.* **Diabetic Exchanges:** *4 lean meat, 1 fat, ½ starch.*

Pesto Veggie Pizza

When I was thinking about what my family likes to eat and what I like to cook, the answer was pizza—especially this one!

—**DANA DIRKS** SAN DIEGO, CA

PREP: 30 MIN. + STANDING • **BAKE:** 10 MIN.
MAKES: 6 SERVINGS

- 1 **package (¼ ounce) active dry yeast**
- 1 **cup warm water (110° to 115°)**
- ⅓ **cup grated Parmesan cheese**
- 2 **tablespoons canola oil**
- 1 **tablespoon sugar**
- 1 **tablespoon dried basil**
- ½ **teaspoon salt**
- ¾ **cup all-purpose flour**
- 1 **to 1½ cups whole wheat flour**
- 3½ **cups fresh baby spinach**
- ¼ **cup prepared pesto**
- 1¾ **cups coarsely chopped fresh broccoli**
- ¾ **cup chopped green pepper**
- 2 **green onions, chopped**
- 4 **garlic cloves, minced**
- 2 **cups (8 ounces) shredded part-skim mozzarella cheese**

1. In a small bowl, dissolve yeast in warm water. Add the Parmesan cheese, oil, sugar, basil, salt, all-purpose flour and ¾ cup whole wheat flour. Beat until smooth. Stir in enough remaining whole wheat flour to form a soft dough (dough will be sticky).

2. Turn onto a lightly floured surface; knead until smooth and elastic, about 6-8 minutes. Cover and let rest for 10 minutes.

3. Roll dough into a 16-in. x 12-in. rectangle. Transfer to a baking sheet coated with cooking spray; build up edges slightly. Prick dough with a fork. Bake at 375° for 8-10 minutes or until lightly browned.

4. Meanwhile, in a large saucepan, bring ½ in. of water to a boil. Add spinach; cover and boil for 3-5 minutes or until wilted. Drain and place in a food processor. Add pesto; cover and process until blended.

5. Spread over pizza crust. Top with broccoli, green pepper, green onions, garlic and mozzarella cheese. Bake for 10-12 minutes longer or until the cheese is melted.

PER SERVING *364 cal., 17 g fat (6 g sat. fat), 29 mg chol., 543 mg sodium, 35 g carb., 5 g fiber, 19 g pro.* **Diabetic Exchanges:** *2 starch, 2 medium-fat meat, 2 fat, 1 vegetable.*

Grilled Tilapia with Raspberry Chipotle Chutney

I eat fish often and am always looking for healthy, tasty ways to prepare it. Making the chutney ahead of time really makes this recipe a quick-dinner solution. I pair it with herbed couscous.

—**MEGAN DICOU** BERKELEY, CA

PREP: 40 MIN. • **GRILL:** 5 MIN.
MAKES: 4 SERVINGS

- 1 medium red onion, chopped
- 1 medium sweet red pepper, chopped
- 2 teaspoons olive oil
- 3 garlic cloves, minced
- 2 teaspoons minced fresh gingerroot
- 1½ cups fresh raspberries
- ¾ cup reduced-sodium chicken broth
- ¼ cup honey
- 2 tablespoons cider vinegar
- 1 tablespoon minced chipotle peppers in adobo sauce
- ½ teaspoon salt, divided
- ½ teaspoon pepper, divided
- 4 tilapia fillets (6 ounces each)

1. In a large saucepan, saute onion and pepper in oil until tender. Add garlic and ginger; cook 1 minute longer. Stir in the raspberries, broth, honey, vinegar, chipotle peppers, ¼ teaspoon salt and ¼ teaspoon pepper. Bring to a boil. Reduce heat; simmer, uncovered, for 25-30 minutes or until thickened.
2. Meanwhile, sprinkle fillets with remaining salt and pepper. Using long-handled tongs, moisten a paper towel with cooking oil and lightly coat the grill rack. Grill fish, covered, over high heat or broil 3-4 in. from the heat for 3-5 minutes or until fish flakes easily with a fork. Serve with chutney.
PER SERVING *277 cal., 4 g fat (1 g sat. fat), 83 mg chol., 491 mg sodium, 29 g carb., 5 g fiber, 33 g pro.* **Diabetic Exchanges:** *5 lean meat, 2 starch, ½ fat.*

Lemon Shrimp Stir-Fry

A friend shared this recipe with me, and I've been enjoying it for more than a decade now. The shrimp and veggies are coated with a mild, lemony sauce to really amplify all the flavors.

—**CAROLINE ELLIOTT** GRANTS PASS, OR

PREP: 25 MIN. • **COOK:** 10 MIN.
MAKES: 2 SERVINGS

- 1 tablespoon cornstarch
- ½ teaspoon sugar
- ½ teaspoon chicken bouillon granules
- ¼ teaspoon grated lemon peel
  Dash pepper
- ½ cup water
- 4½ teaspoons lemon juice
- ½ pound uncooked medium shrimp, peeled and deveined
- 1 tablespoon canola oil
- ¾ cup sliced celery
- ½ medium green pepper, cut into strips
- ½ medium sweet red pepper, cut into strips
- 1 cup sliced fresh mushrooms
- ¾ cup fresh sugar snap peas
- 1 green onion, sliced
- 1 cup hot cooked long grain rice

1. In a small bowl, combine the first five ingredients. Stir in water and lemon juice until blended; set aside.
2. In a large skillet or wok, stir-fry shrimp in oil for 1-2 minutes or until no longer pink. Remove with a slotted spoon and keep warm. In the same pan, stir-fry the celery and peppers for 2 minutes. Add the mushrooms, peas and onion; stir-fry 3-4 minutes longer or until vegetables are crisp-tender.
3. Stir cornstarch mixture and add to the pan. Bring to a boil; cook and stir for 2 minutes or until thickened. Add shrimp; heat through. Serve with rice.
PER SERVING *326 cal., 9 g fat (1 g sat. fat), 168 mg chol., 449 mg sodium, 39 g carb., 4 g fiber, 24 g pro.* **Diabetic Exchanges:** *3 lean meat, 2 starch, 2 vegetable, 1½ fat.*

LEMON SHRIMP STIR-FRY

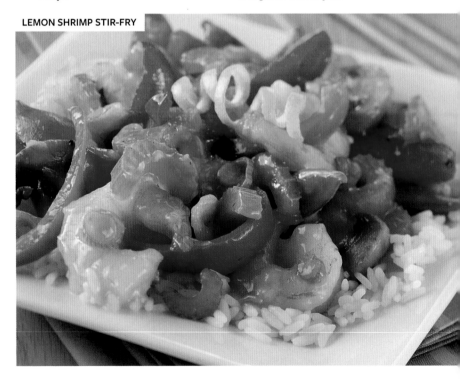

Fiery Stuffed Poblanos

I love Southwestern cuisine, but the dishes are often laden with fat. As a future dietitian, I try to come up with healthy twists on recipes, which is how my stuffed chili dish was born.

—AMBER MASSEY ARGYLE, TX

PREP: 50 MIN. + STANDING • **BAKE:** 20 MIN.
MAKES: 8 SERVINGS

- 8 poblano peppers
- 1 can (15 ounces) black beans, rinsed and drained
- 1 medium zucchini, chopped
- 1 small red onion, chopped
- 4 garlic cloves, minced
- 1 can (15¼ ounces) whole kernel corn, drained
- 1 can (14½ ounces) fire-roasted diced tomatoes, undrained
- 1 cup cooked brown rice
- 1 tablespoon ground cumin
- 1 to 1½ teaspoons ground ancho chili pepper
- ¼ teaspoon salt
- ¼ teaspoon pepper
- 1 cup (4 ounces) shredded reduced-fat Mexican cheese blend, divided
- 3 green onions, chopped
- ½ cup reduced-fat sour cream

1. Broil peppers 3 in. from the heat until skins blister, about 5 minutes. With tongs, rotate peppers a quarter turn. Broil and rotate until all sides are blistered and blackened. Immediately place peppers in a large bowl; cover and let stand for 20 minutes.
2. Meanwhile, in a small bowl, coarsely mash beans; set aside. In a large nonstick skillet coated with cooking spray, cook and stir zucchini and onion until tender. Add garlic; cook 1 minute longer. Add the corn, tomatoes, rice, seasonings and beans. Remove from the heat; stir in ½ cup cheese. Set aside.
3. Peel off and discard charred skins from poblanos. Cut a lengthwise slit down each pepper, leaving the stem intact; remove membranes and seeds. Fill each pepper with ⅔ cup filling.
4. Place peppers in a 13-in. x 9-in. baking dish coated with cooking spray. Bake, uncovered, at 375° for 18-22 minutes or until heated through, sprinkling with green onions and remaining cheese during last 5 minutes of baking. Garnish with sour cream.
PER SERVING *223 cal., 5 g fat (2 g sat. fat), 15 mg chol., 579 mg sodium, 32 g carb., 7 g fiber, 11 g pro.* **Diabetic Exchanges:** *2 vegetable, 1 starch, 1 lean meat, 1 fat.*

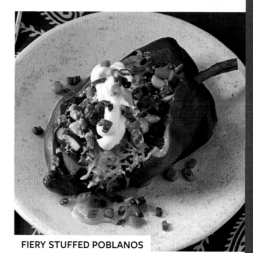

FIERY STUFFED POBLANOS

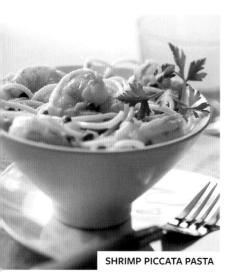

SHRIMP PICCATA PASTA

Shrimp Piccata Pasta

A light and tangy sauce spiked with capers will make this pasta an instant classic in your home. Dig in!

—CAROLE BESS WHITE PORTLAND, OR

START TO FINISH: 20 MIN.
MAKES: 4 SERVINGS

- 6 ounces uncooked spaghetti
- 2 shallots, chopped
- 1 tablespoon olive oil
- 1 pound uncooked medium shrimp, peeled and deveined
- 1 jar (3 ounces) capers, drained
- 3 tablespoons lemon juice
- ½ teaspoon garlic powder

1. Cook spaghetti according to package directions. Meanwhile, in a large nonstick skillet, saute shallots in oil until tender. Add the shrimp, capers, lemon juice and garlic powder; cook and stir for 5-6 minutes or until the shrimp turn pink.
2. Drain spaghetti; toss with the shrimp mixture.
PER SERVING *293 cal., 5 g fat (1 g sat. fat), 168 mg chol., 453 mg sodium, 37 g carb., 2 g fiber, 24 g pro.* **Diabetic Exchanges:** *3 lean meat, 2 starch, ½ fat.*

top tip

Choose the Right Zucchini

When picking out zucchini, handle them carefully—they're thin-skinned and easily damaged. Look for ones that are heavy and have shiny skin.

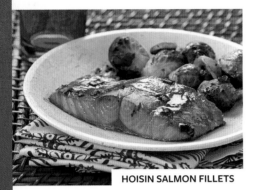

HOISIN SALMON FILLETS

Hoisin Salmon Fillets

Enjoy fabulous Asian flavor in no time—this moist salmon is special enough for guests and easy enough for weekdays. Add steamed brown rice, broccoli and a fresh fruit salad on the side.

—JERI FAROUGH PERRYVILLE, MO

PREP: 10 MIN. + MARINATING • **GRILL:** 10 MIN.
MAKES: 6 SERVINGS

- 3 **green onions, chopped**
- ⅓ **cup reduced-sodium soy sauce**
- ¼ **cup hoisin sauce**
- 3 **tablespoons lemon juice**
- 1 **tablespoon grated lemon peel**
- ½ **teaspoon pepper**
- 6 **salmon fillets (4 ounces each)**

1. In a large resealable plastic bag, combine the first six ingredients. Add the salmon; seal bag and turn to coat. Refrigerate for 30 minutes, turning occasionally.
2. Drain and discard marinade. Using long-handled tongs, moisten a paper towel with cooking oil and lightly coat the grill rack. Place salmon skin side down on grill rack.
3. Grill, covered, over medium heat or broil 4 in. from the heat for 10-12 minutes or until the fish flakes easily with a fork.
PER SERVING *224 cal., 12 g fat (3 g sat. fat), 67 mg chol., 401 mg sodium, 3 g carb., trace fiber, 23 g pro.* **Diabetic Exchanges:** *3 lean meat, 2 fat.*

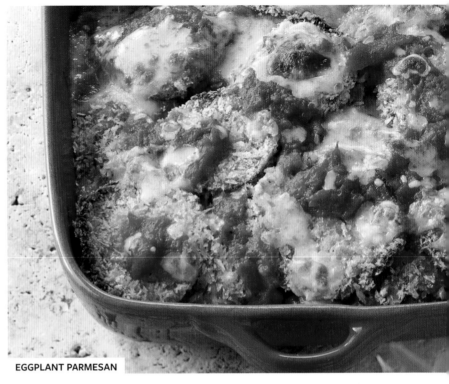

EGGPLANT PARMESAN

Eggplant Parmesan

Because my recipe calls for baking the eggplant instead of frying it, it's much healthier for you. It's worth the extra prep.

—LACI HOOTEN MCKINNEY, TX

PREP: 40 MIN. • **COOK:** 25 MIN.
MAKES: 8 SERVINGS

- 3 **eggs, beaten**
- 2½ **cups panko (Japanese) bread crumbs**
- 3 **medium eggplants, cut into ¼-inch slices**
- 2 **jars (4½ ounces each) sliced mushrooms, drained**
- ½ **teaspoon dried basil**
- ⅛ **teaspoon dried oregano**
- 2 **cups (8 ounces) shredded part-skim mozzarella cheese**
- ½ **cup grated Parmesan cheese**
- 1 **jar (28 ounces) spaghetti sauce**

1. Place eggs and bread crumbs in separate shallow bowls. Dip eggplant in eggs, then coat in crumbs. Place on baking sheets coated with cooking spray. Bake at 350° for 15-20 minutes or until tender and golden brown, turning once.
2. In a small bowl, combine the mushrooms, basil and oregano. In another small bowl, combine the mozzarella and Parmesan cheeses.
3. Spread ½ cup sauce into a 13-in. x 9-in. baking dish coated with cooking spray. Layer with a third of mushroom mixture, eggplant, ¾ cup sauce and a third of the cheese mixture. Repeat layers twice.
4. Bake, uncovered, at 350° for 25-30 minutes or until heated through and cheese is melted.
PER SERVING *305 cal., 12 g fat (5 g sat. fat), 102 mg chol., 912 mg sodium, 32 g carb., 9 g fiber, 18 g pro.* **Diabetic Exchanges:** *2 starch, 2 vegetable, 1 medium-fat meat.*

Tilapia Tostadas

I have family members who don't usually like fish, but this tostada recipe is always a hit. It's a winner in my book.

—JENNIFER KOLB OVERLAND PARK, KS

START TO FINISH: 30 MIN.
MAKES: 4 SERVINGS

- ¼ cup all-purpose flour
- 1 teaspoon chili powder
- ½ teaspoon salt
- ½ teaspoon pepper
- ¼ teaspoon garlic powder
- 4 tilapia fillets (6 ounces each)
- 1 tablespoon butter
- 8 corn tortillas (6 inches)
- 2 cups angel hair coleslaw mix
- 2 tablespoons reduced-fat mayonnaise
- 2 tablespoons reduced-fat sour cream
- 1 tablespoon lime juice
- 1 teaspoon grated lime peel
- 1 cup canned black beans, rinsed and drained
- ½ cup sliced avocado

1. In a large resealable plastic bag, combine the flour, chili powder, salt, pepper and garlic powder. Add tilapia fillets, one at a time, and shake to coat.
2. In a large nonstick skillet over medium heat, cook fillets in butter for 5-6 minutes on each side or until fish flakes easily with a fork. Meanwhile, place tortillas on a baking sheet and spritz with cooking spray. Broil 3-4 in. from the heat for 2-3 minutes on each side or until crisp.
3. In a small bowl, toss the coleslaw mix, mayonnaise, sour cream, lime juice and lime peel. Cut fish into large pieces. On each tortilla, layer coleslaw, black beans, fish and avocado.
PER SERVING *437 cal., 12 g fat (4 g sat. fat), 95 mg chol., 659 mg sodium, 44 g carb., 7 g fiber, 40 g pro.* **Diabetic Exchanges:** *5 lean meat, 3 starch, 1½ fat.*

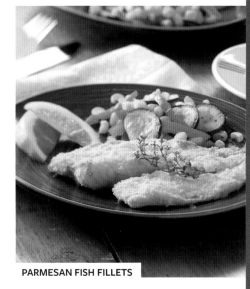

PARMESAN FISH FILLETS

Parmesan Fish Fillets

The hint of Parmesan cheese really seals the deal for this tilapia recipe. It's fast, a cinch to make and diet-friendly.

—PAULA ALF CINCINNATI, OH

START TO FINISH: 30 MIN.
MAKES: 2 SERVINGS

- ¼ cup egg substitute
- 1 tablespoon fat-free milk
- ⅓ cup grated Parmesan cheese
- 2 tablespoons all-purpose flour
- 2 tilapia fillets (5 ounces each)

1. In a shallow bowl, combine egg substitute and milk. In another shallow bowl, combine cheese and flour. Dip fillets in egg mixture, then coat with cheese mixture.
2. Place on a baking sheet coated with cooking spray. Bake at 350° for 20-25 minutes or until the fish flakes easily with a fork.
PER SERVING *196 cal., 5 g fat (3 g sat. fat), 78 mg chol., 279 mg sodium, 5 g carb., trace fiber, 33 g pro.* **Diabetic Exchange:** *4 lean meat.*

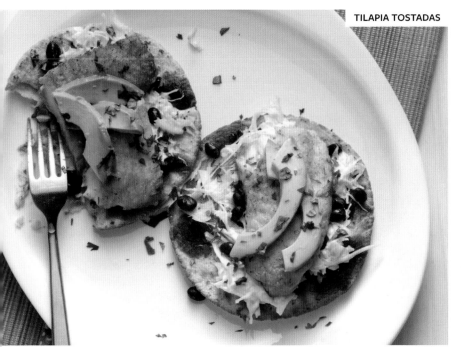

TILAPIA TOSTADAS

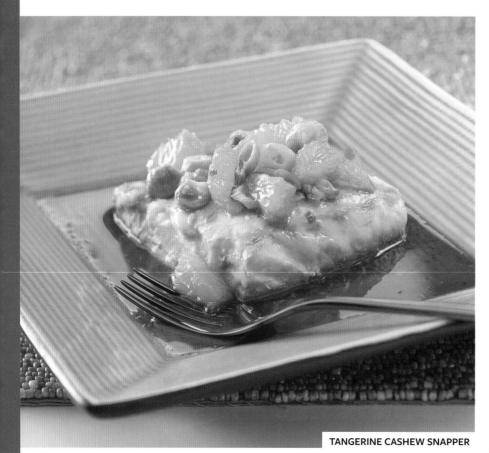

TANGERINE CASHEW SNAPPER

Baked Italian Tilapia

This dish is so simple, you'll want to add it to your list of go-to recipes.

—**KIMBERLY MCGEE** MOSHEIM, TN

PREP: 10 MIN. • **BAKE:** 40 MIN.
MAKES: 4 SERVINGS

- 4 **tilapia fillets (6 ounces each)**
- ¼ **teaspoon pepper**
- 1 **can (14½ ounces) diced tomatoes with basil, oregano and garlic, drained**
- 1 **large onion, halved and thinly sliced**
- 1 **medium green pepper, julienned**
- ¼ **cup shredded Parmesan cheese**

1. Place tilapia in a 13-in. x 9-in. baking dish coated with cooking spray; sprinkle with pepper. Spoon the tomatoes over tilapia; top with onion and green pepper.

2. Cover and bake at 350° for 30 minutes. Uncover; sprinkle with cheese. Bake 10-15 minutes longer or until fish flakes easily with a fork.

PER SERVING *215 cal., 4 g fat (2 g sat. fat), 86 mg chol., 645 mg sodium, 12 g carb., 2 g fiber, 36 g pro.* **Diabetic Exchanges:** *4 lean meat, 2 vegetable.*

BAKED ITALIAN TILAPIA

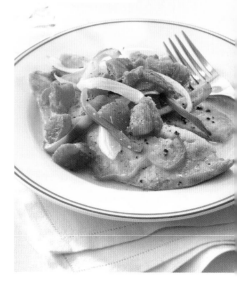

Tangerine Cashew Snapper

Savor the sweetness of tangerines and the crunchiness of cashews. You've probably never had fish quite like this before!

—**CRYSTAL JO BRUNS** ILIFF, CO

START TO FINISH: 30 MIN.
MAKES: 4 SERVINGS

- 4 **tangerines**
- 2 **tablespoons lime juice**
- 2 **tablespoons reduced-sodium soy sauce**
- 1 **tablespoon brown sugar**
- 2 **teaspoons minced fresh gingerroot**
- 1 **teaspoon sesame oil**
- ⅛ **teaspoon crushed red pepper flakes**
- 4 **red snapper fillets (4 ounces each)**
- ⅓ **cup chopped unsalted cashews**
- 2 **green onions, thinly sliced**

1. Peel, slice and remove seeds from 2 tangerines; chop the fruit and place in a small bowl. Squeeze juice from remaining tangerines; add to bowl. Stir in lime juice, soy sauce, brown sugar, ginger, sesame oil and pepper flakes.

2. Place fillets in a 13-in. x 9-in. baking dish coated with cooking spray. Pour tangerine mixture over fillets; sprinkle with cashews and green onions. Bake, uncovered, at 425° for 15-20 minutes or until fish flakes easily with a fork.

PER SERVING *260 cal., 8 g fat (2 g sat. fat), 40 mg chol., 358 mg sodium, 22 g carb., 2 g fiber, 26 g pro.* **Diabetic Exchanges:** *3 lean meat, 1 fruit, 1 fat.*

Moroccan Vegetarian Stew

Ladle this spicy stew over couscous or serve with warm pita bread. If you want to cool it down, add a dollop of yogurt or sour cream.

—SONYA LABBE WEST HOLLYWOOD, CA

PREP: 20 MIN. • **COOK:** 30 MIN.
MAKES: 8 SERVINGS (3 QUARTS)

- 1 **large onion, chopped**
- 1 **tablespoon olive oil**
- 2 **teaspoons ground cinnamon**
- 2 **teaspoons ground cumin**
- 1 **teaspoon ground coriander**
- ½ **teaspoon cayenne pepper**
- ½ **teaspoon ground allspice**
- ¼ **teaspoon salt**
- 3 **cups water**
- 1 **small butternut squash, peeled and cubed**
- 2 **medium potatoes, peeled and cubed**
- 4 **medium carrots, sliced**
- 3 **plum tomatoes, chopped**
- 2 **small zucchini, cut into 1-inch pieces**
- 1 **can (15 ounces) garbanzo beans or chickpeas, rinsed and drained**

1. In a Dutch oven, saute onion in oil until tender. Add spices and salt; cook 1 minute longer.

2. Stir in the water, squash, potatoes, carrots and tomatoes. Bring to a boil. Reduce heat; simmer, uncovered, for 15-20 minutes or until potatoes and squash are almost tender.

3. Add zucchini and chickpeas; return to a boil. Reduce heat; simmer, uncovered, for 5-8 minutes or until vegetables are tender.

PER SERVING *1½ cups equals 172 cal., 3 g fat (trace sat. fat), 0 chol., 174 mg sodium, 34 g carb., 8 g fiber, 5 g pro. Diabetic Exchanges: 2 starch, 1 vegetable.*

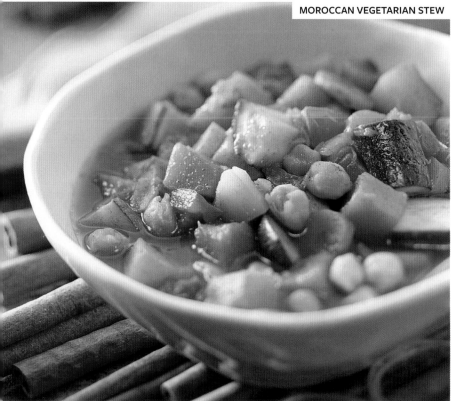

MOROCCAN VEGETARIAN STEW

Crab Macaroni Casserole

This is macaroni and cheese with a twist! Whole wheat macaroni boosts nutrition, while the melted cheese topping makes it satisfyingly ooey-gooey.

—JASON EGNER EDGERTON, WI

PREP: 25 MIN. • **BAKE:** 20 MIN.
MAKES: 6 SERVINGS

- 2 **cups uncooked whole wheat elbow macaroni**
- 3 **tablespoons chopped onion**
- 2 **tablespoons butter**
- 3 **tablespoons all-purpose flour**
- 1½ **cups fat-free milk**
- 2 **cans (6 ounces each) lump crabmeat, drained**
- 1 **cup (8 ounces) reduced-fat sour cream**
- ½ **cup shredded Swiss cheese**
- ½ **teaspoon salt**
- ½ **teaspoon ground mustard**
- 1 **cup (4 ounces) shredded fat-free cheddar cheese, divided**

1. Cook macaroni according to package directions.

2. Meanwhile, in a large skillet, saute onion in butter until tender. Combine flour and milk until smooth; stir into pan. Bring to a boil; cook and stir for 1-2 minutes or until thickened. Remove from the heat. Drain macaroni. Add the crabmeat, sour cream, Swiss cheese, salt, mustard, macaroni and ¼ cup cheddar cheese to the skillet.

3. Transfer to an 11-in. x 7-in. baking dish coated with cooking spray. Sprinkle with remaining cheddar cheese. Bake, uncovered, at 350° for 20-25 minutes or until heated through.

PER SERVING *1 cup equals 380 cal., 11 g fat (6 g sat. fat), 86 mg chol., 619 mg sodium, 38 g carb., 4 g fiber, 31 g pro. Diabetic Exchanges: 3 lean meat, 2 starch, 1½ fat.*

Hearty Shrimp Risotto

Featuring white wine, goat cheese and fresh spinach, this dish will have your guests thinking you picked it up from a restaurant!

—LYDIA BECKER PARKVILLE, MO

PREP: 15 MIN. • **COOK:** 35 MIN.
MAKES: 4 SERVINGS

- 4 cups reduced-sodium chicken broth
- 1 small onion, finely chopped
- 1 tablespoon olive oil
- 1 cup uncooked arborio rice
- 1 fresh thyme sprig
- 1 bay leaf
- ¼ teaspoon pepper
- ¾ cup white wine or additional reduced-sodium chicken broth
- 1 pound uncooked medium shrimp, peeled and deveined
- 2 cups chopped fresh spinach
- 4 ounces fresh goat cheese, crumbled

1. In a small saucepan, heat broth and keep warm. In a large nonstick skillet coated with cooking spray, saute onion in oil until tender. Add the rice, thyme, bay leaf and pepper; cook and stir for 2-3 minutes. Reduce heat; stir in wine. Cook and stir until all of the liquid is absorbed.

2. Add heated broth, ½ cup at a time, stirring constantly. Allow the liquid to absorb between additions. Cook just until risotto is creamy and the rice is almost tender. (Cooking time is about 20 minutes.) Add the shrimp and spinach; cook until shrimp turn pink and spinach is wilted.

3. Stir in cheese. Discard thyme and bay leaf. Serve immediately.

PER SERVING *405 cal., 9 g fat (3 g sat. fat), 157 mg chol., 832 mg sodium, 45 g carb., 1 g fiber, 28 g pro.* **Diabetic Exchanges:** *3 lean meat, 2½ starch, 1 fat.*

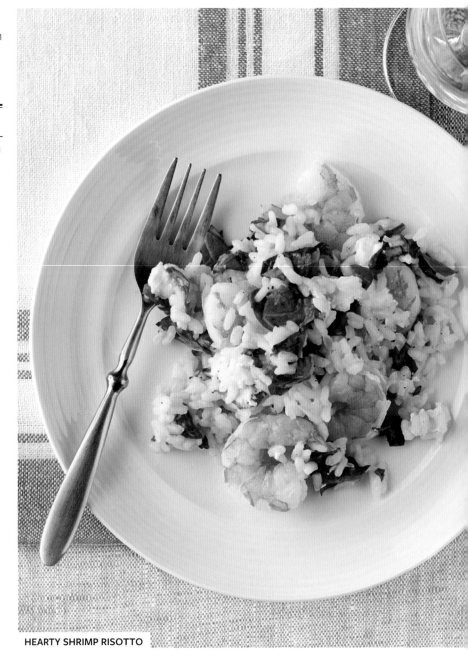

HEARTY SHRIMP RISOTTO

top tip
What's Arborio Rice?

Arborio rice is a medium grain rice used for making risottos. In risottos, the rice has a creamy texture with a chewy center.

Crab-Stuffed Manicotti

I love pasta, and my husband can't ever get enough seafood. So I combined our favorites to create this dish, and he called it the best meal he's ever had!

—**SONYA POLFLIET** ANZA, CA

PREP: 25 MIN. • **BAKE:** 25 MIN.
MAKES: 2 SERVINGS

- 4 uncooked manicotti shells
- 1 tablespoon butter
- 4 teaspoons all-purpose flour
- 1 cup fat-free milk
- 1 tablespoon grated Parmesan cheese
- 1 cup lump crabmeat, drained
- ⅓ cup reduced-fat ricotta cheese
- ¼ cup shredded part-skim mozzarella cheese
- ¼ teaspoon lemon-pepper seasoning
- ¼ teaspoon pepper
- ⅛ teaspoon garlic powder
  Minced fresh parsley

1. Cook manicotti according to package directions. In a small saucepan, melt butter. Stir in flour until smooth; gradually add milk. Bring to a boil; cook and stir for 2 minutes or until mixture is thickened. Remove from the heat; stir in Parmesan cheese.

2. In a small bowl, combine the crab, ricotta cheese, mozzarella cheese, lemon-pepper, pepper and garlic powder. Drain manicotti; stuff with crab mixture. Spread ¼ cup sauce in an 8-in. square baking dish coated with cooking spray. Top with stuffed manicotti. Pour the remaining sauce over top.

3. Cover and bake at 350° for 25-30 minutes or until heated through. Just before serving, sprinkle with parsley.
PER SERVING *359 cal., 12 g fat (7 g sat. fat), 98 mg chol., 793 mg sodium, 38 g carb., 1 g fiber, 26 g pro.* **Diabetic Exchanges:** *2 starch, 2 lean meat, 1 fat, ½ fat-free milk.*

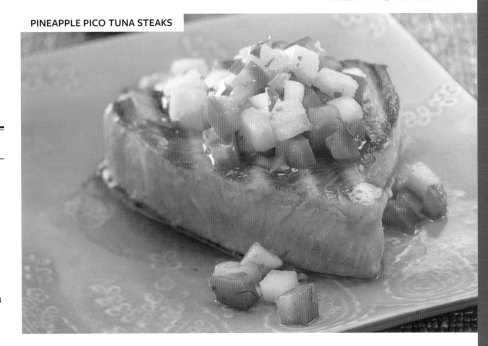

PINEAPPLE PICO TUNA STEAKS

Pineapple Pico Tuna Steaks

Bursting with flavor from a do-it-yourself marinade, these tuna steaks are loaded with pico de gallo made from pineapple, tomatoes, lime juice and a nice but powerful kick of jalapeno.

—**SALLY SIBTHORPE** SHELBY TOWNSHIP, MI

PREP: 10 MIN. + MARINATING • **GRILL:** 10 MIN.
MAKES: 4 SERVINGS

- ½ cup tequila
- 3 tablespoons brown sugar
- 2 tablespoons lime juice
- 1 tablespoon chili powder
- 1 tablespoon olive oil
- 1 teaspoon salt
- 4 tuna steaks (6 ounces each)

PICO DE GALLO

- 1 cup chopped fresh pineapple
- 1 plum tomato, finely chopped
- ⅓ cup finely chopped onion
- ¼ cup minced fresh cilantro
- 2 tablespoons minced seeded jalapeno pepper
- 2 tablespoons lime juice
- 1 tablespoon olive oil
- 2 teaspoons grated lime peel
- ½ teaspoon salt

1. In a large resealable plastic bag, combine the first six ingredients. Add the tuna; seal bag and turn to coat. Refrigerate for 30 minutes. Meanwhile, in a small bowl, combine pico de gallo ingredients. Cover and refrigerate pico de gallo until serving.

2. Drain and discard marinade. Using long-handled tongs, moisten a paper towel with cooking oil and lightly coat the grill rack. For medium-rare, grill tuna, covered, over high heat or broil 3-4 inches from the heat 3-4 minutes on each side or until slightly pink in the center. Serve with pico de gallo.
NOTE *Wear disposable gloves when cutting hot peppers; the oils can burn skin. Avoid touching your face.*
PER SERVING *385 cal., 9 g fat (1 g sat. fat), 77 mg chol., 974 mg sodium, 20 g carb., 2 g fiber, 41 g pro.* **Diabetic Exchanges:** *5 lean meat, 1 starch, 1 fat.*

salads

Whether **green and garden fresh**, packed with people-pleasing pasta or made with **colorful fruits and veggies**, salads are a must for today's healthy families. Simply turn here for some of the best!

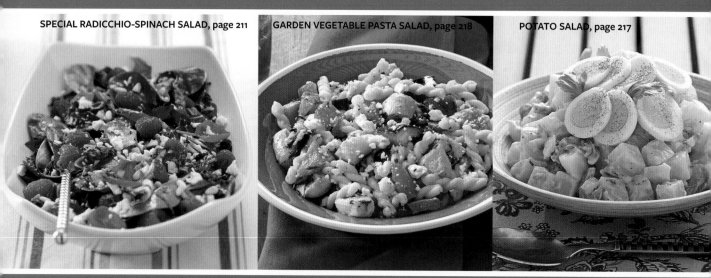

SPECIAL RADICCHIO-SPINACH SALAD, page 211

GARDEN VEGETABLE PASTA SALAD, page 218

POTATO SALAD, page 217

2. In a large bowl, combine the tomato, zucchini, yellow pepper and parsley. Stir in barley. In a small bowl, whisk the oil, vinegar, water, lemon juice, basil, salt and pepper. Pour over barley mixture; toss to coat. Cover and refrigerate for at least 3 hours. Just before serving, stir in almonds.

PER SERVING *¾ cup equals 211 cal., 10 g fat (1 g sat. fat), 0 chol., 334 mg sodium, 27 g carb., 7 g fiber, 6 g pro.* **Diabetic Exchanges:** *2 fat, 1½ starch.*

Cannellini Spinach Pasta Salad

Create a hearty spinach salad when you mix in white beans and pasta shells.

—**VIRGINIA PRAGLOWSKI** TORRANCE, CA

START TO FINISH: 15 MIN.
MAKES: 10 SERVINGS

- 8 **cups fresh spinach, coarsely chopped**
- 3 **cups small shell pasta, cooked and drained**
- 1 **can (15 ounces) cannellini or white kidney beans**
- 3 **tablespoons balsamic vinegar**
- 2 **tablespoons olive oil**
- 2 **teaspoons sugar**
- 2 **garlic cloves, minced**
- ½ **teaspoon salt**
- ¼ **teaspoon pepper**
- ½ **cup shredded Parmesan cheese**

In a large bowl, combine the spinach, pasta and beans. In a jar with a tight-fitting lid, combine the vinegar, oil, sugar, garlic, salt and pepper; shake well. Pour over salad; toss to coat. Sprinkle with cheese. Serve immediately.

PER SERVING *1 cup equals 157 cal., 5 g fat (2 g sat. fat), 3 mg chol., 243 mg sodium, 21 g carb., 3 g fiber, 7 g pro.* **Diabetic Exchanges:** *1 starch, 1 vegetable, 1 fat.*

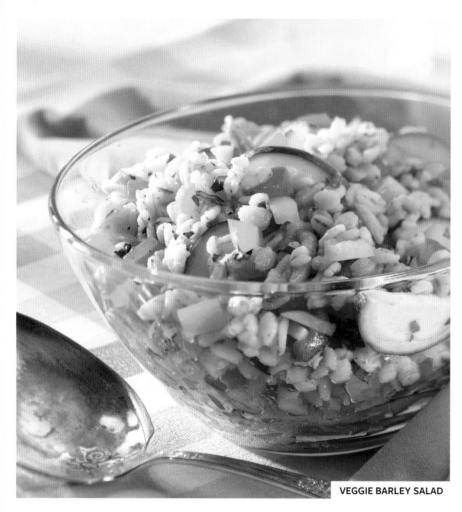

VEGGIE BARLEY SALAD

Veggie Barley Salad

The longer this salads chills, the tastier it becomes. Bring it along to your next potluck and you'll probably go home with an empty dish. I always do!

—**KATHY RAIRIGH** MILFORD, IN

PREP: 30 MIN. + CHILLING
MAKES: 6 SERVINGS

- 1¼ **cups reduced-sodium chicken broth or vegetable broth**
- ¾ **cup water**
- 1 **cup quick-cooking barley**
- 1 **medium tomato, seeded and chopped**
- 1 **small zucchini, halved and thinly sliced**
- 1 **small sweet yellow pepper, chopped**
- 2 **tablespoons minced fresh parsley**

DRESSING

- 3 **tablespoons olive oil**
- 2 **tablespoons white wine vinegar**
- 1 **tablespoon water**
- 1 **tablespoon lemon juice**
- 1 **tablespoon minced fresh basil**
- ½ **teaspoon salt**
- ¼ **teaspoon pepper**
- ¼ **cup slivered almonds, toasted**

1. In a small saucepan, bring the broth, water and barley to a boil. Reduce heat; cover and simmer for 10-12 minutes or until barley is tender. Remove from the heat; let stand for 5 minutes.

Almond Coleslaw

For a twist on my mother's original recipe, I added toasted almonds to this slaw for an extra dose of crunch and nutrition.

—**SARAH NEVIN** GILA, NM

START TO FINISH: 25 MIN.
MAKES: 14 SERVINGS

- 2 **packages (16 ounces each) coleslaw mix**
- 1 **cup reduced-fat mayonnaise**
- 2 **tablespoons cider vinegar**
- 1 **tablespoon sugar**
- ¾ **teaspoon seasoned salt**
- ½ **teaspoon pepper**
- ½ **cup slivered almonds, toasted**

Place coleslaw mix in a serving bowl. In a small bowl, combine the mayonnaise, vinegar, sugar, seasoned salt and pepper. Pour over coleslaw mix; toss to coat. Chill until serving. Just before serving, sprinkle with almonds.

PER SERVING *¾ cup equals 103 cal., 8 g fat (1 g sat. fat), 6 mg chol., 237 mg sodium, 7 g carb., 2 g fiber, 2 g pro.* ***Diabetic Exchanges:** 1½ fat, ½ starch.*

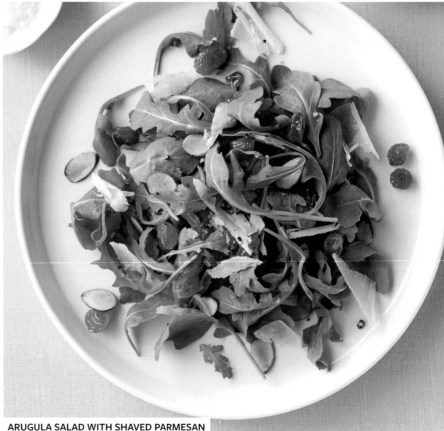

ARUGULA SALAD WITH SHAVED PARMESAN

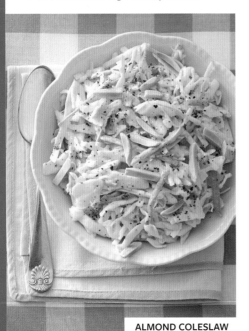

ALMOND COLESLAW

Arugula Salad with Shaved Parmesan

As a treat for my mom, I combined some of her favorite foods, like fresh peppery arugula, golden raisins, crunchy almonds and shredded Parmesan in this simple salad that my whole family ended up liking just as much as she did.

—**NICOLE RASH** BOISE, ID

START TO FINISH: 15 MIN.
MAKES: 4 SERVINGS

- 6 **cups fresh arugula**
- ¼ **cup golden raisins**
- ¼ **cup sliced almonds, toasted**
- 3 **tablespoons olive oil**
- 1 **tablespoon lemon juice**
- ¼ **teaspoon salt**
- ¼ **teaspoon freshly ground pepper**
- ⅓ **cup shaved Parmesan cheese**

In a large bowl, combine the arugula, raisins and almonds. Drizzle with oil and lemon juice. Sprinkle with salt and pepper; toss to coat. Divide among four plates; top with cheese.

NOTE *To toast nuts, spread in a 15x10x1-in. baking pan. Bake at 350° for 5-10 minutes or until lightly browned, stirring occasionally. Or, spread in a dry nonstick skillet and heat over low heat until lightly browned, stirring occasionally.*

PER SERVING *181 cal., 15 g fat (3 g sat. fat), 4 mg chol., 242 mg sodium, 10 g carb., 2 g fiber, 4 g pro.* ***Diabetic Exchanges:** 3 fat, ½ starch.*

Smoked Gouda & Raspberry Salads

An exceptional homemade raspberry vinaigrette tops this refreshing salad. You'll have bursts of flavor and texture from the smoked Gouda, raspberries and crunchy Brazil nuts.

—CHERYL PERRY HERTFORD, NC

START TO FINISH: 20 MIN.
MAKES: 8 SERVINGS

¼ cup champagne vinegar
4½ teaspoons sugar
¼ teaspoon kosher salt
1½ cups fresh raspberries, divided
1 package (5 ounces) spring mix salad greens
4 ounces Gouda cheese, shaved
⅓ cup Brazil nuts, chopped and toasted
2 shallots, thinly sliced

1. Place the vinegar, sugar, salt and ¼ cup raspberries in a food processor; cover and process until pureed.
2. Divide salad greens among eight salad plates; top with cheese, nuts, shallots and remaining raspberries. Drizzle with dressing.
PER SERVING 122 cal., 8 g fat (3 g sat. fat), 16 mg chol., 181 mg sodium, 9 g carb., 2 g fiber, 5 g pro. **Diabetic Exchanges:** 1 medium-fat meat, ½ starch.

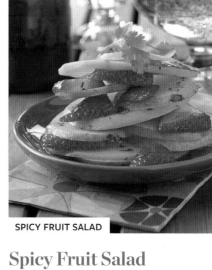

SPICY FRUIT SALAD

Spicy Fruit Salad

If you thought you knew how fruit salads work, think again! This one balances cool fruit and hot spices to perfection.

—REBECCA STURROCK LONGVIEW, TX

START TO FINISH: 15 MIN.
MAKES: 10 SERVINGS

2 medium apples, halved and sliced
2 medium pears, halved and sliced
2 medium mangoes, peeled, halved and sliced
1 pound fresh strawberries, sliced
VINAIGRETTE
¼ cup lime juice
¼ cup orange juice
¼ cup minced fresh cilantro
2 tablespoons champagne vinegar
1½ teaspoons grated lime peel
¼ teaspoon Sriracha Asian hot chili sauce or ⅛ teaspoon hot pepper sauce

In a large bowl, combine the apples, pears, mangoes and strawberries. In a small bowl, whisk the juices, cilantro, vinegar, lime peel and hot chili sauce. Drizzle over fruit mixture; toss to coat.
PER SERVING ¾ cup equals 81 cal., trace fat (trace sat. fat), 0 chol., 6 mg sodium, 21 g carb., 3 g fiber, 1 g pro. **Diabetic Exchange:** 1½ fruit.

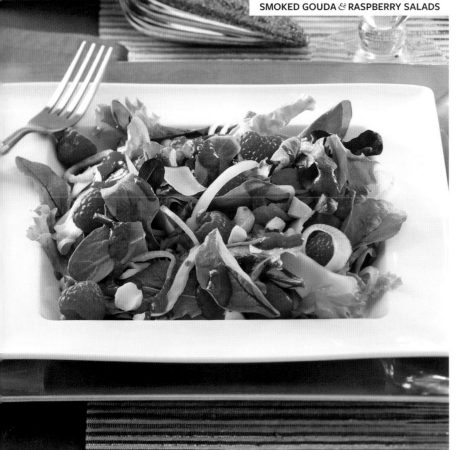

SMOKED GOUDA & RASPBERRY SALADS

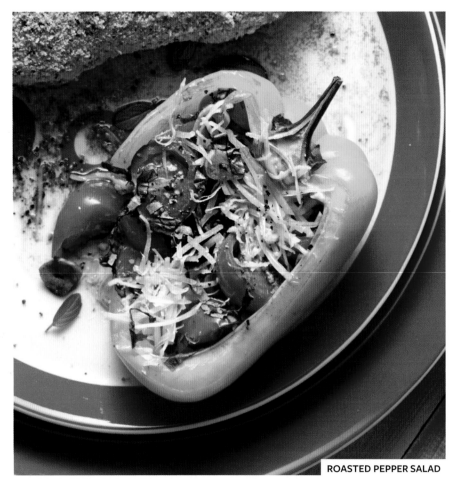
ROASTED PEPPER SALAD

Strawberry Orange Vinegar

Top your next salad with this pretty homemade dressing. Use your favorite salad greens or a ready-to-serve package to keep things even simpler.
—**TASTE OF HOME TEST KITCHEN**

PREP: 10 MIN. • **COOK:** 10 MIN. + STANDING
MAKES: 1⅔ CUPS

- 1 **medium orange**
- 2 **cups white wine vinegar**
- 2 **tablespoons sugar**
- 2 **cups sliced fresh strawberries**

1. Using a citrus zester, peel rind from orange in long narrow strips (being careful not to remove pith). In a large saucepan, heat vinegar and sugar to just below the boiling point. Place strawberries in a warm sterilized quart jar; add heated vinegar mixture and orange peel. Cover and let stand in a cool dark place for 10 days.
2. Strain mixture through a cheesecloth; discard pulp and orange rind. Pour into a sterilized pint jar. Seal tightly. Store in the refrigerator for up to 6 months.
PER SERVING *1 tablespoon equals 15 cal., trace fat (trace sat. fat), 0 chol., trace sodium, 4 g carb., trace fiber, trace pro.* **Diabetic Exchange:** *Free food.*

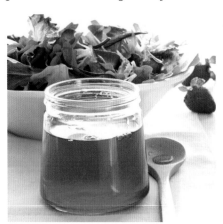
STRAWBERRY ORANGE VINEGAR

Roasted Pepper Salad

Colorful and crunchy, this salad presents peppers in a whole new way. Best of all, kids love it!
—**TRISHA KRUSE** EAGLE, ID

PREP: 15 MIN. • **BAKE:** 25 MIN.
MAKES: 6 SERVINGS

- 2 **cups cherry tomatoes, halved**
- ½ **cup minced fresh basil**
- 8 **garlic cloves, minced**
- 1 **tablespoon balsamic vinegar**
- ½ **teaspoon salt**
- ½ **teaspoon pepper**
- 3 **large sweet yellow peppers, halved and seeded**
- 2 **tablespoons shredded Parmesan cheese**

1. In a small bowl, combine the tomatoes, basil, garlic, vinegar, salt and pepper. Spoon ⅓ cup into each pepper half.
2. Transfer to a 13x9-in. baking dish coated with cooking spray. Cover and bake at 400° for 20 minutes. Uncover; sprinkle with the cheese. Bake for 5-10 minutes longer or until the cheese is melted.
PER SERVING *51 cal., 1 g fat (trace sat. fat), 1 mg chol., 233 mg sodium, 10 g carb., 2 g fiber, 2 g pro.* **Diabetic Exchange:** *2 vegetable.*

Cranberry-Avocado Tossed Salad

When you combine avocado and cranberries in a salad, you've got one vitamin-packed side to look forward to!

—MARSHA POSTAR LUBBOCK, TX

START TO FINISH: 30 MIN.
MAKES: 10 SERVINGS

- ¼ **cup sugar**
- ¼ **cup white wine vinegar**
- ¼ **cup thawed cranberry juice concentrate**
- 4½ **teaspoons ground mustard**
- ½ **teaspoon salt**
- ½ **teaspoon pepper**
- ½ **cup canola oil**
- 1 **medium ripe avocado, peeled and cubed**
- 1 **tablespoon lemon juice**
- 4 **cups torn romaine**
- 4 **cups fresh baby spinach**
- 1 **package (5 ounces) dried cranberries**
- 1 **medium red onion, chopped**
- ⅓ **cup slivered almonds**
- ⅓ **cup sunflower kernels**

1. In a small bowl, combine the first six ingredients. Gradually whisk in the oil; set aside.

2. Combine avocado and lemon juice. In a large bowl, combine the romaine, spinach, cranberries, onion and avocado mixture; drizzle with ½ cup dressing. (Save remaining dressing for another use.) Sprinkle with almonds and sunflower kernels. Serve immediately.

PER SERVING *¾ cup equals 212 cal., 13 g fat (1 g sat. fat), 0 chol., 91 mg sodium, 25 g carb., 4 g fiber, 3 g pro. Diabetic Exchanges: 2 fat, 1 starch, 1 vegetable.*

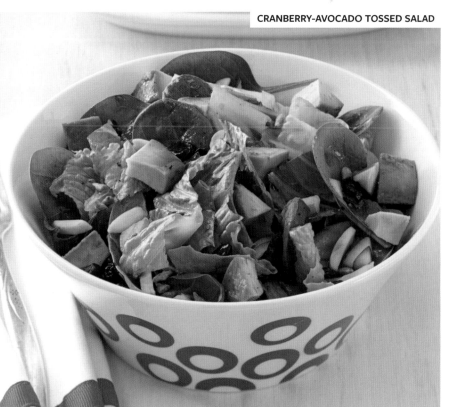

CRANBERRY-AVOCADO TOSSED SALAD

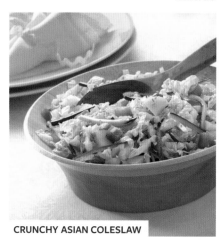

CRUNCHY ASIAN COLESLAW

Crunchy Asian Coleslaw

This flavor-packed twist on traditional creamy coleslaw is a perfect complement to Asian-themed meals. The light, tangy vinaigrette enhances the fresh veggies.

—ERIN CHILCOAT CENTRAL ISLIP, NY

PREP: 15 MIN. + CHILLING
MAKES: 2 SERVINGS

- 1 **cup shredded Chinese or napa cabbage**
- ½ **cup sliced water chestnuts, chopped**
- ½ **small zucchini, julienned**
- 2 **tablespoons chopped green pepper**
- 4½ **teaspoons rice vinegar**
- 1 **teaspoon sugar**
- 1 **teaspoon sesame seeds, toasted**
- 1 **teaspoon reduced-sodium soy sauce**
- ½ **teaspoon sesame oil**
  Dash crushed red pepper flakes

In a small bowl, combine the cabbage, water chestnuts, zucchini and green pepper. In a small bowl, whisk the remaining ingredients. Drizzle over salad; toss to coat. Refrigerate for at least 1 hour.

PER SERVING *1 cup equals 65 cal., 2 g fat (trace sat. fat), 0 chol., 120 mg sodium, 11 g carb., 2 g fiber, 2 g pro. Diabetic Exchange: 2 vegetable.*

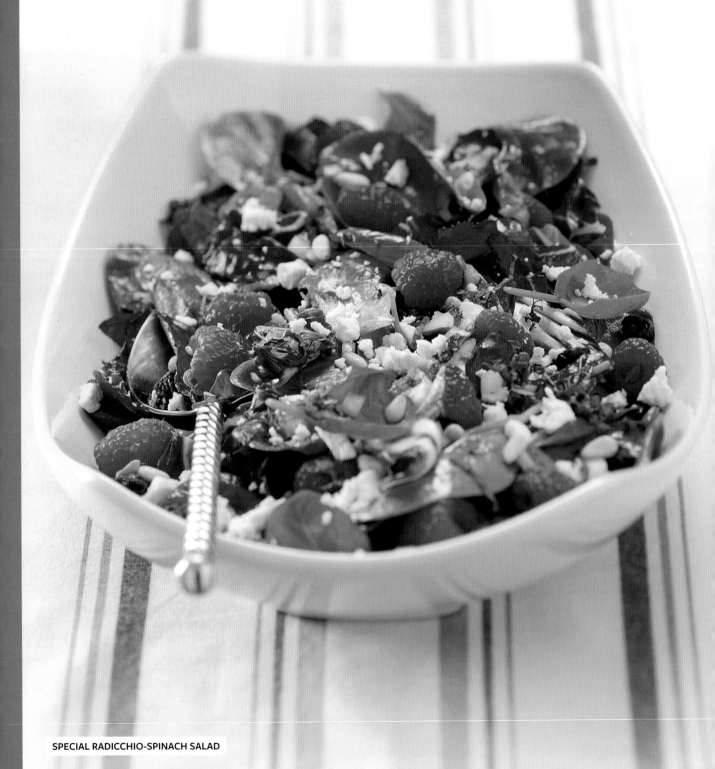

SPECIAL RADICCHIO-SPINACH SALAD

Special Radicchio-Spinach Salad

Enjoy a spicy-sweet salad when you mix mint, chipotle pepper and honey together in my special recipe.

—ROXANNE CHAN ALBANY, CA

START TO FINISH: 20 MIN.
MAKES: 12 SERVINGS

- 6 **cups fresh baby spinach**
- 1 **head radicchio, torn**
- 2 **cups fresh raspberries**
- ½ **cup raisins**
- ¼ **cup pine nuts, toasted**
- ¼ **cup thinly sliced red onion**
- ¼ **cup minced fresh mint**
- 3 **tablespoons lime juice**
- 2 **tablespoons olive oil**
- 2 **teaspoons honey**
- 1½ **to 3 teaspoons chopped chipotle pepper in adobo sauce**
- ¼ **teaspoon salt**
- ½ **cup crumbled feta cheese**

In a large salad bowl, combine the first seven ingredients. In a small saucepan, combine the lime juice, oil, honey, chipotle pepper and salt. Cook and stir until blended and heated through. Immediately pour over salad; toss to coat. Sprinkle with cheese.

PER SERVING *¾ cup equals 92 cal., 5 g fat (1 g sat. fat), 3 mg chol., 117 mg sodium, 11 g carb., 3 g fiber, 3 g pro.* **Diabetic Exchanges:** *1 vegetable, 1 fat, ½ fruit.*

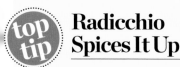

top tip

Radicchio Spices It Up

The crunchy purple leaves of radicchio lend a change-of-pace flavor to salads, offering a nutty, slightly bitter taste.

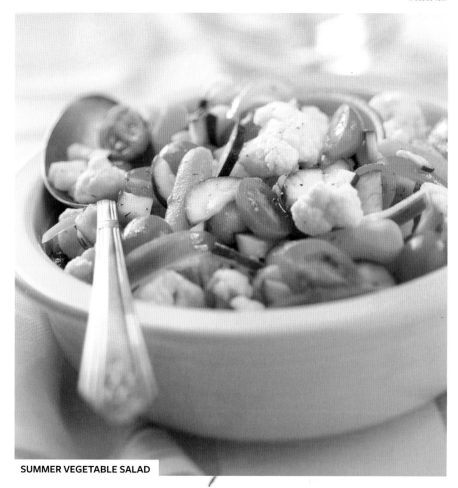

SUMMER VEGETABLE SALAD

Summer Vegetable Salad

We're always looking for ways to use our fresh garden produce, and this salad is great because you can basically include any type of vegetable you have on hand. You'll love the dill dressing.

—MARI ROSEBERRY DUNNING, NE

PREP: 15 MIN. + CHILLING
MAKES: 6 SERVINGS

- 1 **cup fresh cauliflowerets**
- 1 **cup fresh baby carrots**
- 1 **cup sliced red onion**
- 1 **cup halved grape tomatoes**
- 1 **cup chopped zucchini**
- 3 **tablespoons cider vinegar**
- 2 **tablespoons olive oil**
- 1 **teaspoon dill weed**
- ½ **teaspoon salt**
- ½ **teaspoon ground mustard**
- ¼ **to ½ teaspoon garlic powder**
- ¼ **teaspoon pepper**

1. In a large bowl, combine the cauliflower, carrots, onion, tomatoes and zucchini. In a small bowl, whisk the remaining ingredients. Pour over vegetables and toss to coat.
2. Cover and refrigerate for at least 2 hours, stirring occasionally. Serve with a slotted spoon.

PER SERVING *⅔ cup equals 75 cal., 5 g fat (1 g sat. fat), 0 chol., 226 mg sodium, 8 g carb., 2 g fiber, 1 g pro.* **Diabetic Exchanges:** *1 vegetable, 1 fat.*

Zesty Greek Salad

Regardless of what you're serving for your main course, this salad topped with feta cheese and olives makes the ideal side.

—ANGELA LEINENBACH MECHANICSVILLE, VA

START TO FINISH: 25 MIN.
MAKES: 2 SERVINGS

- 2 cups torn red leaf lettuce
- 1 small tomato, cut into wedges
- 4 cucumber slices, halved
- 2 radishes, sliced
- 1 red onion slice, quartered
- 2 tablespoons sliced ripe olives
- 1 tablespoon crumbled feta cheese

DRESSING

- 1 tablespoon red wine vinegar
- 2 teaspoons water
- 2 teaspoons olive oil
- 1 garlic clove, minced
- ¼ teaspoon sugar
- ⅛ teaspoon salt
  Dash pepper

In a small bowl, combine the lettuce, tomato, cucumber, radishes, onion, olives and feta cheese. In a small bowl, whisk the dressing ingredients. Drizzle over salad and toss to coat.

PER SERVING *89 cal., 6 g fat (1 g sat. fat), 2 mg chol., 265 mg sodium, 7 g carb., 2 g fiber, 2 g pro.* **Diabetic Exchanges:** *1 vegetable, 1 fat.*

ZESTY GREEK SALAD

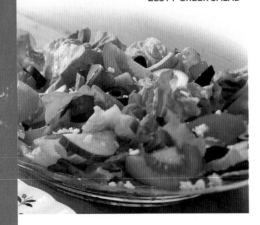

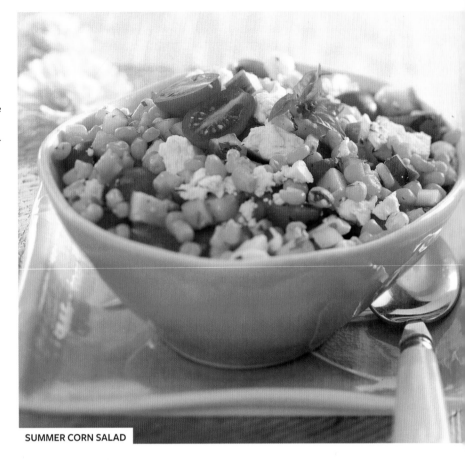

SUMMER CORN SALAD

Summer Corn Salad

This beautiful salad captures the best of summer. Full of fresh veggies, basil and feta cheese, this tangy take on the season's finest will be a hit with the whole family.

—PRISCILLA YEE CONCORD, CA

PREP: 20 MIN. + STANDING
MAKES: 4 SERVINGS

- 5 teaspoons olive oil, divided
- 1 tablespoon lime juice
- ¼ teaspoon salt
- ¼ teaspoon hot pepper sauce
- 1½ cups fresh or frozen corn, thawed
- 1½ cups cherry tomatoes, halved
- ½ cup finely chopped cucumber
- ¼ cup finely chopped red onion
- 2 tablespoons minced fresh basil or 2 teaspoons dried basil
- ¼ cup crumbled feta cheese

1. In a small bowl, whisk 4 teaspoons oil, lime juice, salt and pepper sauce; set aside.

2. In a large skillet, cook and stir corn in remaining oil over medium-high heat until tender. Transfer to a salad bowl; cool slightly. Add the tomatoes, cucumber, onion and basil. Drizzle with dressing and toss to coat.

3. Let stand for 10 minutes before serving or refrigerate until chilled. Sprinkle with the feta cheese just before serving.

PER SERVING *136 cal., 8 g fat (2 g sat. fat), 4 mg chol., 231 mg sodium, 16 g carb., 3 g fiber, 4 g pro.* **Diabetic Exchanges:** *1½ fat, 1 starch.*

Portobello Spinach Salad

You won't miss the meat when you throw some grilled portobellos into this satisfying salad. It makes a great entree, too!

—**THOMAS MC CLEARY** KANSAS CITY, KS

PREP: 15 MIN. + MARINATING • **GRILL:** 10 MIN.
MAKES: 6 SERVINGS

- 1 **cup orange juice**
- ¼ **cup olive oil**
- 4 **teaspoons grated orange peel**
- 1 **teaspoon fennel seed**
- ½ **teaspoon pepper**
- ¼ **teaspoon salt**
- ½ **pound sliced baby portobello mushrooms**
- 1 **package (6 ounces) fresh baby spinach**
- 1 **can (11 ounces) mandarin oranges, drained**
- ½ **medium red onion, thinly sliced**
- ¼ **cup slivered almonds**

1. In a small bowl, combine the first six ingredients. Pour ½ cup marinade into a large resealable plastic bag. Add the mushrooms; seal bag and turn to coat. Refrigerate for 15 minutes. Cover and refrigerate remaining marinade.

2. Drain mushrooms and discard marinade. Transfer mushrooms to a grill wok or basket. Grill, uncovered, over medium heat for 8-12 minutes or until tender, stirring frequently. Cool slightly.

3. Meanwhile, in a large bowl, combine the spinach, oranges, onion, almonds and grilled mushrooms. Drizzle with reserved marinade; toss to coat. Serve immediately.

NOTE *If you do not have a grill wok or basket, use a disposable foil pan. Poke holes in the bottom of the pan with a meat fork to allow liquid to drain.*

PER SERVING *1 cup equals 129 cal., 8 g fat (1 g sat. fat), 0 chol., 90 mg sodium, 12 g carb., 2 g fiber, 3 g pro.* **Diabetic Exchanges:** *1½ fat, 1 vegetable, ½ starch.*

Layered Salad with Curry Dressing

If you love classic seven-layer salads, you'll want to dig into this recipe. Curry powder adds a unique twist, while sliced almonds give it a nice crunch.

—**KERRI PELZ** HENDERSONVILLE, NC

START TO FINISH: 20 MIN.
MAKES: 16 SERVINGS

- 1 **package (10 ounces) ready-to-serve salad greens**
- 2 **celery ribs, chopped**
- ½ **cup chopped green pepper**
- ½ **cup chopped cauliflower**
- 2 **green onions, thinly sliced**
- 1 **package (10 ounces) frozen peas, thawed**
- ¾ **cup fat-free mayonnaise**
- ¾ **cup (6 ounces) reduced-fat plain yogurt**
- 1 **tablespoon lemon juice**
- 1 **teaspoon curry powder**
- ¾ **cup shredded reduced-fat cheddar cheese**
- ½ **cup sliced almonds**

1. In a 3-qt. glass bowl, layer the salad greens, celery, pepper, cauliflower, green onions and peas.

2. In a small bowl, whisk the mayonnaise, yogurt, lemon juice and curry; carefully spread over salad. Sprinkle with cheese. Chill until serving. Just before serving, sprinkle with almonds.

PER SERVING *¾ cup equals 67 cal., 3 g fat (1 g sat. fat), 6 mg chol., 161 mg sodium, 7 g carb., 2 g fiber, 4 g pro.* **Diabetic Exchanges:** *½ starch, ½ fat.*

PORTOBELLO SPINACH SALAD

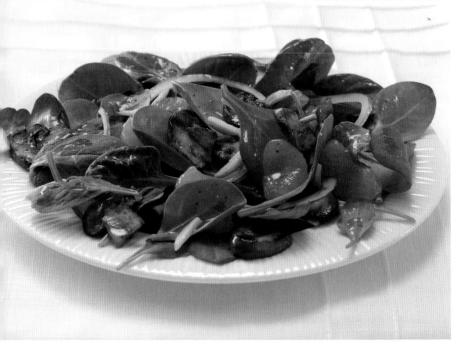

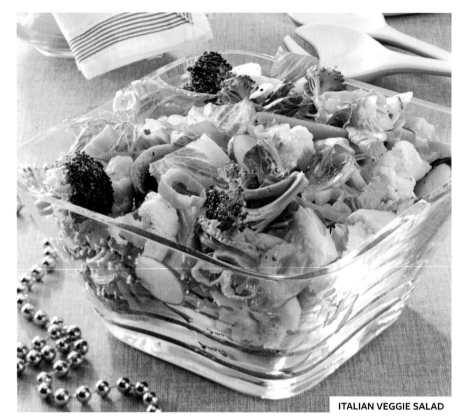

ITALIAN VEGGIE SALAD

Italian Veggie Salad

I first created this recipe for a community charity drive. Now I get recipe requests often and have brought it to at least six events this year.

—**DENISE MURPHY** WATERLOO, IA

PREP: 30 MIN. + CHILLING
MAKES: 16 SERVINGS

- **2 cups fresh baby carrots, quartered lengthwise**
- **1¾ cups thinly sliced radishes**
- **2 celery ribs, sliced**
- **1 small head cauliflower, broken into florets**
- **1 bunch broccoli, cut into florets**
- **6 large fresh mushrooms, thinly sliced**
- **1 can (2¼ ounces) sliced ripe olives, drained**
- **1 package Italian salad dressing mix**
- **⅓ cup water**
- **⅓ cup white vinegar**
- **⅓ cup olive oil**
- **1 package (9 ounces) hearts of romaine salad mix**
  Pepperoncini, optional

1. In a large bowl, combine the first seven ingredients. In a small bowl, whisk the dressing mix, water, vinegar and oil. Pour over the vegetables; toss to coat. Cover and refrigerate for at least 4 hours.

2. Just before serving, place romaine in a large serving bowl. Add vegetables; toss to coat. Top with pepperoncini if desired.

NOTE *Look for pepperoncinis (pickled peppers) in the pickle and olive section of your grocery store.*

PER SERVING *1 cup equals 75 cal., 5 g fat (1 g. sat. fat), 0 chol., 237 mg sodium, 6 g carb., 3 g fiber, 2 g pro.* **Diabetic Exchanges:** *1 vegetable, 1 fat.*

Broccoli & Sweet Potato Salad

You'll experience a medley of flavor when you bite into this refreshing, colorful salad. The veggies are lightly coated with a simple dressing and accented with thyme and a little feta cheese.

—**MARY ANN DELL** PHOENIXVILLE, PA

PREP: 15 MIN. • **BAKE:** 30 MIN. + COOLING
MAKES: 8 SERVINGS

- **4 cups cubed peeled sweet potatoes (about 2 large)**
- **2 medium sweet red peppers, sliced**
- **6 fresh thyme sprigs**
- **7 teaspoons olive oil, divided**
- **4 cups fresh broccoli florets**
- **½ cup crumbled feta cheese**
- **2 tablespoons sunflower kernels**
- **2 tablespoons cider vinegar**
- **½ teaspoon salt**
- **¼ teaspoon pepper**

1. Place the sweet potatoes, red peppers and thyme in a greased 15x10 x1-in. baking pan. Drizzle with 3 teaspoons oil. Bake, uncovered, at 400° for 30-45 minutes or until potatoes are tender, stirring once. Cool; discard thyme sprigs.

2. Fill a large saucepan half full of water; bring to a boil. Add broccoli; cover and boil for 2 minutes. Drain and immediately place in ice water. Drain and pat dry.

3. In a large bowl, combine the roasted vegetables, broccoli, cheese and sunflower kernels. In a small bowl, whisk the vinegar, salt, pepper and remaining oil. Pour over vegetable mixture and gently toss to coat.

PER SERVING *1cup equals 141 cal., 6 g fat (1 g sat. fat), 4 mg chol., 272 mg sodium, 18 g carb., 4 g fiber, 4 g pro.* **Diabetic Exchanges:** *1 starch, 1 vegetable, 1 fat.*

Flavorful Rice Salad

I started with a basic bean, rice and onion medley and added veggies and a lighter dressing to make it a healthy option for dinner. You can substitute brown rice for the long grain.

—KIM COOK DADE CITY, FL

PREP: 15 MIN. + CHILLING
MAKES: 6 SERVINGS

- 1 can (15 ounces) black beans, rinsed and drained
- 1½ cups cold cooked long grain rice
- 1½ cups chopped fresh tomatoes (about 4 medium)
- 4 green onions, chopped
- 1 celery rib, chopped
- ½ cup chopped fresh spinach
- 2 tablespoons minced fresh cilantro
- ½ cup fat-free Italian salad dressing
- 1 cup (4 ounces) crumbled feta cheese

1. In a large bowl, combine the beans, rice, tomatoes, onions, celery, spinach and cilantro. Drizzle with dressing; toss to coat. Cover and refrigerate for 1 hour.

2. Just before serving, sprinkle with the cheese.

PER SERVING *⅔ cup equals 181 cal., 3 g fat (2 g sat. fat), 11 mg chol., 617 mg sodium, 27 g carb., 5 g fiber, 9 g pro. Diabetic Exchanges: 2 starch, 1 lean meat.*

FLAVORFUL RICE SALAD

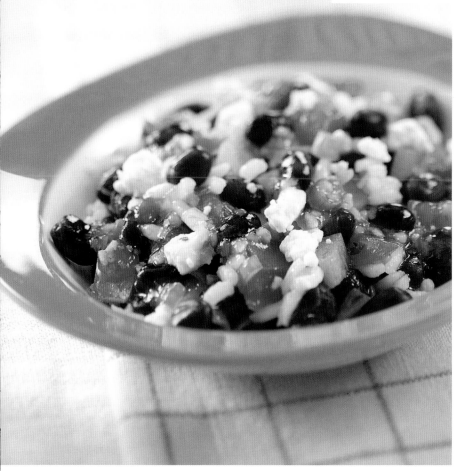

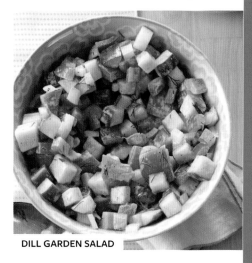

DILL GARDEN SALAD

Dill Garden Salad

Don't be afraid to throw in any fresh veggies you have on hand when making this recipe.

—BETHANY MARTIN LEWISBURG, PA

START TO FINISH: 15 MIN.
MAKES: 6 SERVINGS

- 3 cups chopped English cucumber
- 1 large tomato, seeded and cut into ½-inch pieces
- 1 small sweet red pepper, chopped
- 2 tablespoons chopped sweet onion
- 3 tablespoons reduced-fat mayonnaise
- 4 teaspoons olive oil
- 2 teaspoons rice vinegar
- 2 teaspoons sugar
- ½ teaspoon salt
- ¼ teaspoon garlic powder
- ¼ teaspoon pepper
- 2½ teaspoons snipped fresh dill

In a large bowl, combine cucumbers, tomato, red pepper and onion. In a small bowl, whisk mayonnaise, oil, vinegar, sugar, salt, garlic powder and pepper until blended. Stir in dill. Spoon dressing over salad; toss to coat.

PER SERVING *1 cup equals 75 cal., 6 g fat (1 g sat. fat), 3 mg chol., 260 mg sodium, 6 g carb., 1 g fiber, 1 g pro. Diabetic Exchanges: 1 vegetable, 1 fat.*

Minted Cucumber Salad

Fresh herbs season the cucumbers and tomatoes in this easy salad. I'm a busy mother and pastor's wife and am always looking for new recipes that can be prepared quickly without sacrificing taste or nutritional value. This dish hits all three of the criteria.

—**DEBBIE PURDUE** WESTLAND, MI

START TO FINISH: 20 MIN.
MAKES: 6 SERVINGS

- 2 **large cucumbers, chopped**
- 2 **cups seeded chopped tomatoes**
- ½ **cup chopped fresh mint**
- ½ **cup chopped fresh parsley**
- ½ **cup thinly sliced green onions**
- ¼ **cup lemon juice**
- ¼ **cup olive oil**
- 1 **teaspoon salt**
- ¼ **teaspoon pepper**

In a large bowl, combine the first five ingredients. In a small bowl, whisk the lemon juice, oil, salt and pepper. Add to cucumber mixture; toss to coat.

PER SERVING *¾ cup equals 113 cal., 9 g fat (1 g sat. fat), 0 chol., 403 mg sodium, 7 g carb., 2 g fiber, 2 g pro.* **Diabetic Exchanges:** *2 fat, 1 vegetable.*

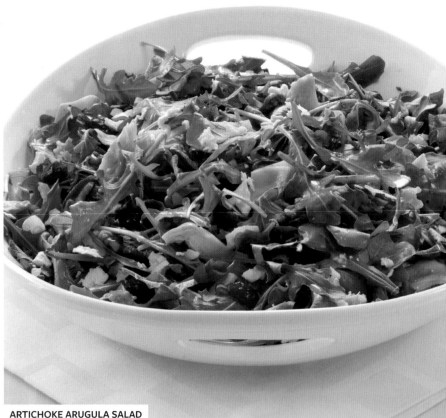

ARTICHOKE ARUGULA SALAD

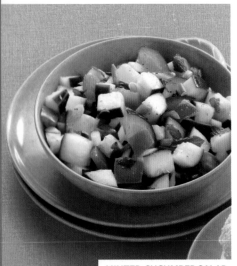

MINTED CUCUMBER SALAD

Artichoke Arugula Salad

Packed with artichokes and dried cranberries, this might be your family's new favorite salad recipe.

—**BARBARA BEGLEY** FAIRFIELD, OH

START TO FINISH: 25 MIN.
MAKES: 10 SERVINGS

- 8 **cups fresh arugula or baby spinach**
- 1 **can (14 ounces) water-packed artichoke hearts, rinsed, drained and chopped**
- 1 **cup dried cranberries**
- ¾ **cup chopped pecans, toasted**
- 4 **green onions, chopped**
- ½ **cup reduced-fat raspberry vinaigrette**
- ¾ **cup crumbled feta cheese**

In a large bowl, combine the first five ingredients. Drizzle with vinaigrette; toss to coat. Sprinkle with cheese.

NOTE *To toast nuts, spread in a 15x10x1-in. baking pan. Bake at 350° for 5-10 minutes or until lightly browned, stirring occasionally. Or, spread in a dry nonstick skillet and heat over low heat until lightly browned, stirring occasionally.*

PER SERVING *1 cup equals 158 cal., 9 g fat (2 g sat. fat), 5 mg chol., 314 mg sodium, 16 g carb., 2 g fiber, 4 g pro.* **Diabetic Exchanges:** *1½ fat, 1 starch.*

Good!

Potato Salad

I made this salad when I worked in a small hospital. It was also served in the cafeteria and to patients who were both diabetic and on regular diets.

—**DOROTHY BAYES** SARDIS, OH

PREP: 30 MIN. + CHILLING
MAKES: 6 SERVINGS

- 4 **cups cubed peeled potatoes**
- 1 **celery rib, thinly sliced**
- ⅓ **cup finely chopped onion**
- ⅓ **cup sweet pickle relish**
- ¾ **cup fat-free mayonnaise**
- 1 **teaspoon ground mustard**
- ½ **teaspoon salt**
- ¼ **teaspoon celery seed**
- ⅛ **teaspoon pepper**
- 2 **hard-cooked eggs, sliced**
- ⅛ **teaspoon paprika**

1. Place potatoes in a large saucepan and cover with water. Bring to a boil. Reduce heat; cover and simmer for 10-15 minutes or until tender. Drain and cool to room temperature.

2. In a large bowl, combine the potatoes, celery, onion and relish. In a small bowl, combine the mayonnaise, mustard, salt, celery seed and pepper. Pour over the potato mixture and toss to coat.

3. Cover and refrigerate until chilled. Top with eggs and sprinkle with paprika.

PER SERVING *¾ cup equals 163 cal., 3 g fat (1 g sat. fat), 74 mg chol., 582 mg sodium, 31 g carb., 3 g fiber, 4 g pro.* **Diabetic Exchanges:** *2 starch, ½ fat.*

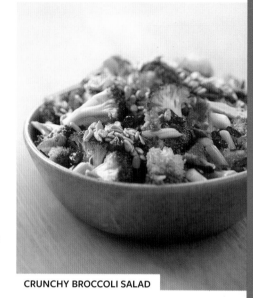

CRUNCHY BROCCOLI SALAD

Crunchy Broccoli Salad

Although I wasn't always a fan of broccoli, I'm now hooked on this salad. It gives broccoli a whole new look and appeal.

—**JESSICA CONREY** CEDAR RAPIDS, IA

START TO FINISH: 25 MIN.
MAKES: 10 SERVINGS

- 8 **cups fresh broccoli florets (about 1 pound)**
- 1 **bunch green onions, thinly sliced**
- ½ **cup dried cranberries**
- 3 **tablespoons canola oil**
- 3 **tablespoons seasoned rice vinegar**
- 2 **tablespoons sugar**
- ¼ **cup sunflower kernels**
- 3 **bacon strips, cooked and crumbled**

In a bowl, combine broccoli, onions and cranberries. In a small bowl, whisk oil, vinegar and sugar until blended; drizzle over broccoli and toss to coat. Refrigerate until serving. Sprinkle with sunflower kernels and bacon.

PER SERVING *¾ cup equals 121 cal., 7 g fat (1 g sat. fat), 2 mg chol., 233 mg sodium, 14 g carb., 3 g fiber, 3 g pro.* **Diabetic Exchanges:** *1 vegetable, 1 fat, ½ starch.*

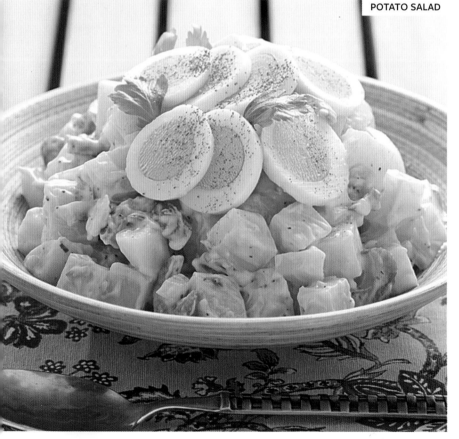

POTATO SALAD

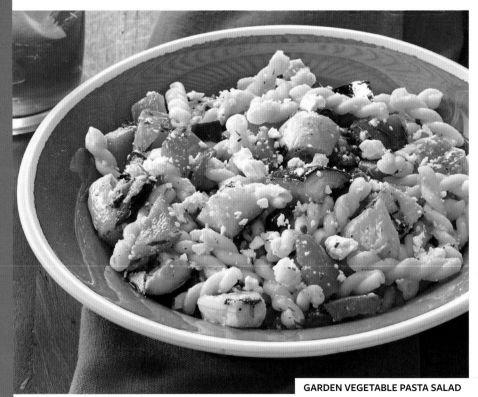
GARDEN VEGETABLE PASTA SALAD

Garden Vegetable Pasta Salad

My family has long enjoyed grilling veggies, so one day I added pasta to make a more filling dish. Then, to give the salad a Mediterranean flair, I tossed in some olives and feta cheese.

—TINA REPAK MIRILOVICH JOHNSTOWN, PA

PREP: 40 MIN. • **GRILL:** 10 MIN.
MAKES: 26 SERVINGS

- 1 **pound fusilli or pasta of your choice**
- 2 **medium eggplant**
- 2 **medium zucchini**
- 2 **medium yellow summer squash**
- 1 **large red onion, cut into ½-inch slices**
- 1 **medium sweet red pepper, cut in half and seeds removed**
- ¼ **cup olive oil**
- ½ **teaspoon salt**
- ¼ **teaspoon pepper**
- 3 **plum tomatoes, chopped**
- 1½ **cups (6 ounces) crumbled feta cheese**
- 2 **cans (2¼ ounces each) sliced ripe olives, drained**
- 2 **tablespoons minced fresh parsley**

PARMESAN VINAIGRETTE
- ¾ **cup olive oil**
- ⅓ **cup grated Parmesan cheese**
- ⅓ **cup white wine vinegar**
- 3 **tablespoons lemon juice**
- 1 **teaspoon sugar**
- 1 **garlic clove, minced**
- 1 **teaspoon salt**
- ½ **teaspoon dried oregano**
- ½ **teaspoon pepper**

1. Cook the pasta according to package directions; drain and rinse in cold water. Place in a large bowl and set aside.

2. Meanwhile, cut the eggplant, zucchini and summer squash lengthwise into ¾-in.-thick slices.

Brush the eggplant, zucchini, summer squash, red onion and red pepper with oil; sprinkle with salt and pepper. Grill vegetables, covered, over medium heat for 4-6 minutes on each side or until crisp-tender. When cool enough to handle, cut into cubes.

3. Add the tomatoes, feta cheese, olives, parsley and grilled vegetables to the pasta. In a small bowl, whisk the vinaigrette ingredients. Pour over salad; toss to coat. Cover and refrigerate until serving.

PER SERVING ¾ cup equals 185 cal., 11 g fat (2 g sat. fat), 4 mg chol., 262 mg sodium, 19 g carb., 3 g fiber, 5 g pro. *Diabetic Exchanges: 1½ fat, 1 starch, 1 vegetable.*

Fruit Cup with Honey-Lime Syrup

I often experiment with fresh fruit for side dishes, and drizzling sweet lime syrup on top of this medley adds a nice zip.

—DAWN E. BRYANT THEDFORD, NE

PREP: 15 MIN. + COOLING
MAKES: 4 SERVINGS

- ⅓ **cup white wine**
- 2 **tablespoons lime juice**
- 2 **tablespoons honey**
- 2 **cups cubed cantaloupe**
- 1 **cup green grapes, halved**
- 1 **cup red grapes, halved**

1. In a small saucepan over medium heat, bring the wine, lime juice and honey to a boil. Reduce heat; simmer, uncovered, until liquid is syrupy and reduced to about ¼ cup. Remove from the heat; cool completely.

2. In a large bowl, combine the fruit. Drizzle with syrup; gently toss to coat.

PER SERVING 1 cup equals 135 cal., 1 g fat (trace sat. fat), 0 chol., 10 mg sodium, 31 g carb., 1 g fiber, 1 g pro. *Diabetic Exchanges: 1½ fruit, ½ starch.*

Quinoa Tabouleh

When my mom and sister developed several food allergies, we had to modify many recipes. I substituted quinoa for couscous in this tabouleh, and now we make it all the time.

—JENNIFER KLANN CORBETT, OR

PREP: 35 MIN. + CHILLING
MAKES: 8 SERVINGS

- 2 cups water
- 1 cup quinoa, rinsed
- 1 can (15 ounces) black beans, rinsed and drained
- 1 small cucumber, peeled and chopped
- 1 small sweet red pepper, chopped
- ⅓ cup minced fresh parsley
- ¼ cup lemon juice
- 2 tablespoons olive oil
- ½ teaspoon salt
- ½ teaspoon pepper

1. In a large saucepan, bring water to a boil. Add quinoa. Reduce heat; cover and simmer for 12-15 minutes or until liquid is absorbed. Remove from the heat; fluff with a fork. Transfer to a bowl; cool completely.

2. Add the beans, cucumber, red pepper and parsley. In a small bowl, whisk the remaining ingredients; drizzle over salad and toss to coat. Refrigerate until chilled.

NOTE *Look for quinoa in the cereal, rice or organic food aisle.*

PER SERVING *¾ cup equals 159 cal., 5 g fat (1 g sat. fat), 0 chol., 255 mg sodium, 24 g carb., 4 g fiber, 6 g pro.* **Diabetic Exchanges:** *1½ starch, 1 fat.*

Fruit & Cream Layered Salad

Being from the South, I love salads, especially fruit salads. I also try to cook healthier foods, so I came up with this take on a layered salad.

—APRIL LANE GREENEVILLE, TN

START TO FINISH: 25 MIN.
MAKES: 13 SERVINGS

- 3 ounces reduced-fat cream cheese
- 1 tablespoon sugar
- 2 teaspoons lemon juice
- ¼ teaspoon almond extract
- ¾ cup (6 ounces) strawberry yogurt
- 2 cups reduced-fat whipped topping
- 3 medium peaches, peeled and sliced
- 2 cups halved fresh strawberries
- 2 cups fresh blueberries
- 2 cups green grapes
- 1 can (11 ounces) mandarin oranges, drained
- ¼ cup sliced almonds, toasted
  Fresh strawberries, optional

1. In a small bowl, beat the cream cheese, sugar, lemon juice and extract until smooth. Add yogurt; beat until blended. Fold in whipped topping.

2. In a 3-qt. trifle bowl, layer the peaches, strawberries and blueberries. Top with half of the whipped topping mixture. Layer with grapes, oranges and remaining whipped topping mixture. Refrigerate until serving.

3. Sprinkle with almonds just before serving. Garnish with strawberries if desired.

PER SERVING *¾ cup equals 124 cal., 4 g fat (2 g sat. fat), 5 mg chol., 37 mg sodium, 22 g carb., 2 g fiber, 2 g pro.* **Diabetic Exchanges:** *1 fruit, ½ starch, ½ fat.*

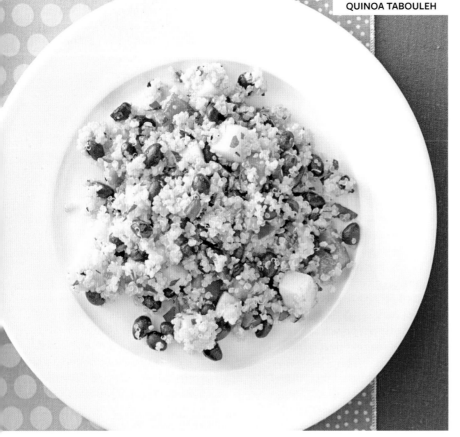

QUINOA TABOULEH

Colorful Gazpacho Salad

A friend first introduced me to this salad, and I'm glad she did! Tomatoes and jicama are topped with cilantro for a specialty you can serve year-round.

—**BRENDA HOFFMAN** STANTON, MI

PREP: 20 MIN. + CHILLING
MAKES: 8 SERVINGS

- 5 medium tomatoes, seeded and chopped
- 1 cup chopped peeled cucumber
- ¾ cup chopped red onion
- 1 small sweet red pepper, chopped
- ½ cup fresh or frozen corn
- 1 tablespoon lime juice
- 1 tablespoon red wine vinegar
- 2 teaspoons water
- 2 garlic cloves, minced
- 1 teaspoon olive oil
- ¼ teaspoon salt
- ¼ teaspoon pepper
- ⅛ teaspoon crushed red pepper flakes
- 8 cups torn romaine
- 1 cup diced peeled jicama
- ½ cup minced fresh cilantro

1. In a large bowl, combine the tomatoes, cucumber, onion, red pepper and corn. In a small bowl, whisk the lime juice, vinegar, water, garlic, oil, salt, pepper and pepper flakes. Drizzle over tomato mixture; toss to coat. Refrigerate until chilled.

2. Just before serving, combine the romaine, jicama and cilantro. Place 1 cup on each of eight salad plates; top each with ⅓ cup tomato mixture.

PER SERVING *58 cal., 1 g fat (trace sat. fat), 0 chol., 87 mg sodium, 12 g carb., 4 g fiber, 2 g pro.* **Diabetic Exchange:** *2 vegetable.*

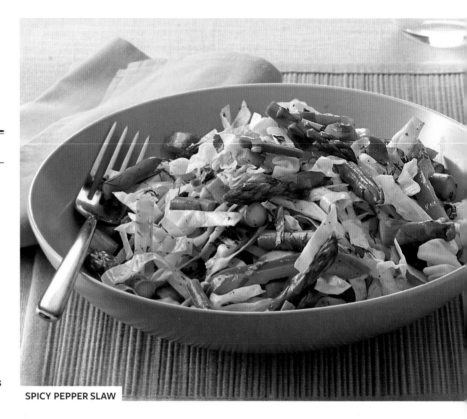

SPICY PEPPER SLAW

Spicy Pepper Slaw

In addition to making a great side, this slaw is wonderful piled on top of a chicken sandwich or burger. Jalapenos give it just the right kick.

—**CHERYL MC CLEARY** KANSAS CITY, KS

PREP: 20 MIN. + CHILLING
MAKES: 8 SERVINGS

- 3 cups shredded cabbage
- 2 celery ribs, chopped
- 1 medium green pepper, julienned
- 1 cup cut fresh green beans (1-inch pieces)
- 1 cup cut fresh asparagus (1-inch pieces)
- 1 bunch green onions, chopped
- 1 banana pepper, seeded and chopped
- 2 jalapeno peppers, seeded and chopped
- 2 serrano peppers, seeded and chopped
- ½ cup cider vinegar
- 3 tablespoons olive oil
- 1 tablespoon lime juice
- 1 tablespoon minced fresh thyme
- 1 tablespoon snipped fresh dill
- 1 tablespoon minced fresh cilantro
- 1 teaspoon salt
- 1 teaspoon pepper

In a large bowl, combine the first nine ingredients. In a small bowl, whisk the remaining ingredients; pour over salad and toss to coat. Refrigerate for at least 1 hour before serving.

NOTE *Wear disposable gloves when cutting hot peppers; the oils can burn skin. Avoid touching your face.*

PER SERVING *1 cup equals 76 cal., 5 g fat (1 g sat. fat), 0 chol., 314 mg sodium, 6 g carb., 3 g fiber, 2 g pro.* **Diabetic Exchanges:** *1 vegetable, 1 fat.*

Mandarin Watermelon Salad

Fruit tossed with feta? You bet! In fact, there's nothing better! Fresh mint, cilantro and parsley add the perfect pop. I'm always looking for something different to serve my vegetarian mom, and she loved this!

—JADE BAUSELL MIAMI, FL

START TO FINISH: 20 MIN.
MAKES: 8 SERVINGS

- 4½ cups cubed seedless watermelon
- 1 can (11 ounces) mandarin oranges, drained
- ½ small red onion, sliced
- ¼ cup crumbled feta cheese
- 2 tablespoons minced fresh mint
- 2 tablespoons minced fresh cilantro
- 2 tablespoons lime juice
- 1 tablespoon minced fresh parsley

Place all ingredients in a large bowl; gently toss to combine. Serve immediately.

PER SERVING *¾ cup equals 48 cal., 1 g fat (trace sat. fat), 2 mg chol., 39 mg sodium, 12 g carb., 1 g fiber, 1 g pro.* **Diabetic Exchange:** *1 fruit.*

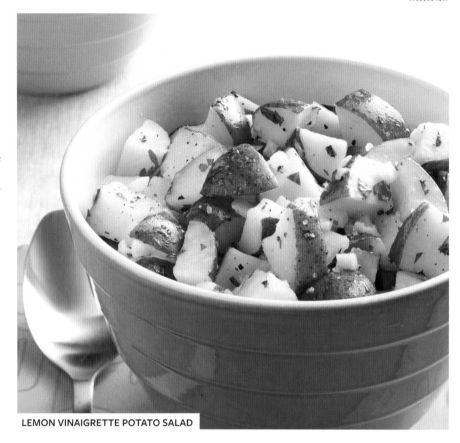

LEMON VINAIGRETTE POTATO SALAD

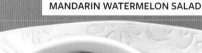

MANDARIN WATERMELON SALAD

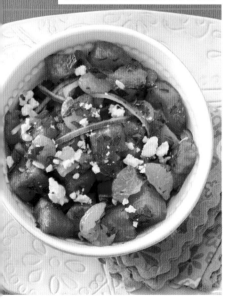

Lemon Vinaigrette Potato Salad

My friend needed a potato salad that could withstand Fourth of July weather, so I developed this recipe for her. The vinaigrette offers a safe and delicious alternative to traditional mayonnaise-based potato salads. I've also substituted fresh thyme for the basil, although any fresh herbs would be great!

—MELANIE CLOYD MULLICA HILL, NJ

PREP: 25 MIN. • **COOK:** 15 MIN.
MAKES: 12 SERVINGS

- 3 pounds red potatoes, cut into 1-inch cubes
- ½ cup olive oil
- 3 tablespoons lemon juice
- 2 tablespoons minced fresh basil
- 2 tablespoons minced fresh parsley
- 1 tablespoon red wine vinegar
- 1 teaspoon grated lemon peel
- ¾ teaspoon salt
- ½ teaspoon pepper
- 1 small onion, finely chopped

1. Place potatoes in a large saucepan and cover with water. Bring to a boil. Reduce heat; cover and simmer for 10-15 minutes or until tender. Meanwhile, in a small bowl, whisk the oil, lemon juice, herbs, vinegar, lemon peel, salt and pepper.

2. Drain potatoes. Place in a large bowl; add onion. Drizzle with vinaigrette; toss to coat. Serve warm or chill until serving.

PER SERVING *¾ cup equals 165 cal., 9 g fat (1 g sat. fat), 0 chol., 155 mg sodium, 19 g carb., 2 g fiber, 2 g pro.* **Diabetic Exchanges:** *2 fat, 1 starch.*

side dishes

Once your main dish has been selected, you'll need **a side or two** to complete the meal. Choose between **dozens of fresh dishes** to take your next dinner to a tasty new level.

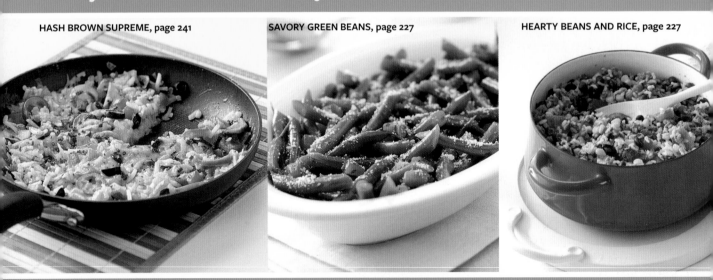

HASH BROWN SUPREME, page 241

SAVORY GREEN BEANS, page 227

HEARTY BEANS AND RICE, page 227

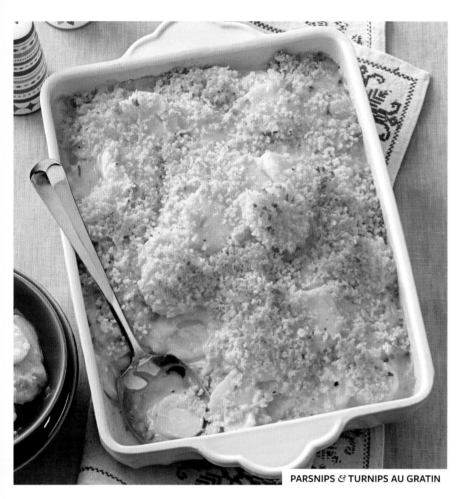

PARSNIPS & TURNIPS AU GRATIN

Parsnips & Turnips au Gratin

You don't need potatoes to make a delicious au gratin dish! I sometimes substitute rutabaga for the turnips. I definitely cherish having this recipe in my collection.

—**PRISCILLA GILBERT**

INDIAN HARBOUR BEACH, FL

PREP: 20 MIN. • **BAKE:** 15 MIN.
MAKES: 8 SERVINGS

- 1½ **pounds parsnips, peeled and sliced**
- 1¼ **pounds turnips, peeled and sliced**
- 1 **can (10¾ ounces) reduced-fat reduced-sodium condensed cream of celery soup, undiluted**
- 1 **cup fat-free milk**
- ½ **teaspoon pepper**
- 1 **cup (4 ounces) shredded sharp cheddar cheese**
- ½ **cup panko (Japanese) bread crumbs**
- 1 **tablespoon butter, melted**

1. Place parsnips and turnips in a large saucepan; cover with water. Bring to a boil. Reduce heat; simmer, uncovered, for 5-7 minutes or until crisp-tender.
2. Meanwhile, in a small saucepan, combine the soup, milk and pepper. Bring to a boil; reduce heat to low. Stir in cheese until melted. Drain the vegetables; transfer to an 11-in. x 7-in. baking dish coated with cooking spray. Pour sauce over vegetables.

3. Combine bread crumbs and butter; sprinkle over top. Bake, uncovered, at 400° for 15-20 minutes or until the vegetables are tender and the crumbs are golden brown.
PER SERVING ¾ cup equals 189 cal., 7 g fat (4 g sat. fat), 21 mg chol., 309 mg sodium, 27 g carb., 4 g fiber, 7 g pro. **Diabetic Exchanges:** 1 starch, 1 high-fat meat, 1 vegetable.

Cheesy Spinach Casserole

Packed with good-for-you spinach, this quichelike side dish will stand out.

—**MARILYN PARADIS** WOODBURN, OR

PREP: 10 MIN. • **BAKE:** 50 MIN.
MAKES: 6 SERVINGS

- ¾ **cup chopped onion**
- 1 **tablespoon butter**
- 2 **eggs**
- 1 **egg white**
- 1 **package (10 ounces) frozen chopped spinach, thawed and squeezed dry**
- 2 **cups (16 ounces) 2% cottage cheese**
- 1 **cup (4 ounces) shredded reduced-fat cheddar cheese**
- 3 **tablespoons all-purpose flour**
- ⅛ **teaspoon salt**

1. In a small nonstick skillet, saute onion in butter until tender. In a large bowl, combine the eggs, egg white and spinach. Stir in the cottage cheese, cheddar cheese, flour, salt and onion mixture. Pour into a 1½-qt. baking dish coated with cooking spray.
2. Bake, uncovered, at 350° for 50-60 minutes or until a thermometer reads 160°.
PER SERVING 199 cal., 9 g fat (5 g sat. fat), 95 mg chol., 440 mg sodium, 10 g carb., 2 g fiber, 20 g pro. **Diabetic Exchanges:** 2 lean meat, 1 vegetable, 1 fat.

Thyme Butternut Squash

Spices, such as cinnamon, nutmeg and mace, turn this butternut squash into a truly appetizing side.

—**ELEANOR DAVIS** SUN LAKES, AZ

PREP: 1¼ HOURS • **BAKE:** 35 MIN.
MAKES: 9 SERVINGS

- 1 **large butternut squash (5 to 6 pounds)**
- 1 **tablespoon brown sugar**
- 1 **tablespoon 2% milk**
- 1 **tablespoon orange juice concentrate**
- 1 **tablespoon butter**
- 1 **tablespoon maple syrup**
- 1 **tablespoon honey**
- 1 **teaspoon grated orange peel**
- 1 **teaspoon dried thyme**
- 1 **teaspoon ground cinnamon**
- ½ **teaspoon salt**
- ¼ **teaspoon ground nutmeg**
- ¼ **teaspoon ground mace**
- ¼ **teaspoon pepper**

1. Cut squash in half; discard seeds. Place squash cut side down in a 13-in. x 9-in. baking pan; add ½ in. of hot water. Cover and bake at 350° for 55-65 minutes or until squash is tender. Cool to room temperature.

2. Meanwhile, in a large bowl, combine the remaining ingredients. Remove squash from shell and add to bowl; mash until smooth. Transfer to an 8-in. square baking dish coated with cooking spray. Bake at 350° for 35-45 minutes or until heated through.

PER SERVING *¾ cup equals 141 cal., 2 g fat (1 g sat. fat), 3 mg chol., 151 mg sodium, 33 g carb., 8 g fiber, 2 g pro. Diabetic Exchange: 1½ starch.*

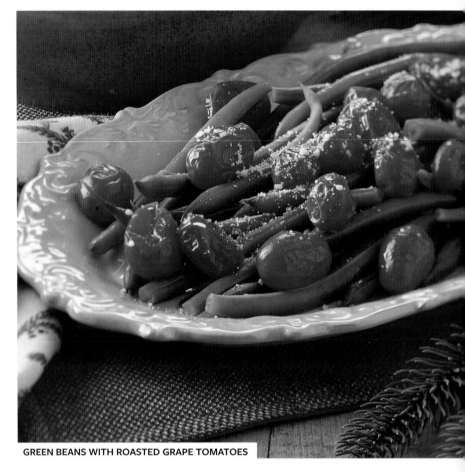

GREEN BEANS WITH ROASTED GRAPE TOMATOES

Green Beans with Roasted Grape Tomatoes

Roasted tomatoes top crisp-tender beans with a bit of sweetness, and grated cheese adds protein and flavor to this lovely dish.

—**MICHAELA ROSENTHAL** INDIO, CA

PREP: 10 MIN. • **BAKE:** 35 MIN.
MAKES: 10 SERVINGS

- 2 **teaspoons olive oil**
- ¼ **teaspoon grated lemon peel**
- 2 **pints grape tomatoes**
- ¼ **teaspoon celery salt**
  Dash white pepper
- 1½ **pounds fresh green beans, trimmed**
- 2 **tablespoons grated Romano or Parmesan cheese**

1. In a small bowl, combine oil and lemon peel. Place tomatoes in a greased 15-in. x 10-in. x 1-in. baking pan; drizzle with oil mixture. Sprinkle with celery salt and pepper; toss to coat. Bake at 350° for 35-40 minutes or until very tender, stirring once.

2. Meanwhile, place beans in a steamer basket; place in a saucepan over 1 in. of water. Bring to a boil; cover and steam for 7-8 minutes or until crisp-tender. Transfer to a serving plate.

3. Place tomatoes over the beans; sprinkle with cheese. Serve warm or at room temperature.

PER SERVING *¾ cup equals 45 cal., 2 g fat (trace sat. fat), 2 mg chol., 72 mg sodium, 7 g carb., 3 g fiber, 2 g pro. Diabetic Exchange: 1 vegetable.*

Hot and Zesty Quinoa

Quinoa, a nutritious grain and a complete protein, is a great substitute for potatoes or rice. This dish is easy to make and has a bit of a kick to it.

—**SANDRA LETIZIA** PROVIDENCE, RI

START TO FINISH: 25 MIN.
MAKES: 4 SERVINGS

- 1 **cup water**
- ½ **cup quinoa, rinsed**
- 1 **small onion, finely chopped**
- 1 **teaspoon olive oil**
- 2 **garlic cloves, minced**
- 1 **can (10 ounces) diced tomatoes and green chilies**
- 2 **tablespoons chopped marinated quartered artichoke hearts**
- 2 **tablespoons grated Parmesan cheese**

1. In a small saucepan, bring water to a boil. Add quinoa. Reduce heat; cover and simmer for 12-15 minutes or until liquid is absorbed. Remove from the heat; fluff with a fork.

2. In a large skillet, saute onion in oil until tender. Add garlic; cook 1 minute longer. Add tomatoes and green chilies. Bring to a boil over medium heat. Reduce heat; simmer, uncovered, for 10 minutes. Stir in the quinoa and artichoke; heat through. Sprinkle with the cheese.

NOTE *Look for quinoa in the cereal, rice or organic food aisle.*

PER SERVING *135 cal., 5 g fat (1 g sat. fat), 2 mg chol., 361 mg sodium, 20 g carb., 2 g fiber, 5 g pro.* **Diabetic Exchanges:** *1 starch, 1 vegetable, 1 fat.*

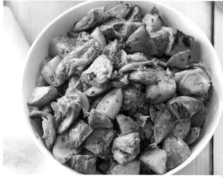

GARLIC AND ARTICHOKE ROASTED POTATOES

Garlic and Artichoke Roasted Potatoes

The artichokes in this side dish lend a gourmet appeal to the potatoes.

—**MARIE RIZZIO** INTERLOCHEN, MI

PREP: 15 MIN. • **BAKE:** 35 MIN.
MAKES: 10 SERVINGS

- 2½ **pounds medium red potatoes, cut into 1½-inch cubes**
- 2 **packages (8 ounces each) frozen artichoke hearts**
- 8 **garlic cloves, halved**
- 3 **tablespoons olive oil**
- ¾ **teaspoon salt**
- ¼ **teaspoon pepper**
- ¼ **cup lemon juice**
- 2 **tablespoons minced fresh parsley**
- 1 **teaspoon grated lemon peel**

1. Place the potatoes, artichokes and garlic in a 15-in. x 10-in. x 1-in. baking pan coated with cooking spray. Combine the oil, salt and pepper; drizzle over vegetables and toss to coat.

2. Bake, uncovered, at 425° for 35-40 minutes or until tender, stirring occasionally. Transfer to a large bowl. Add lemon juice, parsley and lemon peel; toss to coat. Serve warm.

PER SERVING *¾ cup equals 143 cal., 4 g fat (1 g sat. fat), 0 chol., 209 mg sodium, 24 g carb., 4 g fiber, 4 g pro.* **Diabetic Exchanges:** *1 starch, 1 vegetable, 1 fat.*

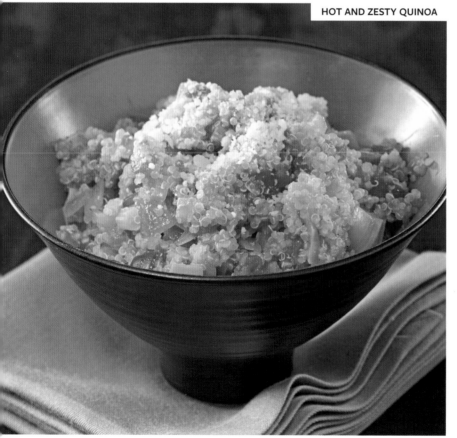

HOT AND ZESTY QUINOA

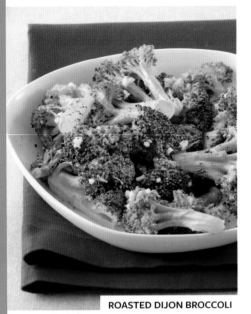

ROASTED DIJON BROCCOLI

Roasted Dijon Broccoli

Treat your taste buds to this twist on broccoli. You'll love the change!

—**AMY WINGENTER** TUSCALOOSA, AL

START TO FINISH: 20 MIN.
MAKES: 4 SERVINGS

- 1 **bunch broccoli, cut into florets**
- 2 **tablespoons olive oil**
- 1 **tablespoon red wine vinegar**
- 1 **teaspoon Dijon mustard**
- 1 **garlic clove, minced**
- ¼ **teaspoon salt**
- ¼ **teaspoon pepper**

1. Place broccoli on a baking sheet. In a small bowl, whisk the remaining ingredients. Drizzle over broccoli; toss to coat.
2. Bake, uncovered, at 425° for 10-15 minutes or until tender.
PER SERVING *106 cal., 7 g fat (1 g sat. fat), 0 chol., 219 mg sodium, 9 g carb., 5 g fiber, 5 g pro.* **Diabetic Exchanges:** *2 vegetable, 1 fat.*

Summer Squash Medley

Turn this side into a main dish, if desired, by adding cooked chicken or turkey sausage.

—**JENNIFER LEIGHTY** WEST SALEM, OH

START TO FINISH: 25 MIN.
MAKES: 6 SERVINGS

- 1 **large sweet onion, chopped**
- 1 **medium yellow summer squash, chopped**
- 1 **large green pepper, chopped**
- 1 **tablespoon olive oil**
- 1 **garlic clove, minced**
- 2 **large tomatoes, seeded and chopped**
- 1½ **teaspoons Italian seasoning**
- 1 **teaspoon salt**
- ½ **teaspoon pepper**
- ⅛ **teaspoon crushed red pepper flakes, optional**

In a large nonstick skillet, saute the onion, squash and green pepper in oil until crisp-tender. Add the garlic; cook 1 minute longer. Stir in the tomatoes, Italian seasoning, salt, pepper and pepper flakes if desired; heat through.
PER SERVING *⅔ cup calculated without crushed red pepper flakes equals 61 cal., 3 g fat (trace sat. fat), 0 chol., 403 mg sodium, 9 g carb., 2 g fiber, 2 g pro.* **Diabetic Exchanges:** *2 vegetable, ½ fat.*

SUMMER SQUASH MEDLEY

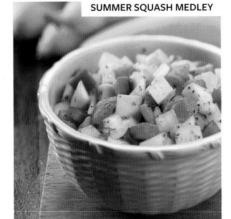

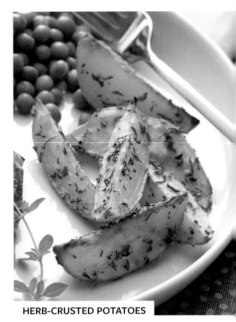

HERB-CRUSTED POTATOES

Herb-Crusted Potatoes

Seasoned with fresh rosemary and herbs, my savory potato wedges bring a pleasantly bold taste to any meal.

—**TASTE OF HOME TEST KITCHEN**

PREP: 10 MIN. • **BAKE:** 40 MIN.
MAKES: 4 SERVINGS

- 1½ **pounds Yukon Gold potatoes, cut into wedges**
- 1 **tablespoon olive oil**
- 1 **tablespoon minced fresh rosemary**
- 1 **teaspoon dried thyme**
- 1 **teaspoon dried oregano**
- ½ **teaspoon salt**
- ¼ **to ½ teaspoon pepper**

1. In a large bowl, toss potatoes with oil. Combine the seasonings; sprinkle over potatoes and toss to coat.
2. Arrange in a single layer in a 15-in. x 10-in. x 1-in. baking pan coated with cooking spray. Bake at 425° for 40-45 minutes or until tender, stirring once.
PER SERVING *155 cal., 4 g fat (1 g sat. fat), 0 chol., 312 mg sodium, 27 g carb., 3 g fiber, 3 g pro.* **Diabetic Exchanges:** *2 starch, ½ fat.*

Hearty Beans and Rice

Be sure to save room for your entree—you just might be tempted to eat all of this filling side dish in one sitting!

—**BARB MUSGROVE** FORT ATKINSON, WI

PREP: 10 MIN. • **COOK:** 25 MIN.
MAKES: 5 SERVINGS

- 1 **pound lean ground beef (90% lean)**
- 1 **can (15 ounces) black beans, rinsed and drained**
- 1 **can (14½ ounces) diced tomatoes with mild green chilies, undrained**
- 1⅓ **cups frozen corn, thawed**
- 1 **cup water**
- ¼ **teaspoon salt**
- 1½ **cups instant brown rice**

In a large saucepan, cook beef over medium heat until no longer pink; drain. Stir in the beans, tomatoes, corn, water and salt. Bring to a boil. Stir in rice; return to a boil. Reduce heat; cover and simmer for 5 minutes. Remove from the heat; let stand, covered, for 5 minutes.

PER SERVING *1¼ cups equals 376 cal., 9 g fat (3 g sat. fat), 56 mg chol., 647 mg sodium, 47 g carb., 7 g fiber, 26 g pro.* **Diabetic Exchanges:** *3 starch, 3 lean meat, 1 vegetable.*

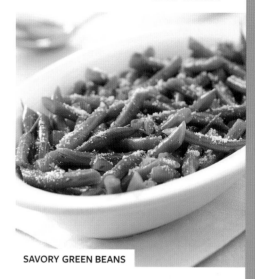

SAVORY GREEN BEANS

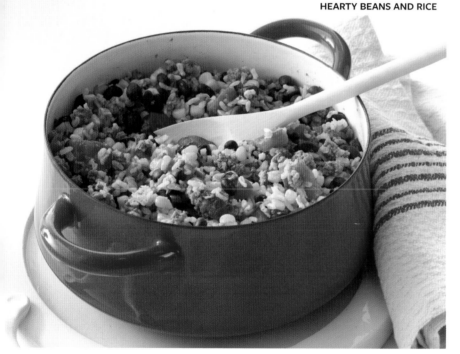

HEARTY BEANS AND RICE

Savory Green Beans

This was my mother's favorite way to fix green beans, always adding her own homegrown savory from the garden.

—**CAROL ANN HAYDEN** EVERSON, WA

START TO FINISH: 30 MIN.
MAKES: 6 SERVINGS

- ¾ **cup chopped sweet red pepper**
- 1 **tablespoon canola oil**
- 1 **garlic clove, minced**
- 1½ **pounds fresh green beans, trimmed and cut into 2-inch pieces**
- ½ **cup water**
- 2 **tablespoons minced fresh savory or 2 teaspoons dried savory**
- 1 **tablespoon minced chives**
- ½ **teaspoon salt**

In a large skillet, saute red pepper in oil for 2-3 minutes or until tender. Add garlic; cook 1 minute longer. Stir in the green beans, water, savory, chives and salt. Bring to a boil. Reduce heat; cover and simmer for 8-10 minutes or until beans are crisp-tender.

PER SERVING *¾ cup equals 59 cal., 3 g fat (trace sat. fat), 0 chol., 203 mg sodium, 9 g carb., 4 g fiber, 2 g pro.* **Diabetic Exchanges:** *2 vegetable, ½ fat.*

top tip

Draining Reduces Salt

Draining canned beans helps remove excess salt from your dish. If you choose not to drain them, be sure to adjust the salt level in your recipe.

Whipped Cauliflower

Need a low-carb substitute for mashed potatoes? This nutritious five-ingredient dish has a mild cauliflower flavor with a smooth, creamy texture.

—TASTE OF HOME TEST KITCHEN

START TO FINISH: 20 MIN.
MAKES: 4 SERVINGS

- 1 medium head cauliflower, cut into florets
- ¼ cup fat-free milk
- 2 tablespoons canola oil
- ¼ teaspoon salt
- ⅛ teaspoon white pepper

1. Place cauliflower in a steamer basket; place in a saucepan over 1 in. of water. Bring to a boil; cover and steam for 8-10 minutes or until tender. Cool cauliflower slightly.

2. Place the milk and oil in a blender. Add the cauliflower, salt and pepper; cover and process until blended. Transfer to a serving bowl.

PER SERVING *105 cal., 7 g fat (1 g sat. fat), 1 mg chol., 199 mg sodium, 8 g carb., 4 g fiber, 3 g pro.* **Diabetic Exchanges:** *1½ fat, 1 vegetable.*

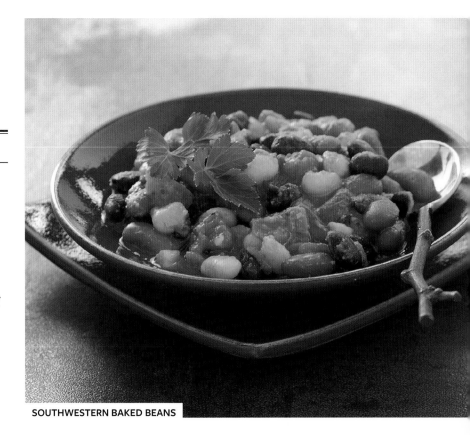

SOUTHWESTERN BAKED BEANS

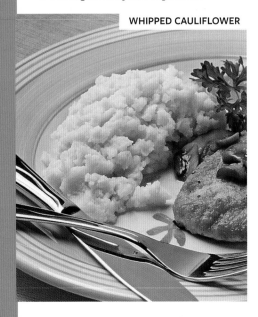

WHIPPED CAULIFLOWER

Southwestern Baked Beans

Three kinds of beans and a host of seasonings make this Southwestern version of baked beans a real standout!

—LESLIE ADAMS SPRINGFIELD, MO

PREP: 20 MIN. • **BAKE:** 1 HOUR
MAKES: 12 SERVINGS

- 2 cans (16 ounces each) kidney beans, rinsed and drained
- 1 can (15½ ounces) great northern beans, rinsed and drained
- 1 can (15 ounces) black beans, rinsed and drained
- 2 cans (14½ ounces each) Italian stewed tomatoes, drained and chopped
- 1 large onion, chopped
- ¼ cup packed brown sugar
- ¼ cup cider vinegar
- 2 tablespoons honey
- 2 teaspoons dried oregano
- 2 teaspoons ground cumin
- 2 teaspoons ground mustard
- 1½ teaspoons ground ginger
- 1 teaspoon garlic powder
- 1 teaspoon chili powder
- ½ teaspoon salt

1. In a large bowl, combine the beans, tomatoes and onion. Combine the remaining ingredients; stir into bean mixture.

2. Transfer to a 3-qt. baking dish coated with cooking spray. Cover and bake at 350° for 45 minutes; stir. Bake, uncovered, 15-30 minutes longer or until heated through.

PER SERVING *¾ cup equals 178 cal., trace fat (trace sat. fat), 0 chol., 502 mg sodium, 35 g carb., 8 g fiber, 9 g pro.* **Diabetic Exchanges:** *2 starch, 1 vegetable.*

Pattypan Saute

The freshness of tomato and sweet red pepper pairs well with sauteed squash for a great sidekick. A bit of shredded Parmesan cheese makes it savory and special.

—TASTE OF HOME TEST KITCHEN

START TO FINISH: 25 MIN.
MAKES: 4 SERVINGS

- 2 cups halved pattypan squash
- 1 medium onion, halved and sliced
- 2 teaspoons canola oil
- 2 garlic cloves, minced
- 1 small sweet red pepper, cut into ½-inch pieces
- 1 cup sliced fresh mushrooms
- 1 medium tomato, chopped
- ½ teaspoon salt
- ½ teaspoon Italian seasoning
- ⅛ teaspoon pepper
- 2 tablespoons shredded Parmesan cheese

1. In a large nonstick skillet coated with cooking spray, saute squash and onion in oil for 2 minutes. Add garlic; cook 1 minute longer. Add red pepper and mushrooms; saute for 5-7 minutes or until vegetables are crisp-tender.

2. Stir in the tomato, salt, Italian seasoning and pepper; heat through. Sprinkle with cheese.

PER SERVING *73 cal., 3 g fat (1 g sat. fat), 2 mg chol., 343 mg sodium, 9 g carb., 2 g fiber, 3 g pro.* **Diabetic Exchanges:** *2 vegetable, ½ fat.*

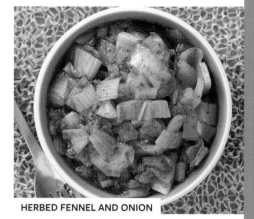

HERBED FENNEL AND ONION

Herbed Fennel and Onion

If you have fennel bulbs but aren't sure what to do with them, try them in this aromatic, rich side dish. Vinegar adds a slight tang.

—MEGHANN MINTON PORTLAND, OR

START TO FINISH: 30 MIN.
MAKES: 3 SERVINGS

- 1 large sweet onion, halved and sliced
- 1 medium fennel bulb, halved and cut into ½-inch slices
- 1 tablespoon olive oil
- 1 cup reduced-sodium chicken broth
- 1 tablespoon minced fresh sage or 1 teaspoon dried sage leaves
- 2 teaspoons minced fresh rosemary or ½ teaspoon dried rosemary, crushed
- 2 teaspoons balsamic vinegar
- ¼ teaspoon salt
- ¼ teaspoon pepper

1. In a large skillet, saute onion and fennel in oil until crisp-tender. Add the broth, sage and rosemary. Bring to a boil; cook until broth is evaporated.

2. Remove from the heat; stir in the vinegar, salt and pepper.

PER SERVING *109 cal., 5 g fat (1 g sat. fat), 0 chol., 437 mg sodium, 15 g carb., 3 g fiber, 3 g pro.* **Diabetic Exchanges:** *2 vegetable, 1 fat.*

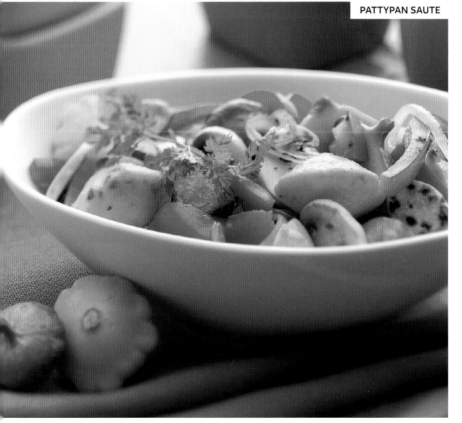

PATTYPAN SAUTE

Grilled Summer Squash

Vegetable lovers will truly enjoy this dish, which is a snap to grill. Fresh-picked squash from your garden will make it even better.

—LISA FINNEGAN FORKED RIVER, NJ

START TO FINISH: 25 MIN.
MAKES: 4 SERVINGS

- 2 **medium yellow summer squash, sliced**
- 2 **medium sweet red peppers, sliced**
- 1 **large sweet onion, halved and sliced**
- 2 **tablespoons olive oil**
- 2 **garlic cloves, minced**
- 1 **teaspoon sugar**
- ¼ **teaspoon salt**
- ¼ **teaspoon pepper**

1. In a large bowl, combine all the ingredients. Divide between two double thicknesses of heavy-duty foil (about 18 in. x 12 in.). Fold foil around vegetable mixture and seal tightly.

2. Grill, covered, over medium heat for 10-15 minutes or until vegetables are tender. Open foil carefully to allow steam to escape.

PER SERVING *124 cal., 7 g fat (1 g sat. fat), 0 chol., 159 mg sodium, 15 g carb., 3 g fiber, 3 g pro.* **Diabetic Exchanges:** *2 vegetable, 1½ fat.*

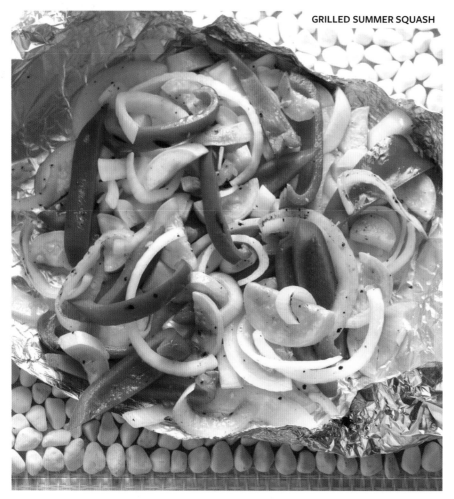

GRILLED SUMMER SQUASH

Broccoli-Cauliflower Cheese Bake

Creamy mozzarella and Swiss cheeses lightly coat the vegetables, while a hint of cayenne pepper gives them some zip. Even the kids will want to eat their veggies now!

—JENN TIDWELL FAIR OAKS, CA

PREP: 35 MIN. • **BAKE:** 20 MIN.
MAKES: 16 SERVINGS

- 7 **cups fresh cauliflowerets**
- 6 **cups fresh broccoli florets**
- 3 **tablespoons butter**
- ⅓ **cup all-purpose flour**
- 1½ **teaspoons spicy brown mustard**
- ¾ **teaspoon salt**
- ¼ **teaspoon ground nutmeg**
- ¼ **teaspoon cayenne pepper**
- ¼ **teaspoon pepper**
- 3¾ **cups fat-free milk**
- 1½ **cups (6 ounces) shredded part-skim mozzarella cheese, divided**
- 1½ **cups (6 ounces) shredded Swiss cheese, divided**

1. Place cauliflower and broccoli in a Dutch oven; add 1 in. of water. Bring to a boil. Reduce heat; cover and simmer for 3-5 minutes or until crisp-tender. Drain; transfer to a 13-in. x 9-in. baking dish coated with cooking spray.

2. In a small saucepan, melt butter. Stir in the flour, mustard, salt, nutmeg, cayenne and pepper until smooth; gradually add milk. Bring to a boil; cook and stir for 1-2 minutes or until thickened.

3. Stir in 1¼ cups each mozzarella and Swiss cheeses until melted. Pour over vegetables. Bake, uncovered, at 400° for 15-20 minutes or until bubbly. Sprinkle with the remaining cheeses. Bake for 5 minutes longer or until golden brown.

PER SERVING *¾ cup equals 132 cal., 7 g fat (4 g sat. fat), 22 mg chol., 252 mg sodium, 9 g carb., 2 g fiber, 9 g pro.* **Diabetic Exchanges:** *1 high-fat meat, 1 vegetable.*

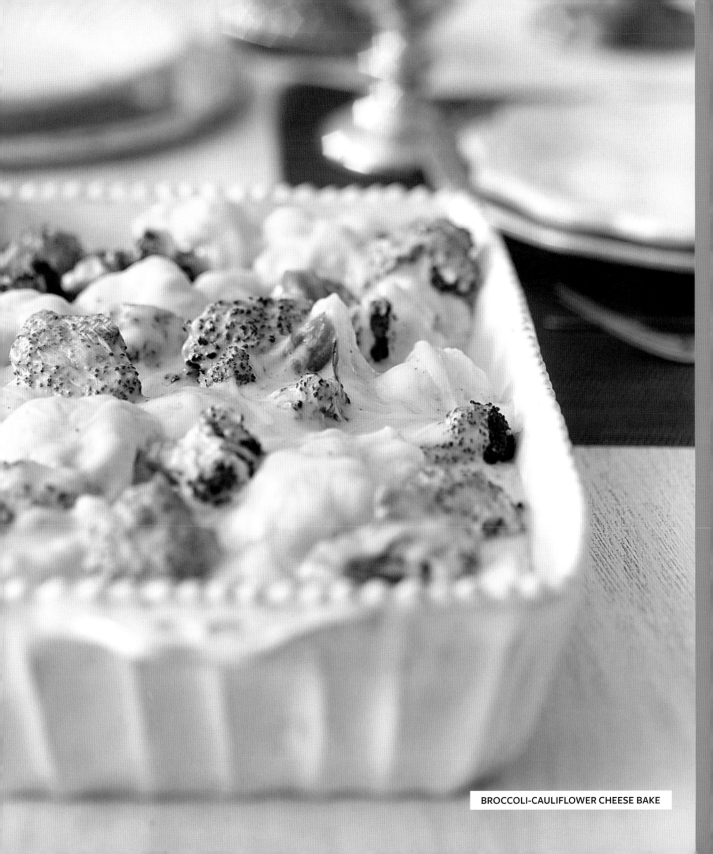

BROCCOLI-CAULIFLOWER CHEESE BAKE

Sesame Broccoli

We turn to this broccoli dish often in my house. It's a breeze to put together.

—JANICE CAWMAN YAKIMA, WA

START TO FINISH: 25 MIN.
MAKES: 6 SERVINGS

- 1 **pound fresh broccoli, cut into spears**
- 1 **tablespoon reduced-sodium soy sauce**
- 2 **teaspoons olive oil**
- 2 **teaspoons balsamic vinegar**
- 1½ **teaspoons honey**
- 2 **teaspoons sesame seeds, toasted**

1. Place broccoli in a steamer basket; place in a saucepan over 1 in. of water. Bring to a boil; cover and steam for 10-15 minutes or until crisp-tender. Meanwhile, in a small saucepan, combine the soy sauce, oil, vinegar and honey; cook and stir over medium-low heat until heated through.

2. Transfer broccoli to a serving bowl; drizzle with soy sauce mixture. Sprinkle with sesame seeds.

PER SERVING *¾ cup equals 48 cal., 2 g fat (trace sat. fat), 0 chol., 127 mg sodium, 6 g carb., 2 g fiber, 3 g pro.* **Diabetic Exchanges:** *1 vegetable, ½ fat.*

Basil Tomato Rice

Whenever my family wants something a little different, I whip up this easy side. It's so fresh-tasting, and I always have the ingredients on hand.

—SARAH RUPE ELDON, IA

START TO FINISH: 25 MIN.
MAKES: 6 SERVINGS

- 2 **cups reduced-sodium chicken broth**
- 2 **cups uncooked instant rice**
- 1 **medium green pepper, diced**
- 1 **small onion, finely chopped**
- 1½ **teaspoons olive oil**
- 2 **medium tomatoes, seeded and chopped**
- 2 **teaspoons dried basil**
- ¼ **teaspoon salt**

1. In a large saucepan, bring broth to a boil. Stir in rice; cover and remove from the heat. Let stand for 5 minutes.

2. Meanwhile, in a small skillet, saute pepper and onion in oil until tender. Add the tomatoes, basil and salt; heat through. Stir into rice.

PER SERVING *¾ cup equals 154 cal., 2 g fat (trace sat. fat), 0 chol., 295 mg sodium, 30 g carb., 2 g fiber, 4 g pro.* **Diabetic Exchange:** *2 starch.*

Acorn Squash Puree

I originally created this recipe to have a healthy option at our Thanksgiving meal. It's now a very popular side even beyond the holiday!

—ANN HENNESSY BURNSVILLE, MN

PREP: 1 HOUR • **BAKE:** 20 MIN.
MAKES: 8 SERVINGS

- 4 **medium acorn squash**
- 8 **ounces fat-free cream cheese, cubed**
- ½ **cup fat-free milk**
- 2 **tablespoons reduced-fat butter, melted**
- 2 **tablespoons dried minced onion**
- 2 **tablespoons minced chives**
- 2 **teaspoons dried basil**
- 3 **tablespoons chopped pecans**

1. Cut squash in half; discard seeds. Place squash cut side down in a 15x10x 1-in. baking pan; add ½ in. of hot water. Bake, uncovered, at 350° for 35 minutes. Drain water from pan; turn squash cut side up. Bake 5-10 minutes longer or until tender. Cool slightly.

2. Carefully scoop out squash; add to food processor. Add the cream cheese, milk, butter, onion, chives and basil; cover and process until blended.

3. Transfer to a 2-qt. baking dish coated with cooking spray; sprinkle with pecans. Cover and bake at 350° for 20-25 minutes or until heated through. **NOTE** *This recipe was tested with Land O'Lakes light stick butter.*

PER SERVING *¾ cup equals 160 cal., 4 g fat (1 g sat. fat), 8 mg chol., 187 mg sodium, 28 g carb., 4 g fiber, 7 g pro.* **Diabetic Exchanges:** *1½ starch, 1 fat.*

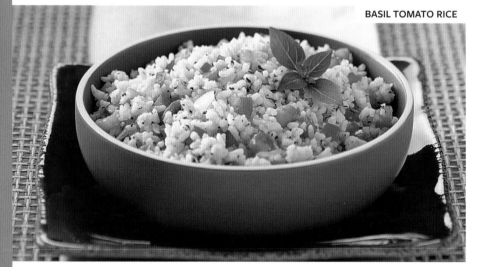

BASIL TOMATO RICE

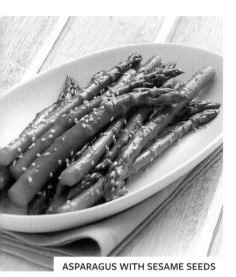

ASPARAGUS WITH SESAME SEEDS

Asparagus with Sesame Seeds

Dress up crisp asparagus with reduced-sodium soy sauce and a sprinkling of sesame seeds for a simple vegetable that will do any dinner entree proud!

—TASTE OF HOME TEST KITCHEN

START TO FINISH: 15 MIN.
MAKES: 2 SERVINGS

- ½ **pound fresh asparagus, trimmed**
- 2 **tablespoons water**
- 1 **teaspoon reduced-sodium soy sauce**
- 1 **teaspoon olive oil**
- ⅛ **teaspoon salt**
   Dash pepper
- 1 **teaspoon sesame seeds, toasted**

Place the asparagus in a steamer basket; place in a saucepan over 1 in. of water. Bring to a boil; cover and steam for 4-5 minutes or until crisp-tender. Transfer to a serving dish. Combine the water, soy sauce, oil, salt and pepper; drizzle over asparagus. Sprinkle with sesame seeds.

PER SERVING *43 cal., 3 g fat (trace sat. fat), 0 chol., 262 mg sodium, 3 g carb., 1 g fiber, 2 g pro.* **Diabetic Exchanges:** *1 vegetable, ½ fat.*

Sweet Corn Gratin

Garlic and onion flavors elevate this dish.

—JENNIFER OLSON PLEASANTON, CA

PREP: 30 MIN. • **BAKE:** 45 MIN. + STANDING
MAKES: 8 SERVINGS

- 1 **medium onion, thinly sliced**
- 2 **tablespoons butter**
- 2 **tablespoons all-purpose flour**
- 2 **garlic cloves, minced**
- 1 **teaspoon salt**
- ½ **teaspoon pepper**
- 1 **cup whole milk**
- 2 **pounds medium Yukon Gold potatoes, peeled and cut into ⅛-inch slices**
- 2 **cups fresh or frozen corn**
- 1 **can (8¼ ounces) cream-style corn**
- ¾ **cup panko (Japanese) bread crumbs**
- 1 **tablespoon butter, melted**

1. In a large saucepan, saute onion in butter until tender. Stir in the flour, garlic, salt and pepper until blended; gradually add milk. Stir in potatoes. Bring to a boil. Reduce heat; cook and stir for 8-10 minutes or until potatoes are crisp-tender.

2. Stir in corn and cream-style corn. Transfer to an 8-in. square baking dish coated with cooking spray.

3. In a small bowl, combine bread crumbs and butter; sprinkle over potatoes. Bake at 350° for 45-50 minutes or until golden brown and potatoes are tender. Let stand for 10 minutes before serving.

PER SERVING *¾ cup equals 213 cal., 6 g fat (3 g sat. fat), 14 mg chol., 452 mg sodium, 37 g carb., 3 g fiber, 5 g pro.* **Diabetic Exchanges:** *2 starch, 1 fat.*

SWEET CORN GRATIN

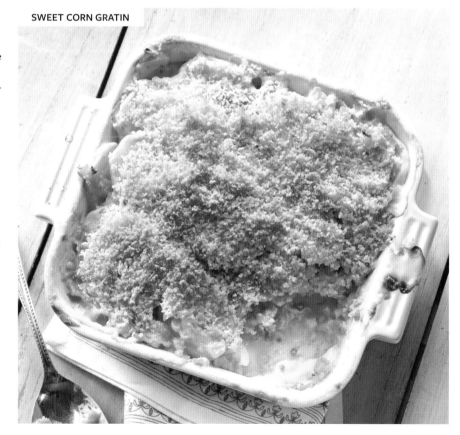

Garlic Roasted Winter Vegetables

These colorful, herby vegetables roast to perfection and are guaranteed to become a family favorite.

—DONNA LAMANO OLATHE, KS

PREP: 20 MIN. • **BAKE:** 45 MIN.
MAKES: 6 SERVINGS

- 2 medium carrots
- 1 medium turnip
- 1 medium parsnip
- 1 cup cubed red potatoes
- 1 cup cubed peeled butternut squash
- 3 whole garlic bulbs, cloves separated and peeled
- 3 shallots, quartered
- 4½ teaspoons olive oil
- ¼ teaspoon salt
- ¼ teaspoon dried thyme
- ¼ teaspoon pepper

1. Peel the carrots, turnip and parsnip; cut into 1-in. pieces. Place in a large bowl; add the potatoes, squash, garlic, shallots, oil, salt, thyme and pepper. Toss to coat. Transfer to a greased 15x10x1-in. baking pan.

2. Bake, uncovered, at 400° for 45-50 minutes or until tender, stirring once.

PER SERVING *⅔ cup equals 135 cal., 4 g fat (1 g sat. fat), 0 chol., 137 mg sodium, 24 g carb., 3 g fiber, 3 g pro.* **Diabetic Exchanges:** *1½ starch, ½ fat.*

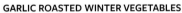

GARLIC ROASTED WINTER VEGETABLES

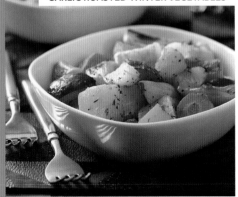

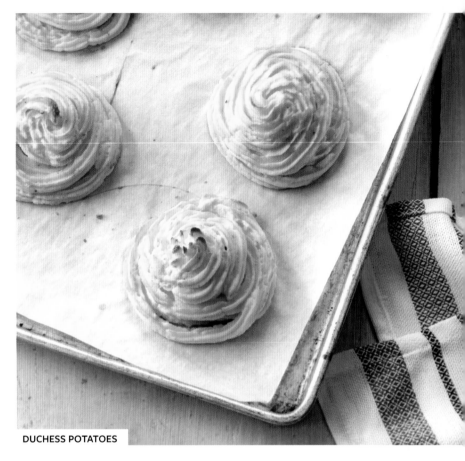

DUCHESS POTATOES

Duchess Potatoes

Present potatoes in an attractive new package! Guests will love these bite-size snacks, so keep recipe copies on hand.

—TASTE OF HOME TEST KITCHEN

PREP: 35 MIN. • **BAKE:** 20 MIN.
MAKES: 6 SERVINGS

- 2 pounds russet potatoes, peeled and quartered
- 3 egg yolks
- 3 tablespoons fat-free milk
- 2 tablespoons butter
- 1 teaspoon salt
- ¼ teaspoon pepper
- ⅛ teaspoon ground nutmeg
- 1 egg, lightly beaten

1. Place potatoes in a large saucepan and cover with water. Bring to a boil. Reduce heat; cover and simmer for 15-20 minutes or until tender. Drain.

2. Over very low heat, stir potatoes for 1-2 minutes or until the steam has evaporated. Press through a potato ricer or strainer into a large bowl. Stir in the egg yolks, milk, butter, salt, pepper and nutmeg.

3. Using a pastry bag or heavy-duty resealable plastic bag and a large star tip, pipe potatoes into six mounds on a parchment paper-lined baking sheet. Brush with beaten egg. Bake at 400° for 20-25 minutes or until golden brown.

PER SERVING *158 cal., 7 g fat (3 g sat. fat), 134 mg chol., 437 mg sodium, 21 g carb., 1 g fiber, 4 g pro.* **Diabetic Exchanges:** *1½ fat, 1 starch.*

Two-Cheese Ziti

My grandkids really like this rich, buttery macaroni and cheese, but it's still light enough for any adults on diets to enjoy.

—**FLO BURTNETT** GAGE, OK

PREP: 25 MIN. • **BAKE:** 25 MIN.
MAKES: 5 SERVINGS

- 3 **cups uncooked ziti or small tube pasta**
- 1 **tablespoon butter**
- 2 **tablespoons all-purpose flour**
- ½ **teaspoon salt**
- ¼ **teaspoon pepper**
- 1¾ **cups fat-free milk**
- ¾ **cup shredded reduced-fat cheddar cheese**
- 2 **tablespoons grated Parmesan cheese**

TOPPING

- 3 **tablespoons dry bread crumbs**
- 1½ **teaspoons butter, melted**
- ¼ **cup shredded reduced-fat cheddar cheese**
- 3 **tablespoons grated Parmesan cheese**

1. Cook ziti according to package directions. Meanwhile, in a large nonstick skillet, melt butter. Stir in the flour, salt and pepper until smooth; gradually add milk. Bring to a boil; cook and stir for 2 minutes or until thickened. Remove from the heat; stir in cheeses until melted.

2. Drain ziti; add to sauce and stir to coat. Transfer to a shallow 1½-qt. baking dish coated with cooking spray. Cover and bake at 350° for 20 minutes.

3. In a small bowl, combine bread crumbs and butter; stir in cheeses. Sprinkle over ziti. Bake, uncovered, for 5-10 minutes or until heated through and topping is lightly browned.

PER SERVING *340 cal., 11 g fat (7 g sat. fat), 31 mg chol., 590 mg sodium, 44 g carb., 2 g fiber, 18 g pro.* **Diabetic Exchanges:** *3 starch, 1 lean meat, 1 fat.*

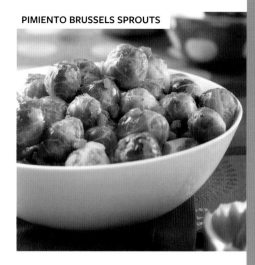

PIMIENTO BRUSSELS SPROUTS

Pimiento Brussels Sprouts

Kids don't normally like Brussels sprouts, but you just might convince them to dig in when you serve them this way. Tarragon and vinegar spruce up the taste, and pimientos give the sprouts a splash of color.

—**CAROLYN HAYES** JOHNSTON CITY, IL

START TO FINISH: 15 MIN.
MAKES: 4 SERVINGS

- 1 **package (16 ounces) frozen Brussels sprouts**
- 4½ **teaspoons butter**
- 4½ **teaspoons white vinegar**
- ¾ **teaspoon dried tarragon**
- ¼ **teaspoon salt**
- 1 **jar (2 ounces) diced pimientos, drained**

1. Cook Brussels sprouts according to package directions. Drain, reserving 1 tablespoon liquid; keep sprouts warm.

2. In a small saucepan, melt butter; stir in the vinegar, tarragon, salt and reserved cooking liquid. Pour over sprouts and toss to coat. Sprinkle with the pimientos.

PER SERVING *88 cal., 5 g fat (3 g sat. fat), 11 mg chol., 191 mg sodium, 10 g carb., 5 g fiber, 5 g pro.* **Diabetic Exchanges:** *2 vegetable, 1 fat.*

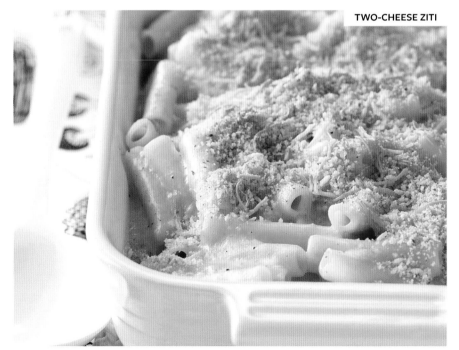

TWO-CHEESE ZITI

Veggie-Topped Polenta Slices

Even though we didn't have too many ingredients in the kitchen at the time, this amazing side dish came from a stroke of genius I had.

—**JENN TIDWELL** FAIR OAKS, CA

PREP: 20 MIN. • **COOK:** 20 MIN.
MAKES: 4 SERVINGS

- 1 tube (1 pound) polenta, cut into 12 slices
- 2 tablespoons olive oil, divided
- 1 medium zucchini, chopped
- 2 shallots, minced
- 2 garlic cloves, minced
- 3 tablespoons reduced-sodium chicken broth
- ½ teaspoon pepper
- ⅛ teaspoon salt
- 4 plum tomatoes, seeded and chopped
- 2 tablespoons minced fresh basil or 2 teaspoons dried basil
- 1 tablespoon minced fresh parsley
- ½ cup shredded part-skim mozzarella cheese

1. In a large nonstick skillet, cook polenta in 1 tablespoon oil over medium heat for 9-11 minutes on each side or until golden brown.

2. Meanwhile, in another large skillet, saute zucchini in remaining oil until tender. Add shallots and garlic; cook 1 minute longer. Add the broth, pepper and salt. Bring to a boil; cook until liquid is almost evaporated.

3. Stir in the tomatoes, basil and parsley; heat through. Serve with polenta; sprinkle with cheese.

PER SERVING *222 cal., 9 g fat (2 g sat. fat), 8 mg chol., 558 mg sodium, 28 g carb., 2 g fiber, 7 g pro.* **Diabetic Exchanges:** *1½ starch, 1½ fat, 1 vegetable.*

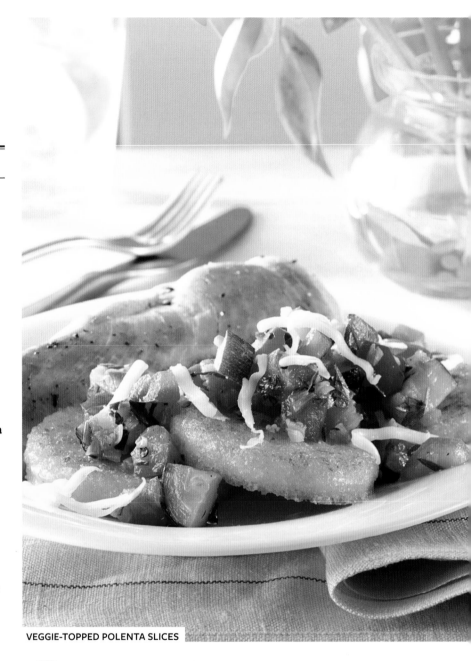

VEGGIE-TOPPED POLENTA SLICES

Polenta Pointers

Polenta is a popular Italian dish made from cornmeal. Tubed polenta is usually found in the produce aisle at the grocery store.

Sweet Potato Delight

I serve this dish at least once a month—it's that popular. The fluffy texture and subtle orange zest make it a standout.

—MARLENE KROLL CHICAGO, IL

PREP: 25 MIN. • **BAKE:** 30 MIN.
MAKES: 10 SERVINGS

- 4 large sweet potatoes, peeled and quartered
- ½ cup orange marmalade
- ½ cup orange juice
- ¼ cup packed brown sugar
- ½ teaspoon almond extract
- 3 egg whites
- ¼ cup slivered almonds

1. Place sweet potatoes in a Dutch oven; cover with water. Bring to a boil. Reduce heat; cover and cook for 15-20 minutes or just until tender. Drain potatoes; place in a large bowl and mash. Stir in orange marmalade, orange juice, brown sugar and extract. Cool slightly.

2. In a small bowl, beat egg whites until stiff peaks form. Fold into sweet potato mixture. Transfer to a 2½-qt. baking dish coated with cooking spray. Sprinkle with almonds. Bake, uncovered, at 350° for 30-35 minutes or until a thermometer reads 160°.

PER SERVING *¾ cup equals 174 cal., 1 g fat (trace sat. fat), 0 chol., 36 mg sodium, 38 g carb., 3 g fiber, 3 g pro. Diabetic Exchange: 2 starch.*

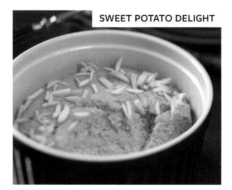
SWEET POTATO DELIGHT

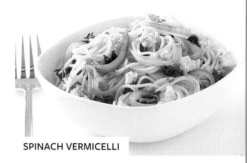
SPINACH VERMICELLI

Spinach Vermicelli

You'll get lots of iron from the spinach in this simple side.

—CHARLEEN BERKERS PALGRAVE, ON

START TO FINISH: 30 MIN.
MAKES: 6 SERVINGS

- 8 ounces uncooked vermicelli
- 1 large red onion, sliced and separated into rings
- 1 tablespoon olive oil
- 2 garlic cloves, minced
- 1 package (10 ounces) fresh spinach, torn
- 2 tablespoons lemon juice
- 1 tablespoon minced fresh tarragon or 1 teaspoon dried tarragon
- ¼ teaspoon salt
- ⅛ teaspoon pepper
- ⅓ cup crumbled Gorgonzola cheese

1. Cook vermicelli according to package directions. Meanwhile, in a large nonstick skillet, saute onion in oil until crisp-tender. Add garlic; saute 1 minute longer. Add spinach, lemon juice, tarragon, salt and pepper; saute for 2 minutes or until spinach is wilted.

2. Drain vermicelli; toss with spinach mixture. Sprinkle with cheese.

PER SERVING *1 cup pasta with about 1 tablespoon cheese equals 220 cal., 6 g fat (3 g sat. fat), 8 mg chol., 296 mg sodium, 33 g carb., 3 g fiber, 9 g pro. Diabetic Exchanges: 2 starch, 1 vegetable, 1 fat.*

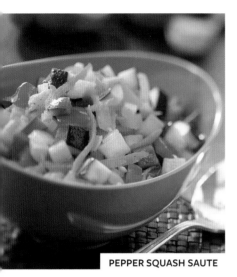
PEPPER SQUASH SAUTE

Pepper Squash Saute

I often double the ingredients when making this recipe because it's just as good when reheated later in the week.

—JANICE MCCLOSKEY HOWARD, PA

START TO FINISH: 25 MIN.
MAKES: 4 SERVINGS

- 1 small onion, chopped
- ⅓ cup each chopped green, sweet red and yellow pepper
- 1 tablespoon butter
- 1 medium zucchini, chopped
- 1 medium yellow summer squash, chopped
- 1 medium carrot, shredded
- 2 garlic cloves, minced
- ½ teaspoon salt
- ¼ teaspoon pepper

In a large nonstick skillet, saute onion and peppers in butter for 3-4 minutes. Stir in the zucchini, summer squash and carrot; saute 3-4 minutes or until vegetables are tender. Add garlic; cook 1 minute longer or until tender. Sprinkle with salt and pepper.

PER SERVING *69 cal., 3 g fat (2 g sat. fat), 8 mg chol., 333 mg sodium, 10 g carb., 3 g fiber, 2 g pro. Diabetic Exchanges: 2 vegetable, ½ fat.*

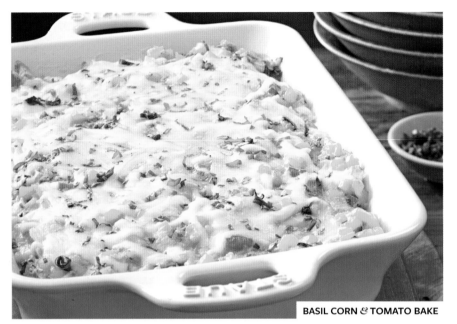

BASIL CORN & TOMATO BAKE

Basil Corn & Tomato Bake

When sweet Jersey corn is in season, I turn to this recipe. Combined with tomatoes, zucchini and basil, this corn bake can be served for brunch, lunch or even dinner.

—**ERIN CHILCOAT** CENTRAL ISLIP, NY

PREP: 30 MIN. • **BAKE:** 45 MIN. + STANDING
MAKES: 10 SERVINGS

- 2 **teaspoons olive oil**
- 1 **medium onion, chopped**
- 2 **eggs**
- 1 **can (10¾ ounces) reduced-fat reduced-sodium condensed cream of celery soup, undiluted**
- 4 **cups fresh or frozen corn**
- 1 **small zucchini, chopped**
- 1 **medium tomato, seeded and chopped**
- ¾ **cup soft whole wheat bread crumbs**
- ⅓ **cup minced fresh basil**
- ½ **teaspoon salt**
- ½ **cup shredded part-skim mozzarella cheese**
  Additional minced fresh basil, optional

1. Preheat oven to 350°. In a small skillet, heat oil over medium heat. Add onion; cook and stir until tender. In a large bowl, whisk eggs and condensed soup until blended. Stir in vegetables, bread crumbs, basil, salt and onion. Transfer mixture to an 11x7-in. baking dish coated with cooking spray.

2. Bake, uncovered, 40-45 minutes or until bubbly. Sprinkle with cheese. Bake 5-10 minutes longer or until cheese is melted. Let stand 10 minutes before serving. If desired, sprinkle with additional basil.

NOTE *To make soft bread crumbs, tear bread into pieces and place in a food processor or blender. Cover and pulse until crumbs form. One slice of bread yields ½ to ¾ cup crumbs.*

PER SERVING *¾ cup equals 131 cal., 4 g fat (1 g sat. fat), 47 mg chol., 299 mg sodium, 20 g carb., 3 g fiber, 6 g pro. Diabetic Exchanges: 1 starch, ½ fat.*

Easy Baked Mushrooms

Bet you've never had mushrooms quite like this! Skipping the deep fryer keeps them low in fat.

—**DENISE DIPACE** MEDFORD, NJ

START TO FINISH: 30 MIN.
MAKES: 4 SERVINGS

- 1 **pound medium fresh mushrooms, halved**
- 2 **tablespoons olive oil**
- ¼ **cup seasoned bread crumbs**
- ¼ **teaspoon garlic powder**
- ¼ **teaspoon pepper**
  Fresh parsley, optional

1. Place mushrooms on a baking sheet. Drizzle with oil; toss to coat. In a small bowl, combine the bread crumbs, garlic powder and pepper; sprinkle over the mushrooms.

2. Bake, uncovered, at 425° for 18-20 minutes or until lightly browned. Garnish with parsley if desired.

PER SERVING *116 cal., 8 g fat (1 g sat. fat), 0 chol., 112 mg sodium, 10 g carb., 2 g fiber, 4 g pro. Diabetic Exchanges: 1½ fat, ½ starch.*

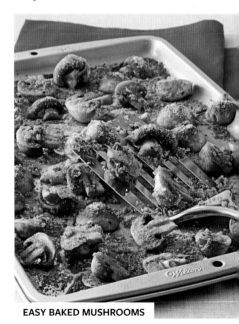

EASY BAKED MUSHROOMS

Quinoa Squash Pilaf

There are so many different veggies packed into this dish, it's almost like eating a really special salad.

—ANNETTE SPIEGLER ARLINGTON HEIGHTS, IL

PREP: 30 MIN. • **COOK:** 20 MIN.
MAKES: 8 SERVINGS

- 1 **cup quinoa, rinsed**
- 1 **can (14½ ounces) vegetable broth**
- ¼ **cup water**
- 2 **medium zucchini, halved lengthwise and sliced**
- 1 **medium yellow summer squash, halved lengthwise and sliced**
- 1 **cup chopped leeks (white portion only)**
- 1 **tablespoon olive oil**
- 2 **garlic cloves, minced**
- 1 **large tomato, chopped**
- 1 **tablespoon minced fresh cilantro**
- ½ **teaspoon salt**
- ½ **teaspoon each dried oregano, ground cumin and chili powder**
- ¼ **teaspoon pepper**
- ⅛ **teaspoon crushed red pepper flakes**
- 2 **cups fresh baby spinach, chopped**

1. In a large nonstick skillet coated with cooking spray, toast the quinoa over medium heat until lightly browned, stirring occasionally.
2. In a small saucepan, bring broth and water to a boil. Add quinoa. Reduce heat; cover and simmer for 12-15 minutes or until liquid is absorbed.
3. In a large nonstick skillet, saute the zucchini, yellow squash and leeks in oil until vegetables are tender. Add garlic; cook 1 minute longer. Stir in the tomato, cilantro, seasonings and quinoa; heat through. Add spinach; cook and stir until spinach is wilted.
NOTE *Look for quinoa in the cereal, rice or organic food aisle.*
PER SERVING *¾ cup equals 126 cal., 3 g fat (trace sat. fat), 0 chol., 377 mg sodium, 21 g carb., 3 g fiber, 5 g pro.* **Diabetic Exchanges:** *1 starch, 1 vegetable, ½ fat.*

QUINOA SQUASH PILAF

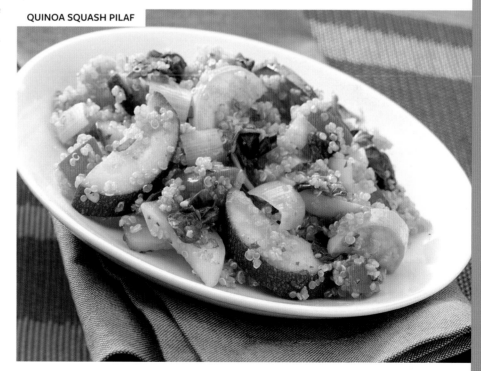

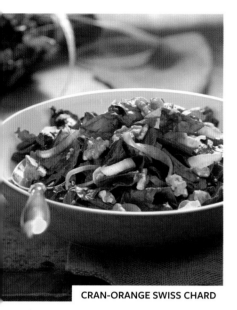

CRAN-ORANGE SWISS CHARD

Cran-Orange Swiss Chard

Maybe you wouldn't think of mixing Swiss chard, cranberries and walnuts, but one bite will have you hooked.

—JOAN JACKAMAN NOBLETON, ON

START TO FINISH: 25 MIN.
MAKES: 4 SERVINGS

- 1 **medium onion, sliced**
- 1 **tablespoon olive oil**
- 10 **cups chopped Swiss chard**
- ¼ **cup orange juice**
- 2 **tablespoons dried cranberries**
  Dash salt and pepper
- 2 **tablespoons coarsely chopped walnuts, toasted**

1. In a large skillet, saute onion in oil until tender. Add chard; saute for 3-5 minutes or just until wilted.
2. Stir in the orange juice, cranberries, salt and pepper; cook for 1-2 minutes or until cranberries are softened. Sprinkle with walnuts.
PER SERVING *104 cal., 6 g fat (1 g sat. fat), 0 chol., 230 mg sodium, 12 g carb., 3 g fiber, 3 g pro.* **Diabetic Exchanges: 2 vegetable, 1 fat.**

Dilly Grilled Veggies

Use any combination of vegetables in this versatile side dish. I'll sometimes include cauliflower, carrots, green peppers and onions, too.

—FRAN SCOTT BIRMINGHAM, MI

START TO FINISH: 30 MIN.
MAKES: 6 SERVINGS

- 2 **cups sliced fresh mushrooms**
- 2 **cups sliced fresh zucchini**
- 2 **cups fresh broccoli florets**
- ½ **medium sweet red pepper, cut into strips**
- 2 **tablespoons olive oil**
- 2 **tablespoons minced fresh dill or 2 teaspoons dill weed**
- ⅛ **teaspoon garlic salt**
- ⅛ **teaspoon pepper**

1. Place vegetables on a double thickness of heavy-duty foil (about 18-in. square). Drizzle with oil; sprinkle with dill, garlic salt and pepper. Fold foil around vegetables and seal tightly.

2. Grill, covered, over medium heat for 15 minutes or until vegetables are tender. Open foil carefully to allow steam to escape.

PER SERVING *¾ cup equals 61 cal., 5 g fat (1 g sat. fat), 0 chol., 49 mg sodium, 4 g carb., 2 g fiber, 2 g pro.* **Diabetic Exchanges:** *1 vegetable, 1 fat.*

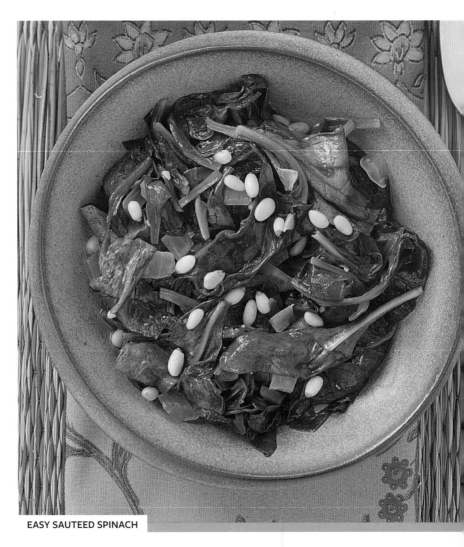

EASY SAUTEED SPINACH

DILLY GRILLED VEGGIES

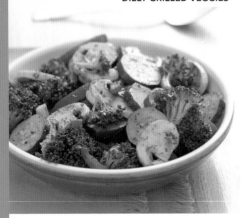

Easy Sauteed Spinach

Spinach doesn't have to be bland—change it up with garlic, onion, a lick of sherry and a sprinkling of pine nuts.

—TASTE OF HOME TEST KITCHEN

START TO FINISH: 20 MIN.
MAKES: 4 SERVINGS

- 1 **small onion, finely chopped**
- 1 **garlic clove, minced**
- 2 **packages (6 ounces each) fresh baby spinach**
- 3 **tablespoons sherry or reduced-sodium chicken broth**
- ¼ **teaspoon salt**
- ⅛ **teaspoon pepper**
- 1 **tablespoon pine nuts**

In a large nonstick skillet coated with cooking spray, saute onion until tender. Add garlic; cook 1 minute longer. Stir in the spinach, sherry, salt and pepper; cook and stir for 4-5 minutes or until the spinach is wilted. Sprinkle with the pine nuts.

PER SERVING *47 cal., 1 g fat (trace sat. fat), 0 chol., 216 mg sodium, 5 g carb., 2 g fiber, 3 g pro.* **Diabetic Exchange:** *1 vegetable.*

Hash Brown Supreme

Toss leftover veggies into the skillet to brighten up this dish! We serve the finished product with a dollop of sour cream.

—JENNIFER BISTLINE CONFLUENCE, PA

PREP: 20 MIN. • **COOK:** 15 MIN.
MAKES: 4 SERVINGS

- 1 small onion, finely chopped
- ½ cup sliced fresh mushrooms
- ½ cup chopped green pepper
- 1 tablespoon canola oil
- 3 cups frozen shredded hash brown potatoes
- 1 medium tomato, finely chopped
- ½ cup shredded reduced-fat cheddar cheese
- 2 tablespoons sliced ripe olives
- 1 jalapeno pepper, seeded and sliced
- ¼ teaspoon seasoned salt
- ⅛ teaspoon pepper
- 1 tablespoon minced chives

1. In a large nonstick skillet, saute the onion, mushrooms and pepper in oil until tender. Add hash browns; cook over medium heat for 8-10 minutes or until the potatoes are browned, stirring occasionally.

2. Stir in the tomato, cheese, olives, jalapeno, seasoned salt and pepper. Cover and cook for 2 minutes or until cheese is melted. Sprinkle with chives; cut into wedges.

NOTE *Wear disposable gloves when cutting hot peppers; the oils can burn skin. Avoid touching your face.*

PER SERVING *142 cal., 7 g fat (2 g sat. fat), 10 mg chol., 233 mg sodium, 15 g carb., 2 g fiber, 6 g pro.* **Diabetic Exchanges:** *1 medium-fat meat, 1 vegetable, ½ starch.*

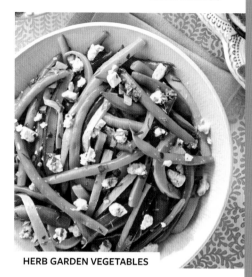

HERB GARDEN VEGETABLES

Herb Garden Vegetables

I have a garden and wanted to highlight what I grow. This medley was the perfect recipe to do just that.

—JULIE STELLA CHAMPLIN, MN

START TO FINISH: 30 MIN.
MAKES: 2 SERVINGS

- ¼ pound fresh green beans, trimmed
- ¾ cup fresh sugar snap peas
- 1 tablespoon olive oil
- ¾ cup julienned zucchini
- ¾ cup julienned yellow summer squash
- ¾ teaspoon each minced fresh rosemary, sage, basil and thyme
- ¼ teaspoon crushed red pepper flakes
- 2 tablespoons crumbled blue cheese

In a small skillet over medium heat, cook the beans and peas in oil for 3 minutes. Add the zucchini, squash, herbs and pepper flakes; cook and stir 3-5 minutes longer or until vegetables are crisp-tender. Sprinkle with cheese just before serving.

PER SERVING *146 cal., 10 g fat (3 g sat. fat), 6 mg chol., 129 mg sodium, 11 g carb., 5 g fiber, 6 g pro.* **Diabetic Exchanges:** *2 vegetable, 2 fat.*

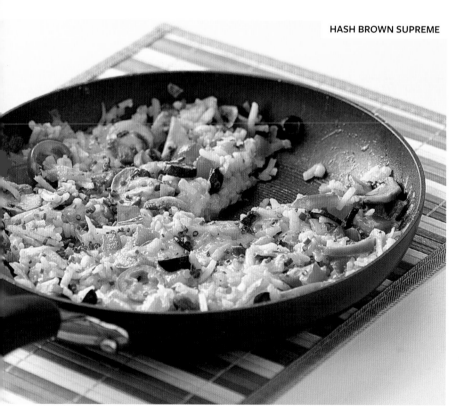

HASH BROWN SUPREME

Parsnip-Carrot Medley

Carrots, rosemary and just a touch of cayenne pepper set off the parsnips here.
—**TARYN KUEBELBECK** PLYMOUTH, MN

START TO FINISH: 25 MIN.
MAKES: 9 SERVINGS

- 2 pounds parsnips, peeled and sliced
- 1½ pounds carrots, peeled and sliced
- ¾ cup chicken broth
- 3 tablespoons butter
- 2 tablespoons honey
- ½ teaspoon salt
- ½ teaspoon dried rosemary, crushed
   Dash cayenne pepper

In a Dutch oven, bring the parsnips, carrots and broth to a boil. Reduce heat; simmer, uncovered, for 6-8 minutes or until vegetables are tender. Add the remaining ingredients; heat through.
PER SERVING *¾ cup equals 152 cal., 4 g fat (2 g sat. fat), 10 mg chol., 302 mg sodium, 28 g carb., 6 g fiber, 2 g pro.* **Diabetic Exchanges:** *1 starch, 1 vegetable, 1 fat.*

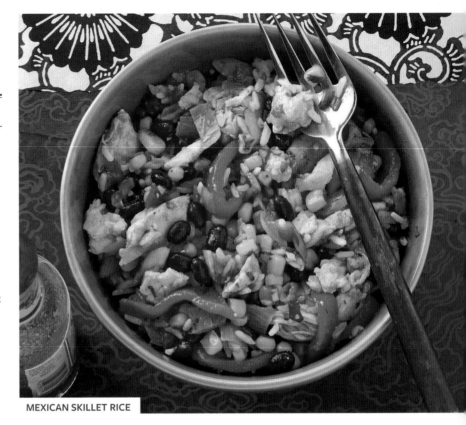

MEXICAN SKILLET RICE

PARSNIP-CARROT MEDLEY

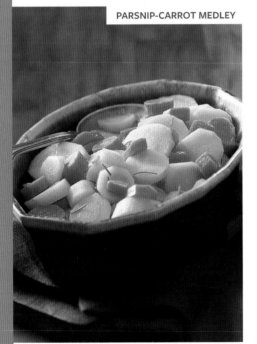

Mexican Skillet Rice

I never come home with leftovers when I take this dish to potlucks and parties, but I usually do bring back a lot of compliments!
—**MARY ANN DELL** PHOENIXVILLE, PA

START TO FINISH: 30 MIN.
MAKES: 6 SERVINGS

- 1 egg, beaten
- 1 pound chicken tenderloins, chopped
- 1 small onion, chopped
- 1 tablespoon olive oil
- 2 garlic cloves, minced
- 2 cups cooked jasmine or long grain rice
- 1 can (15 ounces) black beans, rinsed and drained
- 1 can (11 ounces) Mexicorn, drained
- 1 jar (7 ounces) roasted sweet red peppers, drained and sliced
- 1 jar (8 ounces) taco sauce
- 2 green onions, chopped
- ¼ cup minced fresh cilantro

1. In a large skillet coated with cooking spray, cook and stir the egg over medium-high heat until set. Remove and set aside.
2. In the same skillet, stir-fry chicken and onion in oil until chicken is no longer pink. Add garlic; cook 1 minute longer. Stir in the rice, beans, Mexicorn, peppers, taco sauce and green onions; heat through. Stir in reserved egg. Sprinkle rice with cilantro.
PER SERVING *1⅓ cups equals 302 cal., 4 g fat (1 g sat. fat), 80 mg chol., 793 mg sodium, 40 g carb., 5 g fiber, 25 g pro.* **Diabetic Exchanges:** *3 lean meat, 2 starch, ½ fat.*

Mustard Brussels Sprouts

Mustard boosts the flavor of the sprouts in this side dish. I recommend plating it alongside pork or chicken.

—LEAH-ANNE SCHNAPP GROVE CITY, OH

START TO FINISH: 25 MIN.
MAKES: 5 SERVINGS

- 1½ pounds fresh Brussels sprouts
- ⅓ cup chopped shallots
- 1 tablespoon butter
- ⅓ cup half-and-half cream
- 4½ teaspoons Dijon mustard
- ¼ teaspoon salt
- ¼ teaspoon dried tarragon
- ⅛ teaspoon pepper
- 2 tablespoons grated Parmesan cheese

1. Cut an "X" in the core of each Brussels sprout. In a Dutch oven, bring ½ in. of water to a boil. Add Brussels sprouts; cover and cook for 8-12 minutes or until tender.

2. Meanwhile, in a small saucepan, saute shallots in butter until tender. Add the cream, mustard, salt, tarragon and pepper. Cook and stir over medium heat until thickened. Drain sprouts; add cream mixture and heat through. Sprinkle with cheese.

PER SERVING *121 cal., 5 g fat (3 g sat. fat), 16 mg chol., 316 mg sodium, 16 g carb., 5 g fiber, 6 g pro.* **Diabetic Exchanges:** *2 vegetable, 1 fat.*

Sauteed Spring Vegetables

For an Asian twist, substitute soy sauce for the balsamic vinegar (be sure to adjust the salt level). You can also use red pepper flakes for a little added heat.

—BILLY HENSLEY MOUNT CARMEL, TN

PREP: 20 MIN. + MARINATING
COOK: 10 MIN.
MAKES: 9 SERVINGS

- 2 medium yellow summer squash, sliced
- 1 pound fresh asparagus, trimmed and cut into 1½-inch pieces
- 1 medium zucchini, sliced
- 1 small red onion, cut into thin wedges
- 1 cup green pepper strips
- ½ cup sweet red pepper strips

MARINADE

- ¼ cup olive oil
- 2 tablespoons balsamic vinegar
- 1 tablespoon lemon juice
- 2 garlic cloves, minced
- ½ teaspoon salt
- ½ teaspoon pepper
- ⅛ to ½ teaspoon crushed red pepper flakes

1. Place the vegetables in a large bowl. In a small bowl, whisk the marinade ingredients. Pour over vegetables; toss to coat. Cover and refrigerate for up to 1 hour.

2. In a large skillet, saute vegetable mixture in batches for 3-6 minutes or until crisp-tender.

PER SERVING *¾ cup equals 82 cal., 6 g fat (1 g sat. fat), 0 chol., 139 mg sodium, 6 g carb., 2 g fiber, 2 g pro.* **Diabetic Exchanges:** *1 vegetable, 1 fat.*

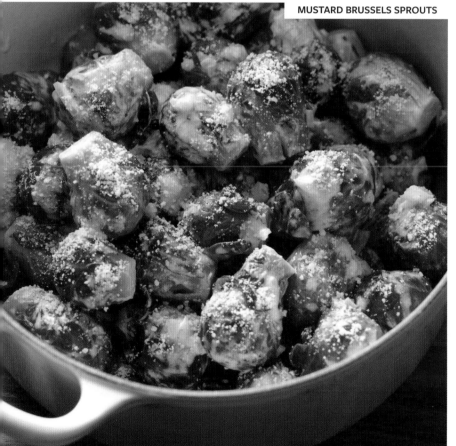

MUSTARD BRUSSELS SPROUTS

breads, rolls & muffins

Watching what you eat doesn't mean you have to give up the goodness of **freshly baked** treats! Turn here next time you're craving **golden loaves** or other bakeshop favorites.

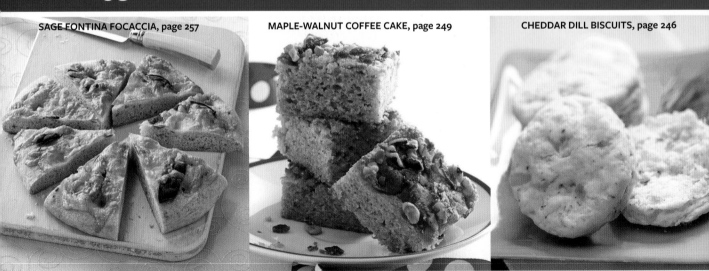

SAGE FONTINA FOCACCIA, page 257

MAPLE-WALNUT COFFEE CAKE, page 249

CHEDDAR DILL BISCUITS, page 246

4. Bake at 350° for 35-40 minutes or until golden brown. Remove from pans to wire racks to cool completely.

PER SERVING *141 cal., 2 g fat (1 g sat. fat), 17 mg chol., 239 mg sodium, 27 g carb., 1 g fiber, 4 g pro.* **Diabetic Exchange:** *1½ starch.*

Low-Fat Chocolate Muffins

Even if you have family members who aren't particularly fond of low-fat foods, these muffins will win them over. You can freeze them, too.

—**MONA KRUSE** MILAN, IL

PREP: 10 MIN. • **BAKE:** 15 MIN. + COOLING
MAKES: 1 DOZEN

- 1½ cups all-purpose flour
- ¾ cup sugar
- ¼ cup baking cocoa
- 2 teaspoons baking powder
- 1 teaspoon baking soda
- ½ teaspoon salt
- ⅔ cup fat-free vanilla yogurt
- ⅔ cup fat-free milk
- ½ teaspoon vanilla extract
  Confectioners' sugar, optional

1. In a large bowl, combine the first six ingredients. Stir in the yogurt, milk and vanilla just until moistened. Coat muffin cups with cooking spray; fill two-thirds full.
2. Bake at 400° for 15-20 minutes or until a toothpick inserted near the center comes out clean. Cool for 5 minutes before removing from pan to a wire rack; sprinkle with confectioners' sugar if desired.

PER SERVING *128 cal., trace fat (trace sat. fat), 1 mg chol., 258 mg sodium, 29 g carb., 1 g fiber, 3 g pro.* **Diabetic Exchange:** *2 starch.*

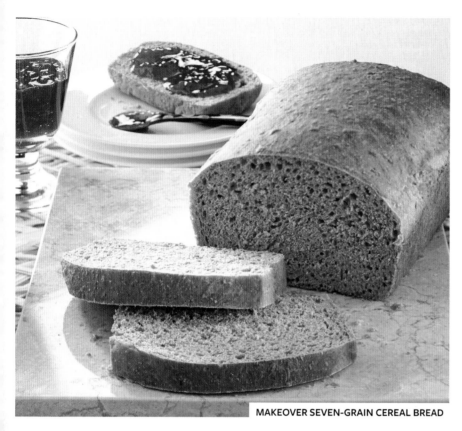

MAKEOVER SEVEN-GRAIN CEREAL BREAD

Makeover Seven-Grain Cereal Bread

Baking bread needn't be an all-day event. Quick-rise yeast helps these tender, mildly sweet loaves come together in just half the time.

—**LAURA REESE** FLAGSTAFF, AZ

PREP: 35 MIN. + RISING
BAKE: 35 MIN. + COOLING
MAKES: 2 LOAVES (16 SLICES EACH)

- ½ cup seven-grain cereal
- 2½ cups water
- ⅓ cup molasses
- ¼ cup butter, cubed
- 6 to 6¼ cups all-purpose flour
- 1 cup whole wheat flour
- ⅓ cup packed brown sugar
- 3 teaspoons salt
- 2 packages (¼ ounce each) quick-rise yeast
- 2 eggs

1. In a large microwave-safe bowl, combine cereal and water. Cover and cook on high for 4 minutes (mixture will be liquidy). Stir in molasses and butter. Let stand until mixture cools to 120°-130°, stirring occasionally.
2. In a large bowl, combine 4 cups all-purpose flour, whole wheat flour, brown sugar, salt and yeast. Add cereal mixture to dry ingredients; beat just until moistened. Add eggs; beat until smooth. Stir in enough remaining flour to form a firm dough (dough will be sticky).
3. Turn dough onto a floured surface; knead until smooth and elastic, about 6-8 minutes. Cover and let dough rest for 10 minutes. Divide dough in half. Shape into loaves. Place in two 9x5-in. loaf pans coated with cooking spray. Cover and let rise until doubled, about 45 minutes.

Buttermilk Onion Bread

Prepare this oniony bread in the bread machine, then serve it warm with dinner or use it to make hearty sandwiches.

—JOAN POWERS EAST WENATCHEE, WA

PREP: 10 MIN. • **BAKE:** 3 HOURS
MAKES: 1 LOAF (16 SLICES)

- 1 **cup plus 2 tablespoons warm buttermilk (70° to 80°)**
- 1 **tablespoon butter**
- 2½ **cups bread flour**
- ½ **cup whole wheat flour**
- 3 **tablespoons sugar**
- 1 **tablespoon dried minced onion**
- 1 **tablespoon dried parsley flakes**
- 1½ **teaspoons salt**
- 1 **teaspoon dill weed**
- 2¼ **teaspoons active dry yeast**

In bread machine pan, place all ingredients in order suggested by manufacturer. Select basic bread setting. Choose crust color and loaf size if available. Bake according to bread machine directions (check dough after 5 minutes of mixing; add 1 to 2 tablespoons of water or flour if needed).

PER SERVING *99 cal., 1 g fat (1 g sat. fat), 3 mg chol., 245 mg sodium, 20 g carb., 1 g fiber, 4 g pro.* **Diabetic Exchange:** *1 starch.*

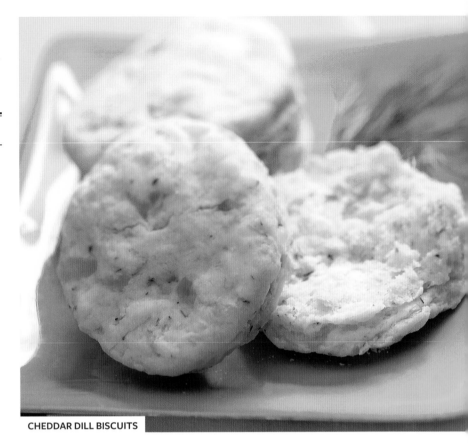

CHEDDAR DILL BISCUITS

Cheddar Dill Biscuits

My husband and I try to eat healthy, decreasing fat and calories wherever possible. These homemade biscuits are low-cal and great for breakfast or served alongside dinner.

—CAROL BRALY SOUTH FORK, CO

START TO FINISH: 30 MIN.
MAKES: 1 DOZEN

- 2 **cups all-purpose flour**
- 2 **teaspoons sugar**
- 1 **teaspoon dill weed**
- ½ **teaspoon baking soda**
- ½ **teaspoon cream of tartar**
- ½ **teaspoon salt**
- ¼ **cup cold butter, cubed**
- ⅔ **cup buttermilk**
- ¼ **cup egg substitute**
- ½ **cup shredded reduced-fat cheddar cheese**

1. In a large bowl, combine the first six ingredients. Cut in butter until mixture resembles coarse crumbs. Combine buttermilk and egg substitute; stir into flour mixture just until moistened. Stir in cheese.

2. Turn onto a lightly floured surface; knead 8-10 times. Pat to ¾-in. thickness; cut with a floured 2½-in. biscuit cutter.

3. Place 1 in. apart on an ungreased baking sheet. Bake at 400° for 12-16 minutes or until golden brown. Serve warm.

PER SERVING *134 cal., 5 g fat (3 g sat. fat), 14 mg chol., 245 mg sodium, 18 g carb., 1 g fiber, 4 g pro.* **Diabetic Exchanges:** *1 starch, 1 fat.*

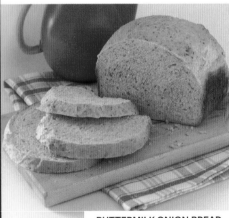

BUTTERMILK ONION BREAD

Swiss Cheese Muffins

Enjoy these muffins for snack or a quick breakfast. You won't be able to resist the cheesy goodness.

—**MARY RELYEA** CANASTOTA, NY

START TO FINISH: 30 MIN.
MAKES: 1 DOZEN

- 2 **cups all-purpose flour**
- 1 **tablespoon sugar**
- ¾ **teaspoon salt**
- ½ **teaspoon baking soda**
- 2 **eggs**
- 1 **cup (8 ounces) reduced-fat sour cream**
- 2 **tablespoons canola oil**
- ½ **cup shredded Swiss cheese**
- 2 **green onions, chopped**

1. In a small bowl, combine the flour, sugar, salt and baking soda. In another bowl, combine the eggs, sour cream and oil. Stir into dry ingredients just until moistened. Fold in cheese and onions.
2. Coat muffin cups with cooking spray or use paper liners; fill three-fourths full with batter. Bake at 375° for 15-18 minutes or until a toothpick inserted in muffin comes out clean. Cool muffins for 5 minutes before removing from pan to a wire rack. Serve warm.
PER SERVING *157 cal., 6 g fat (2 g sat. fat), 46 mg chol., 237 mg sodium, 19 g carb., 1 g fiber, 6 g pro.* **Diabetic Exchanges:** *1 starch, 1 fat.*

SWISS CHEESE MUFFINS

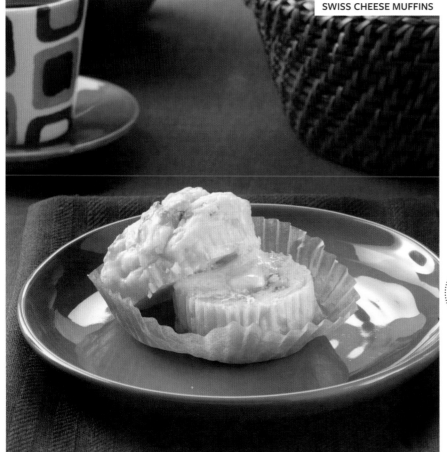

Dilly Spoon Rolls

I prepare a big batch and freeze the extras.

—**ELLEN THOMPSON** SPRINGFIELD, OH

PREP: 30 MIN. + RISING • **BAKE:** 15 MIN.
MAKES: 1½ DOZEN

- 1 **package (¼ ounce) active dry yeast**
- 1½ **cups warm fat-free milk (110° to 115°)**
- 3 **to 3½ cups all-purpose flour**
- ¼ **cup sugar**
- 1 **teaspoon dill weed**
- ¾ **teaspoon salt**
- 1 **egg, lightly beaten**
- ¼ **cup canola oil**

1. In a large bowl, dissolve yeast in warm milk. Stir in 1½ cups flour, sugar, dill, salt, egg and oil. Beat until smooth. Beat in enough remaining flour to achieve a slightly sticky, thick batter. Do not knead. Cover and let rise in a warm place until doubled, about 45 minutes.
2. Spoon batter into muffin cups coated with cooking spray. Cover and let rise until doubled, about 30 minutes.
3. Bake at 400° for 13-18 minutes or until golden brown. Remove from pans to wire racks. Serve warm.
PER SERVING *127 cal., 4 g fat (trace sat. fat), 12 mg chol., 113 mg sodium, 20 g carb., 1 g fiber, 3 g pro.* **Diabetic Exchanges:** *1 starch, 1 fat.*

top tip
Freezing Yeast Dough

Divide the dough into desired amounts and flatten into disks 1 inch thick. Set disks on baking sheets; freeze for 1 hour. Wrap frozen dough tightly with plastic wrap; place in resealable storage bags. Freeze for up to 4 weeks.

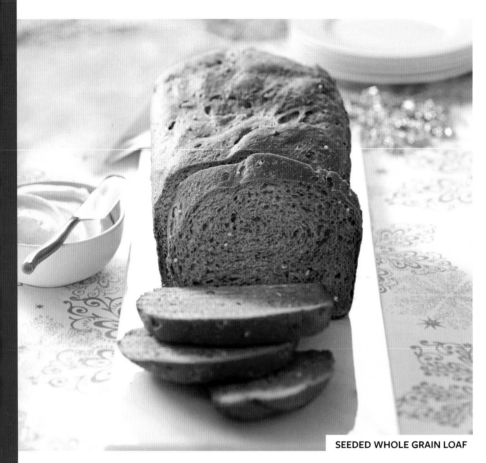

SEEDED WHOLE GRAIN LOAF

Morning Cinnamon Rolls

Convenient crescent roll dough hurries along these yummy glazed rolls. They're great with a cup of hot coffee.

—HELEN LIPKO MARTINSBURG, PA

START TO FINISH: 25 MIN.
MAKES: 8 SERVINGS

- 1 tube (8 ounces) refrigerated reduced-fat crescent rolls
- ½ teaspoon ground cinnamon Sugar substitute equivalent to ½ cup sugar, divided
- ¼ cup confectioners' sugar
- 1 tablespoon fat-free milk

1. Unroll crescent dough into a rectangle; seal seams and perforations. Combine the cinnamon and half of the sugar substitute; sprinkle over dough. Roll up jelly-roll style, starting with a long side; seal edge. Cut into eight slices.

2. Place rolls cut side down in a 9-in. round baking pan coated with cooking spray. Bake at 375° for 12-15 minutes or until golden brown.

3. In a small bowl, combine the confectioners' sugar, milk and remaining sugar substitute; drizzle over warm rolls.

TO FREEZE *Cool unfrosted rolls and wrap in foil. Freeze for up to 3 months.*
TO USE FROZEN ROLLS *Thaw at room temperature; warm if desired. Follow directions for icing.*
NOTE *This recipe was tested with Splenda sugar blend.*
PER SERVING *123 cal., 5 g fat (1 g sat. fat), trace chol., 234 mg sodium, 18 g carb., trace fiber, 2 g pro.* **Diabetic Exchanges:** *1 starch, 1 fat.*

Seeded Whole Grain Loaf

My husband and I wanted to eat more whole grain bread, but we didn't like the spongy texture of some store-bought varieties. I ended up drastically altering one of my favorite batter bread recipes to create this earthy loaf. The add-ins are simply suggestions—sometimes I use pepitas, sesame seeds or even ¼ cup of a multigrain hot cereal mix.

—AMBER RIFE COLUMBUS, OH

PREP: 20 MIN. • **BAKE:** 4 HOURS
MAKES: 1 LOAF (1½ POUNDS, 16 SLICES)

- 1⅓ cups warm 2% milk (70° to 80°)
- 3 tablespoons honey
- 2 tablespoons canola oil
- 1¼ teaspoons salt
- 2⅔ cups whole wheat flour
- 2 tablespoons old-fashioned oats
- 4 teaspoons vital wheat gluten
- 1 tablespoon millet
- 1 tablespoon sunflower kernels
- 1 tablespoon flaxseed
- 1 tablespoon cracked wheat or additional flaxseed
- 1 package (¼ ounce) active dry yeast

In bread machine pan, place all the ingredients in order suggested by manufacturer. Select basic bread setting. Choose the crust color and loaf size if available. Bake according to bread machine directions (check dough after 5 minutes of mixing; add 1 to 2 tablespoons of water or flour if needed).
PER SERVING *128 cal., 3 g fat (1 g sat. fat), 2 mg chol., 199 mg sodium, 21 g carb., 3 g fiber, 5 g pro.* **Diabetic Exchanges:** *1 starch, ½ fat.*

Maple-Walnut Coffee Cake

Sleepyheads will roll out of bed when they smell this sweet and savory coffee cake baking. Bacon and nuts in the crumbly topping blend beautifully with maple, nutmeg and cinnamon.

—ANGELA SPENGLER CLOVIS, NM

PREP: 25 MIN. • **BAKE:** 35 MIN. + COOLING
MAKES: 24 SERVINGS

- 2½ cups all-purpose flour
- 1 cup packed brown sugar
- ½ teaspoon salt
- ⅓ cup cold butter
- 2 teaspoons baking powder
- ½ teaspoon baking soda
- ½ teaspoon ground cinnamon
- ¼ teaspoon ground nutmeg
- 2 eggs
- 1½ cups buttermilk
- ½ cup maple syrup
- ⅓ cup unsweetened applesauce
- 5 bacon strips, cooked and crumbled
- ½ cup chopped walnuts

1. In a large bowl, combine the flour, brown sugar and salt. Cut in butter until crumbly. Set aside ½ cup for topping. Combine the baking powder, baking soda, cinnamon and nutmeg; stir into remaining flour mixture.

2. In a small bowl, whisk the eggs, buttermilk, syrup and applesauce until well blended. Gradually stir into flour mixture until combined.

3. Spread into a 13x9-in. baking pan coated with cooking spray. Sprinkle with reserved topping, then with the bacon and walnuts. Bake at 350° for 35-40 minutes or until a toothpick inserted near the center comes out clean. Cool on a wire rack.

PER SERVING *1 piece equals 160 cal., 5 g fat (2 g sat. fat), 27 mg chol., 183 mg sodium, 25 g carb., 1 g fiber, 3 g pro.* **Diabetic Exchanges:** *1½ starch, 1 fat.*

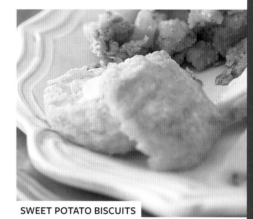

SWEET POTATO BISCUITS

Sweet Potato Biscuits

Using sweet potatoes in a bread recipe may sound a little odd, but the results are divinely delicious.

—DELYNNE RUTLEDGE LOVELADY, TX

START TO FINISH: 30 MIN.
MAKES: 17 BISCUITS

- 2 cups all-purpose flour
- ⅓ cup yellow cornmeal
- 2½ teaspoons baking powder
- ½ teaspoon salt
- ⅓ cup cold butter, cubed
- 1 cup mashed sweet potato
- ½ cup fat-free milk
- 2 tablespoons honey

1. In a large bowl, combine the flour, cornmeal, baking powder and salt. Cut in butter until the mixture resembles coarse crumbs. Stir in the sweet potato, milk and honey just until moistened. Turn onto a lightly floured surface; knead 5-8 times. Pat out to ½-in. thickness; cut with a floured 2-in. biscuit cutter.

2. Place 2 in. apart on an ungreased baking sheet. Bake at 400° for 14-18 minutes or until lightly browned. Serve warm.

PER SERVING *120 cal., 4 g fat (2 g sat. fat), 10 mg chol., 162 mg sodium, 19 g carb., 1 g fiber, 2 g pro.* **Diabetic Exchanges:** *1 starch, 1 fat.*

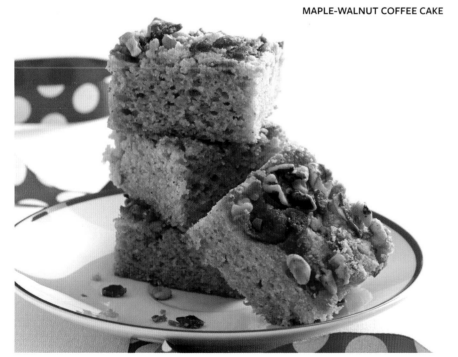

MAPLE-WALNUT COFFEE CAKE

Parmesan Herb Loaf

Take frozen bread dough to a new level when you try this good-for-you recipe.

—**SHIRLEY SIBIT RUDDER** BURKEVILLE, TX

PREP: 10 MIN. + RISING • **BAKE:** 20 MIN.
MAKES: 1 LOAF (12 SLICES)

- 1 **loaf (1 pound) frozen whole wheat bread dough**
- ¼ **cup shredded Parmesan cheese**
- 1½ **teaspoons dried parsley flakes**
- 1½ **teaspoons dried minced garlic**
- ¼ **teaspoon dill weed**
- ¼ **teaspoon salt**
- 1 **tablespoon butter, melted**

1. Place dough in an 8x4-in. loaf pan coated with cooking spray. Thaw according to package directions. In a small bowl, combine the cheese, parsley, garlic, dill and salt. Brush dough with butter; sprinkle with cheese mixture. Cover and let rise in a warm place until nearly doubled, about 2½ hours.

2. Bake at 350° for 20-25 minutes or until golden brown. Remove from pan to a wire rack to cool.

PER SERVING *111 cal., 3 g fat (1 g sat. fat), 4 mg chol., 250 mg sodium, 18 g carb., 2 g fiber, 6 g pro.* **Diabetic Exchange:** *1 starch.*

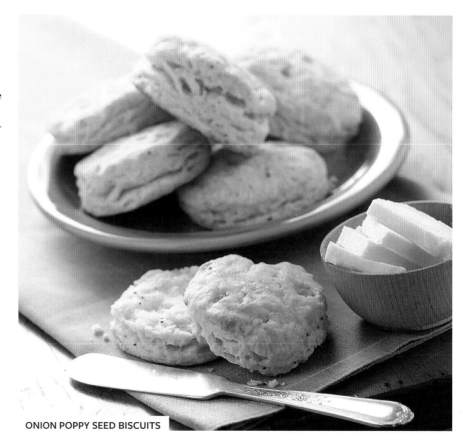

ONION POPPY SEED BISCUITS

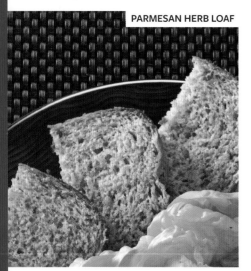

PARMESAN HERB LOAF

Onion Poppy Seed Biscuits

Perfect alongside a salad or casserole, these buttermilk biscuits are ready in no time. Golden on the outside but soft on the inside, they offer a mild onion taste with every bite.

—**TASTE OF HOME TEST KITCHEN**

START TO FINISH: 30 MIN.
MAKES: 1 DOZEN

- 1 **medium onion, finely chopped**
- 2 **cups all-purpose flour**
- 1 **teaspoon baking powder**
- 1 **teaspoon brown sugar**
- ¾ **teaspoon poppy seeds**
- ½ **teaspoon salt**
- ½ **teaspoon baking soda**
- ¼ **cup cold butter, cubed**
- 1 **cup buttermilk**

1. In a small nonstick skillet coated with cooking spray, saute the onion until tender; set aside. In a large bowl, combine the flour, baking powder, brown sugar, poppy seeds, salt and baking soda. Cut in butter until mixture resembles coarse crumbs. Stir in onions. Stir in buttermilk just until moistened.

2. Turn dough onto a lightly floured surface; knead 6-8 times. Pat to ½-in. thickness; cut with a floured 2½-in. biscuit cutter. Place 2 in. apart on baking sheets coated with cooking spray.

3. Bake at 450° for 9-12 minutes or until golden brown. Serve warm.

PER SERVING *125 cal., 4 g fat (3 g sat. fat), 11 mg chol., 245 mg sodium, 18 g carb., 1 g fiber, 3 g pro.* **Diabetic Exchanges:** *1 starch, 1 fat.*

Sweet Potato Yeast Rolls

Mashed sweet potatoes add a hint of color and flavor to these home-baked dinner rolls. The tempting knots are topped with a sprinkling of sesame seeds.

—TASTE OF HOME TEST KITCHEN

PREP: 35 MIN. + RISING • **BAKE:** 15 MIN.
MAKES: 2½ DOZEN

- 1 **package (¼ ounce) active dry yeast**
- 1 **cup warm fat-free milk (110° to 115°)**
- 1 **teaspoon plus ⅓ cup sugar, divided**
- ⅓ **cup cold mashed sweet potatoes**
- 2 **eggs, separated**
- 2 **tablespoons butter, softened**
- ¾ **teaspoon salt**
- 3½ **to 4 cups all-purpose flour**
- 4 **teaspoons cold water**
- 1 **tablespoon sesame seeds**

1. In a large bowl, dissolve yeast in warm milk. Add 1 teaspoon sugar; let stand for 5 minutes. Add the sweet potatoes, egg yolks, butter, salt, remaining sugar and 2 cups flour. Beat until smooth. Stir in enough remaining flour to form a soft dough.

2. Turn onto a floured surface; knead until smooth and elastic, about 6-8 minutes. Place in a bowl coated with cooking spray, turning once to coat top. Cover and let rise in a warm place until doubled, about 1½ hours.

3. Punch dough down. Turn onto a lightly floured surface; divide into 30 balls. Roll each ball into a 10-in. rope; tie each rope into a loose knot. Place 2 in. apart on baking sheets coated with cooking spray. Cover and let rise until doubled, about 30 minutes.

4. In a small bowl, beat egg whites and cold water; brush over rolls. Sprinkle with sesame seeds. Bake at 350° for 15-17 minutes or until lightly browned. Remove from pans to cool on wire racks.

PER SERVING *92 cal., 1 g fat (1 g sat. fat), 16 mg chol., 76 mg sodium, 16 g carb., 1 g fiber, 3 g pro.* **Diabetic Exchange:** *1 starch.*

Dilled Wheat Bread

I like to serve this everyday bread with just about any meal, especially alongside hearty soups and stews.

—**JENNY WITCRAFT** CLEVELAND, OH

PREP: 10 MIN. • **BAKE:** 3 HOURS
MAKES: 1 LOAF (1¾ POUNDS, 12 SLICES)

- 1¼ **cups water (70° to 80°)**
- 1 **tablespoon butter, softened**
- 2 **tablespoons sugar**
- 2 **teaspoons dill weed**
- 1½ **teaspoons salt**
- 2 **cups whole wheat flour**
- 1¼ **cups all-purpose flour**
- 1½ **teaspoons active dry yeast**

In bread machine pan, place all ingredients in order suggested by manufacturer. Select basic bread setting. Choose crust color and loaf size if available. Bake according to bread machine directions (check the dough after 5 minutes of mixing; add 1 to 2 tablespoons of water or flour if needed).

PER SERVING *134 cal., 1 g fat (1 g sat. fat), 3 mg chol., 307 mg sodium, 27 g carb., 3 g fiber, 4 g pro.* **Diabetic Exchange:** *1½ starch.*

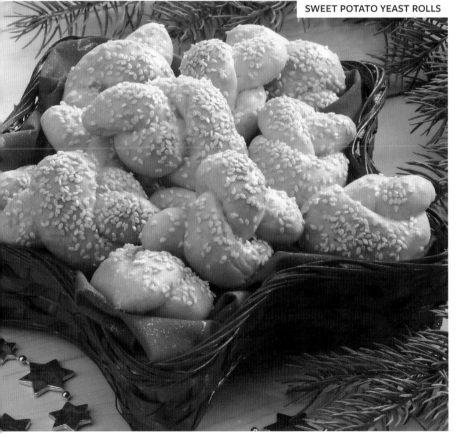

SWEET POTATO YEAST ROLLS

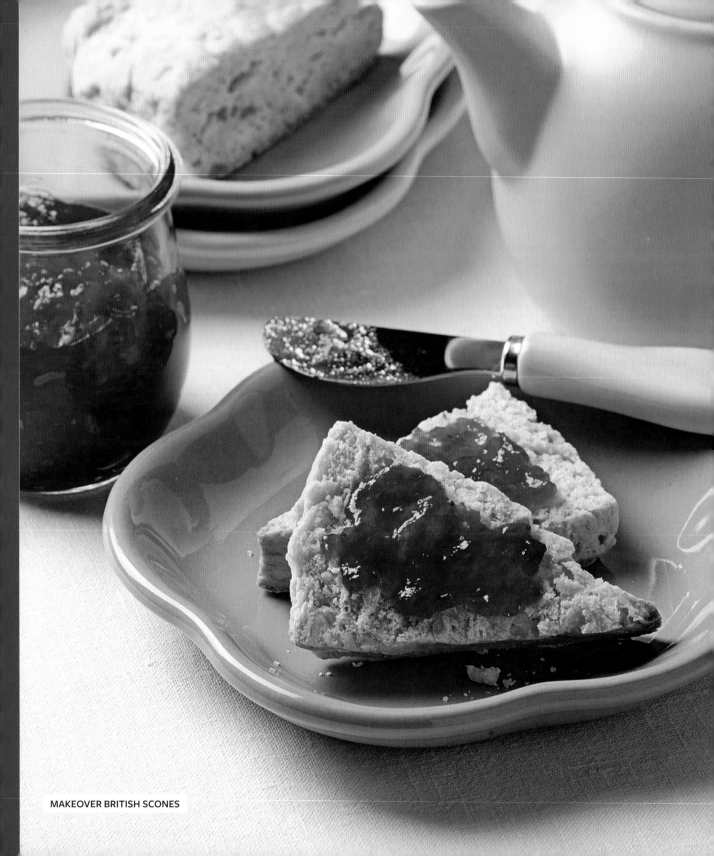

MAKEOVER BRITISH SCONES

Makeover British Scones

Enjoy these lightened-up scones—they come in at 54 fewer calories and 75 percent less saturated fat per serving than the original recipe!

—**CAROLE JASLER** LECANTO, FL

START TO FINISH: 30 MIN.
MAKES: 8 SCONES

- 1¼ cups all-purpose flour
- 1 cup cake flour
- 2 tablespoons brown sugar
- 1½ teaspoons baking powder
- ½ teaspoon salt
- ¼ teaspoon baking soda
- 3 tablespoons cold butter
- 1 egg, lightly beaten
- ⅓ cup buttermilk
- 2 tablespoons canola oil
- ½ teaspoon vanilla extract
- 1 tablespoon 2% milk
- 1 teaspoon sugar

1. In a large bowl, combine the flours, brown sugar, baking powder, salt and baking soda. Cut in butter until mixture resembles coarse crumbs. Combine the egg, buttermilk, oil and vanilla; add to crumb mixture and stir until a soft dough forms. Turn onto a floured surface; gently knead 6-8 times.
2. Pat dough into a 6-in. circle. Cut into eight wedges. Separate wedges and place 1 in. apart on an ungreased baking sheet. Brush tops with milk; sprinkle with sugar. Bake at 400° for 12-14 minutes or until lightly browned. Remove to a wire rack. Serve warm.
PER SERVING *219 cal., 9 g fat (3 g sat. fat), 39 mg chol., 343 mg sodium, 30 g carb., 1 g fiber, 4 g pro. **Diabetic Exchanges:** 2 starch, 1½ fat.*

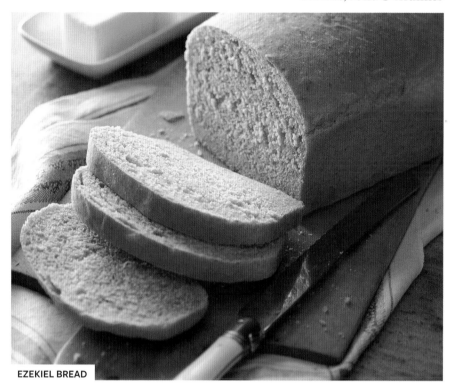
EZEKIEL BREAD

Ezekiel Bread

My bread bakes up tender and chewy with a hint of sweetness. It's great to give as a gift or to accompany your Sunday dinner.

—**ROGER HAWLEY** VALLEY PARK, MO

PREP: 45 MIN. + RISING
BAKE: 30 MIN. + COOLING
MAKES: 4 LOAVES (16 SLICES EACH)

- 3 packages (¼ ounce each) active dry yeast
- 5 cups warm water (110° to 115°), divided
- 1 tablespoon plus ⅔ cup honey, divided
- ⅔ cup canola oil
- ½ cup sugar
- 2 teaspoons salt
- 4 cups whole wheat flour
- 1 cup toasted wheat germ
- 6 to 8 cups bread flour

1. In a large bowl, dissolve yeast in ¾ cup warm water and 1 tablespoon honey. Add the remaining water and honey, oil, sugar, salt, whole wheat flour, wheat germ and 3 cups bread flour. Beat until smooth. Stir in enough remaining bread flour to form a soft dough (dough will be sticky).
2. Turn onto a lightly floured surface; knead until smooth and elastic, about 6-8 minutes. Place in a bowl coated with cooking spray, turning once to coat the top. Cover and let rise in a warm place until doubled, about 1 hour.
3. Punch dough down. Shape into four loaves. Place in 9x5-in. loaf pans coated with cooking spray. Cover and let rise until nearly doubled, about 30 minutes.
4. Bake at 350° for 30-35 minutes or until golden brown. Remove from pans to wire racks to cool.
PER SERVING *108 cal., 3 g fat (trace sat. fat), 0 chol., 75 mg sodium, 19 g carb., 1 g fiber, 3 g pro. **Diabetic Exchange:** 1½ starch.*

Honey Wheat Breadsticks

Not only are these breadsticks delicious, but they come together easily. Whole wheat flour and a little honey keep them on the healthy side.

—TED VAN SCHOICK JERSEY SHORE, PA

PREP: 30 MIN. + RISING • **BAKE:** 10 MIN.
MAKES: 16 BREADSTICKS

1⅓ cups water (70° to 80°)
3 tablespoons honey
2 tablespoons canola oil
1½ teaspoons salt
2 cups bread flour
2 cups whole wheat flour
3 teaspoons active dry yeast

1. In bread machine pan, place all ingredients in order suggested by manufacturer. Select dough setting (check dough after 5 minutes of mixing; add 1 to 2 tablespoons of water or flour if needed.
2. When cycle is completed, turn dough onto a lightly floured surface. Divide into 16 portions; shape each into a ball. Roll each into an 8-in. rope. Place 2 in. apart on greased baking sheets.
3. Cover and let rise in a warm place until doubled, about 30 minutes. Bake at 375° for 10-12 minutes or until golden brown. Remove to wire racks.
PER SERVING *131 cal., 2 g fat (trace sat. fat), 0 chol., 222 mg sodium, 25 g carb., 2 g fiber, 4 g pro.* **Diabetic Exchanges:** *1½ starch.*

top tip
Bread Flour

Bread flour is made from high-gluten hard wheat flour, giving strength and elasticity to yeast doughs. Bread flour can also be used for yeast-raised doughs, strudel, puff pastry and popovers.

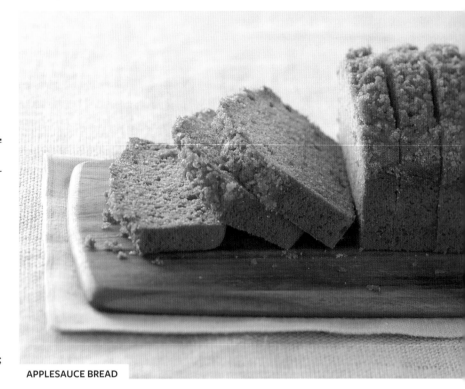

APPLESAUCE BREAD

Applesauce Bread

The abundant applesauce in this bread recipe provides natural sweetness, so you use less sugar. You also won't need to use much oil.

—SHERRY CRAW MATTOON, IL

PREP: 20 MIN. • **BAKE:** 50 MIN. + COOLING
MAKES: 1 LOAF (16 SLICES)

1 cup all-purpose flour
1 cup whole wheat flour
½ cup sugar
1½ teaspoons ground cinnamon, divided
1 teaspoon baking soda
½ teaspoon salt
½ teaspoon baking powder
¼ teaspoon ground nutmeg
2 egg whites
1 egg
1¼ cups unsweetened applesauce
¼ cup canola oil
3 tablespoons fat-free milk
¼ cup packed brown sugar

1. In a large bowl, combine the flours, sugar, 1 teaspoon cinnamon, baking soda, salt, baking powder and nutmeg. In a small bowl, whisk the egg whites, egg, applesauce, oil and milk. Stir into dry ingredients just until moistened.
2. Transfer to a 9x5-in. loaf pan coated with cooking spray. Combine brown sugar and remaining cinnamon; sprinkle over the top.
3. Bake at 350° for 50-60 minutes or until a toothpick inserted near the center comes out clean. Cool bread for 10 minutes before removing from pan to a wire rack.
PER SERVING *139 cal., 4 g fat (trace sat. fat), 13 mg chol., 180 mg sodium, 24 g carb., 1 g fiber, 3 g pro.* **Diabetic Exchanges:** *1½ starch, ½ fat.*

Jalapeno Garlic Bread

My mother loves spicy foods, so I created this crusty rustic loaf for her. Now my whole family requests it.

—NATALIE ANN GALLAGHER CLOVIS, CA

PREP: 30 MIN. + RISING
BAKE: 40 MIN. + COOLING
MAKES: 2 LOAVES (12 SLICES EACH)

- 1 cup warm fat-free milk (70° to 80°)
- ½ cup egg substitute
- 2 tablespoons butter, melted
- 1 teaspoon salt
- 2 cups bread flour
- 2 cups whole wheat flour
- ¼ cup sugar
- 2 teaspoons active dry yeast

FILLING

- ¾ cup chopped seeded jalapeno peppers
- 3 garlic cloves, minced
- 5 teaspoons butter, softened, divided
- 1 teaspoon garlic salt
- 3 tablespoons grated Parmesan cheese, divided

1. In bread machine pan, place the first eight ingredients in order suggested by manufacturer. Select dough setting (check dough after 5 minutes of mixing; add 1 to 2 tablespoons of water or flour if needed).

2. In a small bowl, combine the jalapenos and garlic; set aside. When cycle is completed, turn dough onto a lightly floured surface. Divide dough in half.

3. For each loaf, roll one portion of dough into a 14x9-in. rectangle. Spread dough with 1½ teaspoons butter. Sprinkle with ½ teaspoon garlic salt, 1 tablespoon cheese and ⅓ cup of the jalapeno mixture. Roll up jelly-roll style, starting with a short side; pinch seam to seal. Place in a 9x5-in. loaf pan coated with cooking spray. Cover and let rise in a warm place until doubled, about 40 minutes.

4. Melt remaining butter; brush over loaves. Sprinkle with remaining cheese and jalapeno mixture.

5. Bake at 350° for 40-50 minutes or until golden brown. Remove from pans to wire racks to cool.

NOTE *Wear disposable gloves when cutting hot peppers; the oils can burn skin. Avoid touching your face.*

PER SERVING *102 cal., 2 g fat (1 g sat. fat), 5 mg chol., 220 mg sodium, 18 g carb., 2 g fiber, 4 g pro.* **Diabetic Exchanges:** *1 starch, ½ fat.*

Pumpkin Oat Bran Muffins

These muffins freeze well, are very nutritious and taste incredible—so they disappear fast!

—IRENE ROBINSON CINCINNATI, OH

PREP: 15 MIN. • **BAKE:** 20 MIN.
MAKES: 9 MUFFINS.

- 1½ cups oat bran
- ½ cup all-purpose flour
- ½ cup packed brown sugar
- 2 teaspoons baking powder
- 1 teaspoon pumpkin pie spice
- ½ teaspoon salt
- 2 egg whites
- 1 cup canned pumpkin
- ½ cup fat-free milk
- 2 tablespoons canola oil

1. In a small bowl, combine the first six ingredients. In another bowl, whisk the egg whites, pumpkin, milk and oil until well blended. Stir into dry ingredients just until moistened.

2. Coat muffin cups with cooking spray; fill half full. Bake at 400° for 20-25 minutes or until a toothpick inserted near the center comes out clean. Cool muffins for 5 minutes before removing from pan to a wire rack. Serve warm.

PER SERVING *155 cal., 4 g fat (trace sat. fat), trace chol., 246 mg sodium, 30 g carb., 4 g fiber, 5 g pro.* **Diabetic Exchanges:** *2 starch, ½ fat.*

JALAPENO GARLIC BREAD

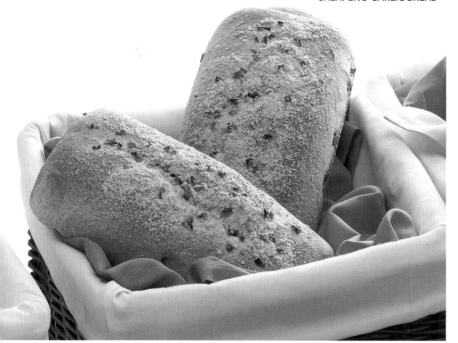

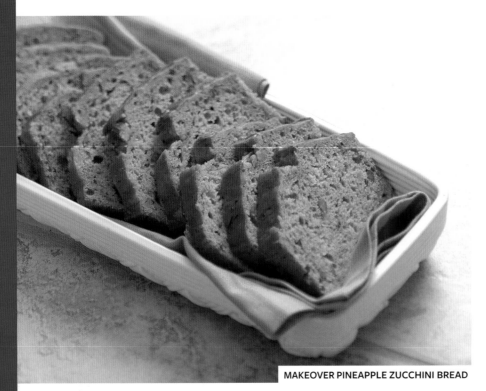

Makeover Pumpkin Spice Bread

With less than half the fat and just one-fourth the calories of my original recipe, this new favorite allows even those who are watching what they eat to enjoy a slice or two without guilt.

—**HEIDI FIGIEL** BRIDGEPORT, WV

PREP: 20 MIN. • **BAKE:** 45 MIN. + COOLING
MAKES: 2 LOAVES (16 SLICES EACH)

- 2¼ cups sugar
- 2 cups all-purpose flour
- 1⅓ cups cake flour
- 2 teaspoons baking soda
- 2 teaspoons ground cinnamon
- 1 teaspoon salt
- 1 teaspoon baking powder
- ¾ teaspoon ground cloves
- ½ teaspoon ground nutmeg
- 4 eggs
- 1 can (15 ounces) solid-pack pumpkin
- 1 cup buttermilk
- ½ cup unsweetened applesauce
- ⅓ cup canola oil

1. In a large bowl, combine the first nine ingredients. In another bowl, whisk the eggs, pumpkin, buttermilk, applesauce and oil. Stir into dry ingredients just until moistened.
2. Transfer to two 9x5-in. loaf pans coated with cooking spray. Bake at 350° for 45-55 minutes or until golden brown and a toothpick inserted near the center comes out with moist crumbs. Cool for 10 minutes before removing from pans to wire racks.
PER SERVING *143 cal., 3 g fat (trace sat. fat), 27 mg chol., 183 mg sodium, 27 g carb., 1 g fiber, 3 g pro.* **Diabetic Exchanges:** *2 starch, ½ fat.*

Makeover Pineapple Zucchini Bread

This makeover recipe has the delectable taste and wonderful texture of my original loaf, but with less than half the fat and one-third fewer calories.

—**NANCY SKRAMSTED** BILLINGS, MT

PREP: 20 MIN. • **BAKE:** 50 MIN. + COOLING
MAKES: 2 LOAVES (12 SLICES EACH)

- 1½ cups sugar
- ⅔ cup unsweetened applesauce
- ⅓ cup canola oil
- 2 egg whites
- 1 egg
- 2 teaspoons vanilla extract
- 3 cups all-purpose flour
- 2 teaspoons ground cinnamon
- 1½ teaspoons baking powder
- 1 teaspoon salt
- ¾ teaspoon ground nutmeg
- ½ teaspoon baking soda
- 2 cups shredded zucchini
- 1 can (8 ounces) unsweetened crushed pineapple, drained
- ⅓ cup chopped walnuts

1. In a large bowl, beat the sugar, applesauce, oil, egg whites, egg and vanilla until well blended. Combine the flour, cinnamon, baking powder, salt, nutmeg and baking soda; gradually beat into sugar mixture until blended. Stir in the zucchini, pineapple and walnuts.
2. Transfer to two 8x4-in. loaf pans coated with cooking spray. Bake at 350° for 50-60 minutes or until a toothpick inserted near the center comes out clean. Cool for 10 minutes before removing from pans to wire racks to cool completely.
PER SERVING *159 cal., 5 g fat (trace sat. fat), 9 mg chol., 158 mg sodium, 27 g carb., 1 g fiber, 3 g pro.* **Diabetic Exchanges:** *2 starch, 1 fat.*

Sage Fontina Focaccia

Add sage to your bread and it'll complement almost any main dish.
—**BETH DAUENHAUER** PUEBLO, CO

PREP: 30 MIN. + RISING • **BAKE:** 10 MIN.
MAKES: 1 LOAF (8 WEDGES)

- 1¼ **teaspoons active dry yeast**
- ½ **cup warm water (110° to 115°)**
- ½ **teaspoon honey**
- ¾ **to 1 cup all-purpose flour**
- ¼ **cup whole wheat flour**
- 1 **tablespoon olive oil**
- 2 **teaspoons minced fresh sage**
- ¼ **teaspoon salt**

TOPPING

- 1½ **teaspoons olive oil, divided**
- 8 **fresh sage leaves**
- ½ **cup shredded fontina cheese**

1. In a large bowl, dissolve yeast in warm water. Stir in honey; let stand for 5 minutes. Add ¾ cup all-purpose flour, whole wheat flour, oil, minced sage and salt. Beat on medium speed for 3 minutes or until smooth. Stir in enough remaining flour to form a soft dough (dough will be sticky).

2. Turn onto a lightly floured surface; knead until smooth and elastic, about 6-8 minutes. Place in a large bowl coated with cooking spray, turning once to coat the top. Cover and let rise in a warm place until doubled, about 1 hour.

3. Punch dough down. Cover and let rest for 5 minutes. Shape into an 8-in. circle; place on a baking sheet coated with cooking spray. Cover and let rise until doubled, about 30 minutes. Using the end of a wooden spoon handle, make several ¼-in. indentations in the loaf.

4. For topping, brush dough with 1 teaspoon oil. Top with sage leaves; brush leaves with remaining oil. Sprinkle with cheese. Bake at 400° for 8-10 minutes or until golden brown. Remove to a wire rack.

PER SERVING *112 cal., 5 g fat (2 g sat. fat), 8 mg chol., 131 mg sodium, 12 g carb., 1 g fiber, 4 g pro.* **Diabetic Exchanges:** *1 starch, 1 fat.*

Seven-Grain Bread

Flavorful and stuffed with grains, this lovely loaf is the best thing I've ever made in my bread machine.
—**LISE THOMSON** MAGRATH, AB

PREP: 10 MIN. • **BAKE:** 3 HOURS
MAKES: 1 LOAF (16 SLICES)

- 1⅔ **cups water (70° to 80°)**
- 3 **tablespoons nonfat dry milk powder**
- 2 **tablespoons shortening**
- 2 **tablespoons honey**
- 2 **teaspoons salt**
- 2½ **cups all-purpose flour**
- 1 **cup whole wheat flour**
- ¾ **cup five-grain cereal**
- 1¼ **teaspoons active dry yeast**

In bread machine pan, place all ingredients in order suggested by manufacturer. Select basic bread setting. Choose crust color and loaf size if available. Bake according to bread machine directions (check dough after 5 minutes of mixing; add 1 to 2 tablespoons of water or flour if needed).

NOTE *This recipe was tested with Red Mill brand five-grain cereal. You may substitute Oatmeal Crisp Raisin Cereal. Remove raisins and crush enough cereal to measure ¾ cup.*

PER SERVING *134 cal., 2 g fat (trace sat. fat), trace chol., 298 mg sodium, 26 g carb., 2 g fiber, 4 g pro.* **Diabetic Exchange:** *1½ starch.*

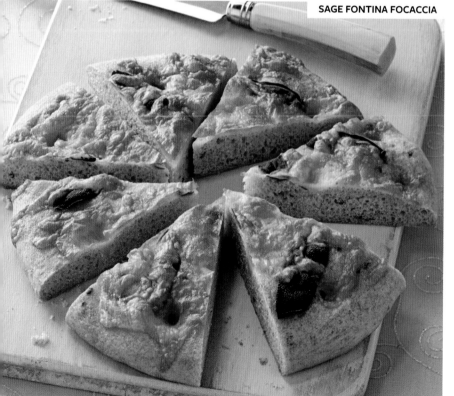

SAGE FONTINA FOCACCIA

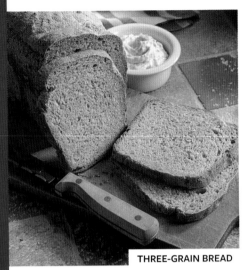

THREE-GRAIN BREAD

Three-Grain Bread

My grandchildren really like this hearty loaf's crunchy crust and chewy texture. I like how nutritious it is because it contains more fiber than many other loaves.

—**JOHN REED** LEES SUMMIT, MO

PREP: 10 MIN. • **BAKE:** 3 HOURS
MAKES: 1 LOAF (2 POUNDS, 20 SLICES)

- 1½ cups water (70° to 80°)
- ½ cup honey
- 1½ teaspoons salt
- 2 cups bread flour
- 1 cup whole wheat flour
- ¾ cup rye flour
- ¾ cup cornmeal
- 2¼ teaspoons active dry yeast

1. In bread machine pan, place all ingredients in order suggested by manufacturer. Select basic bread setting. Choose crust color and loaf size if available.

2. Bake according to bread machine directions (check dough after 5 minutes of mixing; add 1 to 2 tablespoons of water or flour if needed).

PER SERVING *108 cal., trace fat (trace sat. fat), 0 chol., 148 mg sodium, 24 g carb., 2 g fiber, 3 g pro.* **Diabetic Exchange:** *1½ starch.*

Tart Cranberry Quick Bread

My mother loved to bake this cranberry bread. I usually stock up on cranberries when they're in season and freeze them so I can prepare the loaf year-round.

—**KAREN CZECHOWICZ** OCALA, FL

PREP: 20 MIN. • **BAKE:** 45 MIN. + COOLING
MAKES: 1 LOAF (12 SLICES)

- 1½ cups all-purpose flour
- ¾ cup sugar
- 1 teaspoon baking powder
- ¼ teaspoon salt
- ¼ teaspoon baking soda
- 1 egg
- ½ cup orange juice
- 2 tablespoons butter, melted
- 1 tablespoon water
- 1½ cups fresh or frozen cranberries, halved

TART CRANBERRY QUICK BREAD

1. In a large bowl, combine the first five ingredients. In a small bowl, whisk the egg, orange juice, butter and water. Stir into the dry ingredients just until moistened. Fold in cranberries.

2. Transfer to an 8x4-in. loaf pan coated with cooking spray and sprinkled with flour. Bake at 350° for 45-50 minutes or until a toothpick inserted near the center comes out clean. Cool for 10 minutes before removing from pan to a wire rack.

PER SERVING *138 cal., 2 g fat (1 g sat. fat), 23 mg chol., 129 mg sodium, 27 g carb., 1 g fiber, 2 g pro.* **Diabetic Exchange:** *2 starch.*

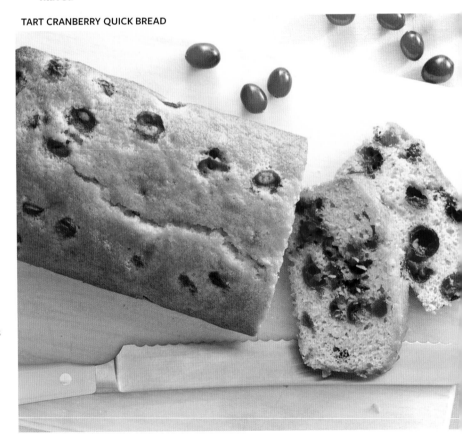

Savory Breakfast Muffins

After taking a bite, few people can resist gobbling up more of these out-of-the-ordinary muffins. They're packed with cheese, ham, pepper and onions.

—**VAN MAANEN MICHELLE** LETHBRIDGE, AB

PREP: 25 MIN. • **BAKE:** 20 MIN.
MAKES: 16 MUFFINS.

- 1½ **cups whole wheat flour**
- ½ **cup all-purpose flour**
- 2 **teaspoons baking powder**
- ½ **teaspoon baking soda**
- ½ **teaspoon salt**
- ½ **teaspoon pepper**
- 2 **eggs**
- 1¼ **cups buttermilk**
- 2 **tablespoons butter, melted**
- 1 **tablespoon canola oil**
- ¾ **cup cubed Havarti cheese with jalapeno or pepper Jack cheese**
- ¾ **cup finely chopped fully cooked ham**
- 1 **medium sweet red pepper, finely chopped**
- 4 **green onions, finely chopped**

1. In a large bowl, combine the flours, baking powder, baking soda, salt and pepper. In another bowl, combine the eggs, buttermilk, butter and oil. Stir into the dry ingredients just until moistened. Fold in the remaining ingredients.

2. Fill greased or paper-lined muffin cups three-fourths full. Bake at 400° for 18-22 minutes or until a toothpick inserted in muffin comes out clean. Cool for 5 minutes before removing from pans to wire racks. Serve warm.

PER SERVING *124 cal., 6 g fat (2 g sat. fat), 40 mg chol., 319 mg sodium, 13 g carb., 2 g fiber, 6 g pro.* **Diabetic Exchanges:** *1 starch, 1 fat.*

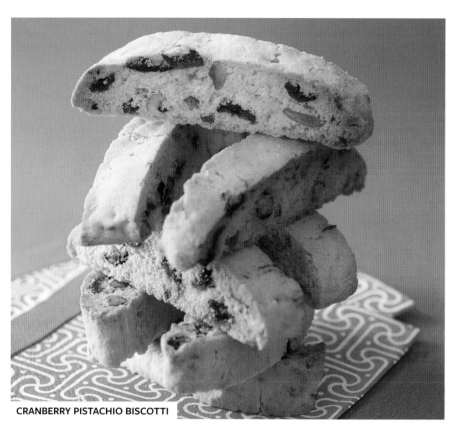

CRANBERRY PISTACHIO BISCOTTI

Cranberry Pistachio Biscotti

Studded with dried cranberries and crunchy pistachios, this delicious biscotti goes well with tea or coffee.

—**DIANE GRUBER** SIOUX CITY, IA

PREP: 25 MIN. • **BAKE:** 30 MIN.
MAKES: ABOUT 2½ DOZEN

- ¾ **cup sugar**
- ¼ **cup canola oil**
- 2 **eggs**
- 2 **teaspoons vanilla extract**
- 1 **teaspoon almond extract**
- 1¾ **cups all-purpose flour**
- 1 **teaspoon baking powder**
- ¼ **teaspoon salt**
- ⅔ **cup chopped pistachios**
- ½ **cup dried cranberries**

1. In a small bowl, beat sugar and oil until blended. Beat in eggs, then extracts. Combine the flour, baking powder and salt; gradually add to sugar mixture and mix well (dough will be stiff). Stir in pistachios and cranberries.

2. Divide dough in half. With floured hands, shape each half into a 12x2-in. rectangle on a parchment paper-lined baking sheet. Bake at 350° for 18-22 minutes or until set.

3. Place pan on wire rack. When cool enough to handle, transfer to a cutting board; cut diagonally with a serrated knife into ¾-in. slices. Place cut side down on ungreased baking sheets. Bake for 12-14 minutes or until firm. Remove to wire racks to cool. Store in an airtight container.

PER SERVING *85 cal., 3 g fat (trace sat. fat), 13 mg chol., 46 mg sodium, 12 g carb., 1 g fiber, 2 g pro.* **Diabetic Exchange:** *1 starch.*

Irish Soda Bread

My husband's family is Irish. Hoping to impress my future mother-in-law, I baked this bread and took it along with me when I met her the first time. She gave it a big thumbs-up!

—**PADMINI ROY-DIXON** COLUMBUS, OH

PREP: 20 MIN. • **BAKE:** 50 MIN. + COOLING
MAKES: 1 LOAF (16 SLICES)

- ¾ cup raisins
- 1 cup boiling water
- 2 cups all-purpose flour
- 1 cup whole wheat flour
- ⅓ cup sugar
- 3 teaspoons baking powder
- 1 teaspoon baking soda
- 1 teaspoon salt
- 1 egg
- 2 cups buttermilk
- ¼ cup butter, melted

1. Place raisins in a small bowl. Cover with boiling water; let raisins stand for 5 minutes. Drain and pat dry.
2. In a large bowl, combine the flours, sugar, baking powder, baking soda and salt. In a small bowl, whisk the egg, buttermilk and butter. Stir into dry ingredients just until moistened. Fold in raisins.
3. Transfer to a 9x5-in. loaf pan coated with cooking spray. Bake at 350° for 50-60 minutes or until a toothpick inserted near the center comes out clean. Cool for 10 minutes before removing from pan to a wire rack.

PER SERVING *161 cal., 4 g fat (2 g sat. fat), 22 mg chol., 359 mg sodium, 28 g carb., 2 g fiber, 4 g pro.* ***Diabetic Exchanges:*** *2 starch, 1 fat.*

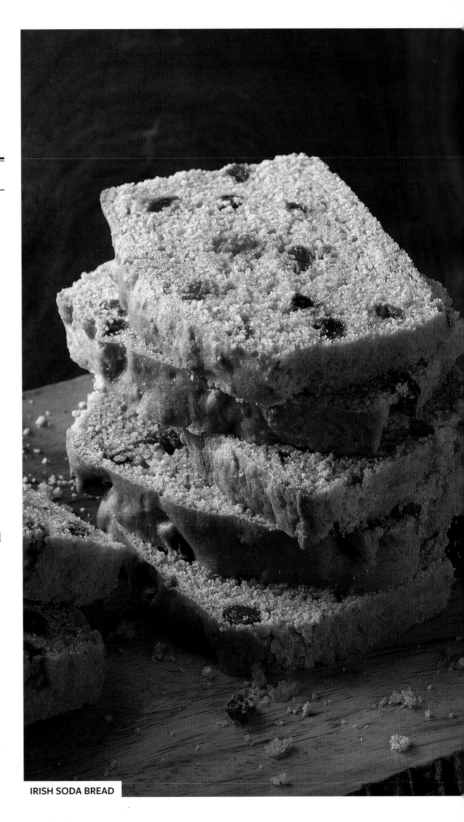

IRISH SODA BREAD

Wild Rice Bread

I add texture and a subtle nutty flavor to homemade bread by mixing in wild rice.

—BONNIE GROH MANISTIQUE, MI

PREP: 20 MIN. + RISING
BAKE: 40 MIN. + COOLING
MAKES: 2 LOAVES (16 SLICES EACH)

- 3 **cups whole wheat flour**
- 3 **cups all-purpose flour**
- 2 **packages (¼ ounce each) active dry yeast**
- 2½ **teaspoons salt**
- 1 **cup water**
- 1 **cup fat-free milk**
- ¼ **cup butter, cubed**
- ¼ **cup honey**
- 2 **cups cooked wild rice**

1. In a large bowl, combine the whole wheat flour, 1 cup all-purpose flour, yeast and salt. In a small saucepan, heat the water, milk, butter and honey to 120°-130°. Add to dry ingredients; beat until smooth. Stir in the wild rice and enough remaining all-purpose flour to form a stiff dough.
2. Turn onto a lightly floured surface; knead until smooth and elastic, about 6-8 minutes. Place in a bowl coated with cooking spray, turning once to coat top. Cover and let rise in a warm place until doubled, about 40 minutes.
3. Punch dough down. Turn onto a lightly floured surface; divide in half. Shape into loaves. Place in two 9x5-in. loaf pans coated with cooking spray. Cover and let rise until doubled, about 30 minutes.
4. Bake at 375° for 40-45 minutes or until golden brown. Remove from pans to wire racks to cool completely.

PER SERVING *116 cal., 2 g fat (1 g sat. fat), 4 mg chol., 203 mg sodium, 22 g carb., 2 g fiber, 4 g pro.* **Diabetic Exchange:** *1½ starch.*

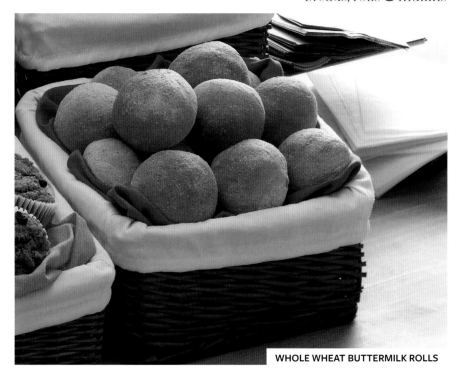

WHOLE WHEAT BUTTERMILK ROLLS

Whole Wheat Buttermilk Rolls

I'm always looking for recipes tailored to my husband's low-fat, low-sugar diet. These rolls have just a hint of sweetness, and we both love them.

—IRENE CLIETT CEDAR BLUFF, MS

PREP: 35 MIN. + RISING • **BAKE:** 10 MIN.
MAKES: 1½ DOZEN

- 1½ **cups self-rising flour**
- 1½ **cups whole wheat flour**
- ⅓ **cup sugar**
- 1 **package (¼ ounce) quick-rise yeast**
- 1 **cup buttermilk**
- ¼ **cup canola oil**

1. In a large bowl, combine the self-rising flour, ¾ cup whole wheat flour, sugar and yeast. In a small saucepan, heat buttermilk and oil to 120°-130° (mixture will appear curdled). Add to dry ingredients; beat just until smooth. Stir in remaining whole wheat flour.
2. Turn onto a lightly floured surface; knead until smooth and elastic, about 6-8 minutes. Cover and let dough rest for 10 minutes.
3. Roll dough to ½-in. thickness; cut with a floured 2½-in. biscuit cutter. Place 2 in. apart on baking sheets coated with cooking spray. Cover and let rise in a warm place until doubled, about 35-40 minutes.
4. Bake at 375° for 8-12 minutes or until golden brown. Serve warm.

NOTE *As a substitute for 1½ cups self-rising flour, place 2¼ teaspoons baking powder and ¾ teaspoon salt in a measuring cup. Add all-purpose flour to measure 1 cup. Combine with an additional ½ cup all-purpose flour.*

PER SERVING *116 cal., 3 g fat (trace sat. fat), 1 mg chol., 135 mg sodium, 19 g carb., 1 g fiber, 3 g pro.* **Diabetic Exchanges:** *1 starch, 1 fat.*

desserts

Yes, you can eat dessert! Even when you crave something sweet, you can still stick to your diet. **It's the best of both worlds.** Sometimes you can have your cake, and eat it, too!

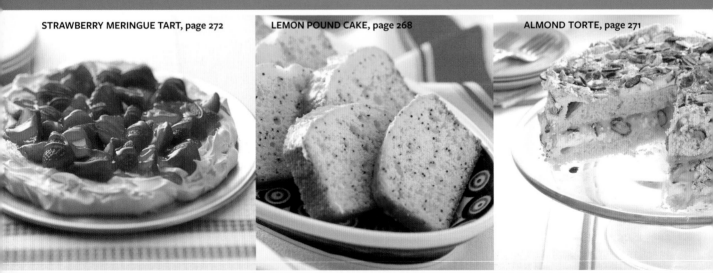

STRAWBERRY MERINGUE TART, page 272

LEMON POUND CAKE, page 268

ALMOND TORTE, page 271

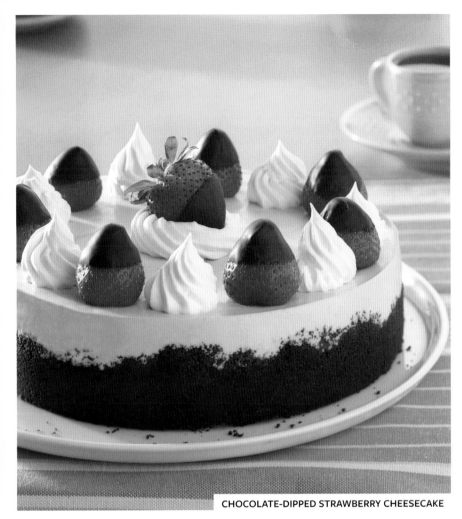

CHOCOLATE-DIPPED STRAWBERRY CHEESECAKE

1. In a small bowl, combine cracker crumbs and butter. Press onto the bottom and 1 in. up the sides of a 9-in. springform pan coated with cooking spray. Place on a baking sheet. Bake at 350° for 10 minutes or until set. Cool on a wire rack.

2. Hull strawberries if necessary; puree in a food processor. Remove and set aside. In a small saucepan, sprinkle gelatin over cold water; let stand for 1 minute. Heat over low heat, stirring until gelatin is completely dissolved. Transfer to the food processor; add the cream cheese, cottage cheese and sugar substitute. Cover and process until smooth.

3. Add strawberry puree; cover and process until blended. Transfer to a large bowl; fold in 2 cups whipped topping. Pour into crust. Cover and refrigerate for 2-3 hours or until set.

4. For garnish, wash strawberries and gently pat with paper towels until completely dry. Cut tops off berries. In a microwave, melt chocolate; stir until smooth. Dip each berry tip until half of the berry is coated, allowing excess to drip off. Place with tips pointing up on a waxed paper-lined baking sheet; refrigerate for at least 30 minutes.

5. Carefully run a knife around edge of springform pan to loosen; remove sides of pan. Garnish cheesecake with chocolate-dipped strawberries and remaining whipped topping.

NOTE *This recipe was tested with Splenda no-calorie sweetener.*

PER SERVING *1 slice equals 245 cal., 11 g fat (7 g sat. fat), 14 mg chol., 377 mg sodium, 26 g carb., 2 g fiber, 10 g pro. Diabetic Exchanges: 2 starch, 2 fat.*

Chocolate-Dipped Strawberry Cheesecake

This light and airy cheesecake is great for entertaining. The chocolate crust lends a unique flavor that complements the sweet strawberry filling. It always earns praise and adds a touch of elegance to the table.

—**KATHY BERGER** DRY RIDGE, KY

PREP: 45 MIN. + CHILLING
MAKES: 12 SERVINGS

- 1¾ cups chocolate graham cracker crumbs (about 9 whole crackers)
- ¼ cup butter, melted
- 1 pound fresh or frozen strawberries, thawed
- 2 envelopes unflavored gelatin
- ½ cup cold water
- 2 packages (8 ounces each) fat-free cream cheese, cubed
- 1 cup (8 ounces) fat-free cottage cheese
  Sugar substitute equivalent to ¾ cup sugar
- 1 carton (8 ounces) frozen reduced-fat whipped topping, thawed, divided
- 12 medium fresh strawberries
- 4 ounces semisweet chocolate, chopped

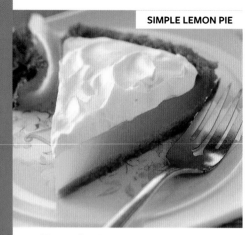

SIMPLE LEMON PIE

Simple Lemon Pie

Lemon meringue pie is one of my favorite desserts, and this yummy, sweet-tart version is so good that no one will suspect that it's light.

—FRANCES VANFOSSAN WARREN, MI

PREP: 20 MIN. + CHILLING
MAKES: 8 SERVINGS

- 1 **package (.8 ounce) sugar-free cook-and-serve vanilla pudding mix**
- 1 **package (.3 ounce) sugar-free lemon gelatin**
- 2⅓ **cups water**
- ⅓ **cup lemon juice**
- 1 **reduced-fat graham cracker crust (8 inches)**
- 1½ **cups reduced-fat whipped topping**

1. In a small saucepan, combine pudding mix and gelatin. Add water and lemon juice; stir until smooth. Cook and stir over medium heat until mixture comes to a boil. Cook and stir 1-2 minutes longer or until thickened.
2. Remove from the heat; cool slightly. Pour into crust. Cover and refrigerate for 6 hours or overnight. Spread with whipped topping.
PER SERVING *1 piece equals 146 cal., 5 g fat (3 g sat. fat), 0 chol., 174 mg sodium, 22 g carb., trace fiber, 2 g pro.* **Diabetic Exchanges:** *1½ starch, 1 fat.*

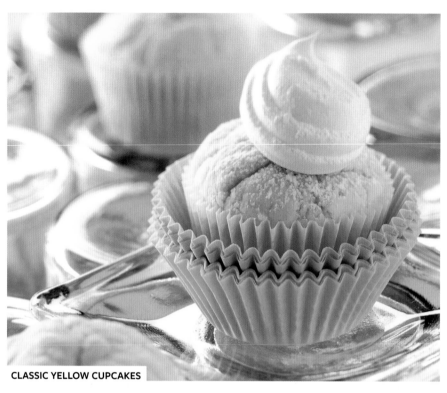

CLASSIC YELLOW CUPCAKES

Classic Yellow Cupcakes

Sugar substitute makes these dreamy cupcakes a divine treat, whether they're eaten for dessert or as a fast snack. Light and buttery, the bites make a perfect contribution to a baby shower or casual ending to lunch with friends.

—TASTE OF HOME TEST KITCHEN

PREP: 15 MIN. • **BAKE:** 20 MIN. + COOLING
MAKES: 1½ DOZEN

- ⅔ **cup butter, softened**
- ¾ **cup sugar blend**
- 3 **eggs**
- 1½ **teaspoons vanilla extract**
- 2¼ **cups cake flour**
- 2 **teaspoons baking powder**
- ¼ **teaspoon salt**
- ¾ **cup fat-free milk**
   Fat-free whipped topping, optional
- 1 **teaspoon confectioners' sugar**

1. In a large bowl, cream butter and sugar substitute until light and fluffy.

Add eggs, one at a time, beating well after each addition. Beat in vanilla. Combine the flour, baking powder and salt; add to creamed mixture alternately with milk, mixing well after each addition.
2. Fill paper-lined muffin cups three-fourths full. Bake at 350° for 20-25 minutes or until lightly browned and a toothpick inserted near the center comes out clean. Cool for 5 minutes before removing from pans to wire racks to cool completely.
3. Top with a dollop of whipped topping if desired, then dust with confectioners' sugar.
NOTE *This recipe was tested with Splenda sugar blend.*
PER SERVING *1 cupcake (calculated without whipped topping) equals 171 cal., 8 g fat (4 g sat. fat), 54 mg chol., 171 mg sodium, 22 g carb., trace fiber, 3 g pro.* **Diabetic Exchanges:** *1½ starch, 1½ fat.*

Cran-Orange Gelatin Salad

Serve this sweet treat as an after-dinner treat or as a fruit salad alongside brunch.

—EVA DEWOLF ERWIN, TN

PREP: 45 MIN. + CHILLING
MAKES: 15 SERVINGS

- 1 can (15 ounces) mandarin oranges
- 2 packages (.3 ounce each) sugar-free cranberry gelatin
- 1½ cups boiling water
- 1 can (14 ounces) whole-berry cranberry sauce
- 1½ cups crushed salt-free pretzels
- 6 tablespoons butter, melted
  Sugar substitute equivalent to
  5 tablespoons sugar, divided
- 1 package (8 ounces) fat-free cream cheese
- 1 carton (8 ounces) frozen reduced-fat whipped topping, thawed

1. Drain oranges, reserving juice in a 2-cup measuring cup; set oranges and juice aside.

2. In a large bowl, dissolve gelatin in boiling water. Stir in cranberry sauce until melted. Add enough cold water to the reserved juice to measure 1½ cups; add to gelatin mixture. Stir in oranges. Chill until partially set.

3. Meanwhile, in a large bowl, combine the pretzels, butter and 2 tablespoons sugar substitute. Press into an ungreased 13-in. x 9-in. dish; chill.

4. In a small bowl, beat cream cheese and remaining sugar substitute until smooth. Fold in whipped topping. Spread over crust. Spoon gelatin mixture over cream cheese layer. Chill for at least 3 hours or until set.

NOTE *This recipe was tested with Splenda no-calorie sweetener.*
PER SERVING *1 piece equals 183 cal., 7 g fat (5 g sat. fat), 13 mg chol., 185 mg sodium, 26 g carb., 1 g fiber, 4 g pro.* **Diabetic Exchanges:** *2 starch, 1 fat.*

CRAN-ORANGE GELATIN SALAD

Mini Neapolitan Baked Alaskas

Surprise—there's ice cream inside! This recipe is a showstopper.

—TASTE OF HOME TEST KITCHEN

PREP: 30 MIN. • **BROIL:** 5 MIN.
MAKES: 4 SERVINGS

- 4 foil muffin liners
- 4 chocolate wafers
- 1 cup reduced-fat strawberry ice cream
- 3 egg whites
- 6 tablespoons sugar
- ⅛ teaspoon cream of tartar
- ½ teaspoon vanilla extract

1. Flatten muffin liners; place on a baking sheet. Place a wafer on each. Scoop ¼ cup of ice cream onto each wafer; freeze.

2. Meanwhile, in a small heavy saucepan, combine the egg whites, sugar and cream of tartar; beat on low speed with a portable mixer for 1 minute. Continue beating over low heat until mixture reaches 160°, about 12 minutes. Remove from the heat; add vanilla. Beat until stiff peaks form and sugar is dissolved, about 4 minutes.

3. Remove baking sheet from freezer; immediately spread meringue over ice cream, sealing to edges of wafers. Broil 4-6 in. from the heat for 1-2 minutes or until meringues are lightly browned. Serve immediately.

PER SERVING *163 cal., 2 g fat (1 g sat. fat), 8 mg chol., 99 mg sodium, 32 g carb., trace fiber, 5 g pro.* **Diabetic Exchange:** *2 starch.*

top tip

Keep Cool

Avoid making meringue on a humid day—the excess moisture may cause beading.

Glazed Roasted Pineapple

If you've never tried roasted pineapple before, you need to! Raspberry sorbet is an ideal accompaniment, but you could serve the pineapple with other sorbets, too.

—AGNES WARD STRATFORD, ON

PREP: 15 MIN. • **BAKE:** 35 MIN.
MAKES: 6 SERVINGS

- 1 **fresh pineapple**
- 2 **tablespoons butter, melted**
- ¼ **cup packed brown sugar**
- 2 **tablespoons honey**
- ½ **teaspoon pumpkin pie spice or ground cinnamon**
- ¼ **teaspoon rum extract**
- ¾ **cup raspberry sorbet**

1. Peel pineapple; cut into six wedges. Cut wedges lengthwise to remove core; cut each widthwise into four pieces. Pour butter into a 2-qt. baking dish; top with pineapple. Combine the brown sugar, honey, pie spice and extract; spoon over pineapple.

2. Bake, uncovered, at 400° for 35-40 minutes or until golden brown. Spoon cooking juices over the top. Serve warm with sorbet.

PER SERVING *4 pineapple pieces with 2 tablespoons sorbet equals 159 cal., 4 g fat (2 g sat. fat), 10 mg chol., 43 mg sodium, 32 g carb., 1 g fiber, trace pro. Diabetic Exchanges: 1 starch, 1 fruit, 1 fat.*

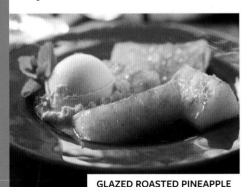

GLAZED ROASTED PINEAPPLE

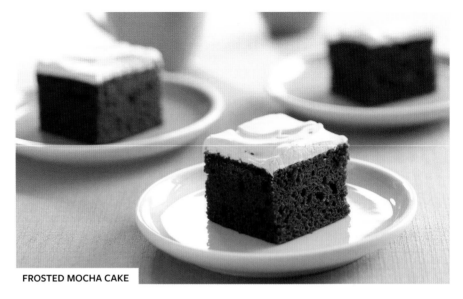

FROSTED MOCHA CAKE

Frosted Mocha Cake

The mixture of both sugar and sugar substitute helps keep the sweetness while still cutting calories and carbs. If you want to make this recipe even better for you, try using a reduced-fat whipped topping in the frosting.

—TASTE OF HOME TEST KITCHEN

PREP: 20 MIN. • **BAKE:** 30 MIN. + COOLING
MAKES: 24 SERVINGS

- ¾ **cup sugar blend**
- ½ **cup sugar**
- 2 **eggs**
- ¼ **cup canola oil**
- 1 **container (2½ ounces) prune baby food**
- 3 **teaspoons white vinegar**
- 1 **teaspoon vanilla extract**
- 1 **cup fat-free milk**
- 1 **cup cold strong brewed coffee**
- 3 **cups all-purpose flour**
- ⅓ **cup baking cocoa**
- 2 **teaspoons baking soda**
- 1 **teaspoon salt**

FROSTING
- 1 **teaspoon instant coffee granules**
- 1 **teaspoon hot water**
- ½ **teaspoon vanilla extract**
- 2 **cups whipped topping**

1. In a large bowl, combine the first seven ingredients; beat until well blended. In a small bowl, combine the milk and coffee. Combine the flour, cocoa, baking soda and salt; gradually beat into egg mixture alternately with milk mixture.

2. Pour into a 13-in. x 9-in. baking pan coated with cooking spray. Bake at 350° for 30-35 minutes or until a toothpick inserted near the center comes out clean. Cool on a wire rack.

3. In a small bowl, dissolve coffee granules in hot water. Stir in vanilla. Place whipped topping in a large bowl; gently fold in coffee mixture. Frost cake. Store in the refrigerator.

NOTE *This recipe was tested with Splenda Sugar Blend for Baking. Look for it in the baking aisle of your grocery store.*

PER SERVING *1 piece equals 151 cal., 4 g fat (1 g sat. fat), 18 mg chol., 214 mg sodium, 25 g carb., 1 g fiber, 3 g pro. Diabetic Exchanges: 1½ starch, 1 fat.*

No-Bake Strawberry Dessert

Convenience items make the prep work for this refrigerated delight as simple as can be. Serve it in a glass dish for added elegance.

—SHERRI DANIELS CLARK, SD

PREP: 20 MIN. + CHILLING
MAKES: 20 SERVINGS

- 1 loaf (10½ ounces) angel food cake, cut into 1-inch cubes
- 2 packages (.3 ounce each) sugar-free strawberry gelatin
- 2 cups boiling water
- 1 package (20 ounces) frozen unsweetened whole strawberries, thawed
- 2 cups cold 1% milk
- 1 package (1 ounce) sugar-free instant vanilla pudding mix
- 1 carton (8 ounces) frozen reduced-fat whipped topping, thawed Chopped fresh strawberries, optional

1. Arrange cake cubes in a single layer in a 13-in. x 9-in. dish. In a bowl, dissolve gelatin in boiling water; stir in strawberries. Pour over cake and gently press cake down. Refrigerate until set, about 1 hour.

2. In a large bowl, whisk milk and pudding mix for 2 minutes. Let stand for 2 minutes or until soft-set.

3. Spoon over gelatin layer. Spread with whipped topping. Refrigerate until serving. Garnish with chopped fresh strawberries if desired.

PER SERVING *1 piece equals 92 cal., 2 g fat (1 g sat. fat), 2 mg chol., 172 mg sodium, 16 g carb., 1 g fiber, 2 g pro.* **Diabetic Exchange:** *1 starch.*

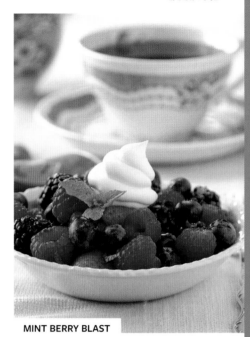

MINT BERRY BLAST

Mint Berry Blast

What's better than a bowl of fresh-picked berries? A bowl of berries enhanced with mint, lemon juice and a dollop of whipped topping! It's so refreshing.

—DIANE HARRISON MECHANICSBURG, PA

START TO FINISH: 10 MIN.
MAKES: 4 SERVINGS

- 1 cup each fresh raspberries, blackberries, blueberries and halved strawberries
- 1 tablespoon minced fresh mint
- 1 tablespoon lemon juice Whipped topping, optional

In a large bowl, combine the berries, mint and lemon juice; gently toss to coat. Cover and refrigerate until serving. Garnish with whipped topping if desired.

PER SERVING *65 cal., 1 g fat (trace sat. fat), 0 chol., 1 mg sodium, 16 g carb., 6 g fiber, 1 g pro.* **Diabetic Exchange:** *1 fruit.*

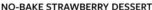

NO-BAKE STRAWBERRY DESSERT

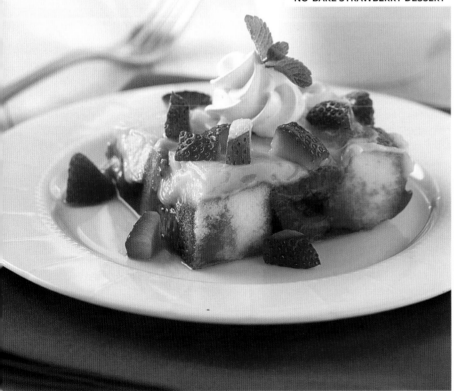

Iced Tea Parfaits

Next time you're hosting a patio party, be sure to serve this! Tea adds a wonderfully unexpected flavor to gelatin, and kids will have fun finding the cherry at the bottom.

—TEENA PETRUS JOHNSTOWN, PA

PREP: 15 MIN. + CHILLING
MAKES: 4 SERVINGS

- 2 **cups water**
- 3 **individual tea bags**
- 1 **package (3 ounces) lemon gelatin**
- 4 **maraschino cherries**
- 1½ **cups whipped topping, divided**
- 4 **lemon slices**

1. In a small saucepan, bring the water to a boil. Remove from the heat; add tea bags. Cover and steep for 5 minutes. Discard the tea bags. Stir the gelatin into tea until completely dissolved. Cool slightly.

2. Pour ¼ cup gelatin mixture into each of four parfait glasses. Place a cherry in each glass; refrigerate until set but not firm, about 1 hour. Transfer remaining gelatin mixture to a small bowl; refrigerate for 1 hour or until soft-set.

3. Whisk reserved gelatin mixture for 2-3 minutes or until smooth. Stir in ½ cup whipped topping; spoon into parfait glasses. Refrigerate for at least 2 hours. Just before serving, top with remaining whipped topping and garnish with lemon slices.

PER SERVING *162 cal., 5 g fat (5 g sat. fat), 0 chol., 48 mg sodium, 27 g carb., 0 fiber, 2 g pro.* ***Diabetic Exchanges:*** *1½ starch, 1 fat.*

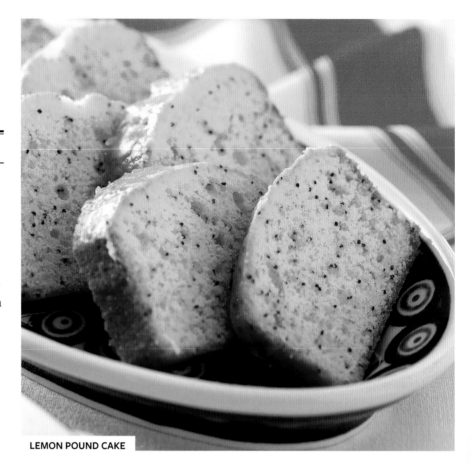
LEMON POUND CAKE

Lemon Pound Cake

When you are in the mood for a sweet but don't want a large cake or batch of cookies, turn to my pound cake recipe. It bakes in a small loaf pan and makes six delicious slices.

—CORKEY ADDCOX MT. SHASTA, CA

PREP: 20 MIN. **• BAKE:** 30 MIN. + COOLING
MAKES: 1 MINI LOAF (6 SLICES)

- ⅓ **cup sugar**
- 1 **egg**
- 3 **tablespoons canola oil**
- 3 **tablespoons orange juice**
- ½ **teaspoon lemon extract**
- ⅔ **cup all-purpose flour**
- ¾ **teaspoon baking powder**
- ⅛ **teaspoon salt**
- 1 **teaspoon poppy seeds, optional**
- ⅓ **cup confectioners' sugar**
- 2 **tablespoons lemon juice**

1. In a small bowl, combine the sugar, egg, oil, orange juice and extract. Combine the flour, baking powder and salt; add to egg mixture and mix well. Stir in poppy seeds if desired.

2. Pour into a greased and floured 5¾-in. x 3-in. x 2-in. loaf pan. Bake at 350° for 30-35 minutes or until a toothpick inserted near the center comes out clean. Cool for 10 minutes before removing from pan to a wire rack to cool completely.

3. For glaze, in a small bowl, whisk confectioners' sugar and lemon juice until smooth; drizzle over cake.

PER SERVING *1 slice equals 200 cal., 8 g fat (1 g sat. fat), 35 mg chol., 111 mg sodium, 30 g carb., trace fiber, 3 g pro.* ***Diabetic Exchanges:*** *2 starch, 1 fat.*

Mini Apple Strudels

Present strudel in a whole new way! Phyllo dough surrounds tender slices of apple in this version. One strudel is only 100 calories, so you can have dessert!

—TASTE OF HOME TEST KITCHEN

PREP: 30 MIN. • **BAKE:** 20 MIN.
MAKES: 6 SERVINGS

- 1½ cups chopped peeled tart apples
- 2 tablespoons plus 2 teaspoons sugar
- 2 tablespoons chopped walnuts
- 1 tablespoon all-purpose flour
- ¼ teaspoon ground cinnamon
- 6 sheets phyllo dough (14 inches x 9 inches)
   Butter-flavored cooking spray
   Confectioners' sugar, optional

1. In a small bowl, combine the apples, sugar, walnuts, flour and cinnamon. Set mixture aside.

2. Place one sheet of phyllo dough on a work surface (keep remaining dough covered with plastic wrap and a damp towel to prevent it from drying out). Spray with butter-flavored spray.

3. Fold in half widthwise; spray again with butter-flavored spray. Spoon a scant ⅓ cup filling onto phyllo about 2 in. from a short side. Fold side and edges over filling and roll up. Place seam side down on a baking sheet coated with cooking spray. Repeat.

4. With a sharp knife, cut diagonal slits in tops of strudels. Spray the strudels with butter-flavored spray. Bake at 350° for 20-22 minutes or until golden brown. Sprinkle with confectioners' sugar if desired.

CINNAMON APPLE STRUDELS *Omit confectioner's sugar. Before baking, spray strudels with butter-flavored cooking spray, then sprinkle with a mixture of 1 teaspoon sugar and a dash of ground cinnamon. Bake as directed.*

PER SERVING *1 strudel equals 100 cal., 3 g fat (trace sat. fat), 0 chol., 45 mg sodium, 17 g carb., 1 g fiber, 2 g pro.* **Diabetic Exchanges:** *1 starch, ½ fat.*

MINI APPLE STRUDELS

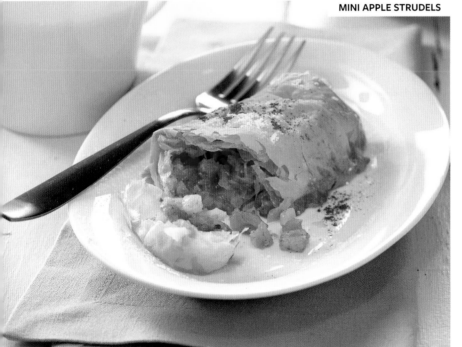

Strawberry-Banana Graham Pudding

I sometimes add in more fruit than the recipe calls for to get more daily servings of fruit. Try using different flavored puddings and fruits to switch up the recipe.

—JACKIE TERMONT RUTHER GLEN, VA

PREP: 20 MIN. + CHILLING
MAKES: 12 SERVINGS

- 9 whole reduced-fat cinnamon graham crackers
- 1¾ cups cold fat-free milk
- 1 package (1 ounce) sugar-free instant cheesecake or vanilla pudding mix
- 1 large firm banana, sliced
- ½ teaspoon lemon juice
- 2 cups sliced fresh strawberries, divided
- 2½ cups reduced-fat whipped topping, divided
   Mint sprigs, optional

1. Line the bottom of a 9-in. square pan with 4½ graham crackers; set aside.

2. In a small bowl, whisk milk and pudding mix for 2 minutes. Let stand for 2 minutes or until soft-set. Place banana slices in another small bowl; toss with lemon juice. Stir bananas and 1 cup strawberries into the pudding. Fold in 1¾ cups whipped topping.

3. Spread half of pudding over the graham crackers; repeat layers. Cover and refrigerate overnight. Refrigerate remaining berries and whipped topping. Just before serving, top with remaining berries and topping. Garnish with mint if desired.

PER SERVING *1 piece equals 117 cal., 2 g fat (2 g sat. fat), 1 mg chol., 171 mg sodium, 23 g carb., 1 g fiber, 2 g pro.* **Diabetic Exchanges:** *1 starch, ½ fruit.*

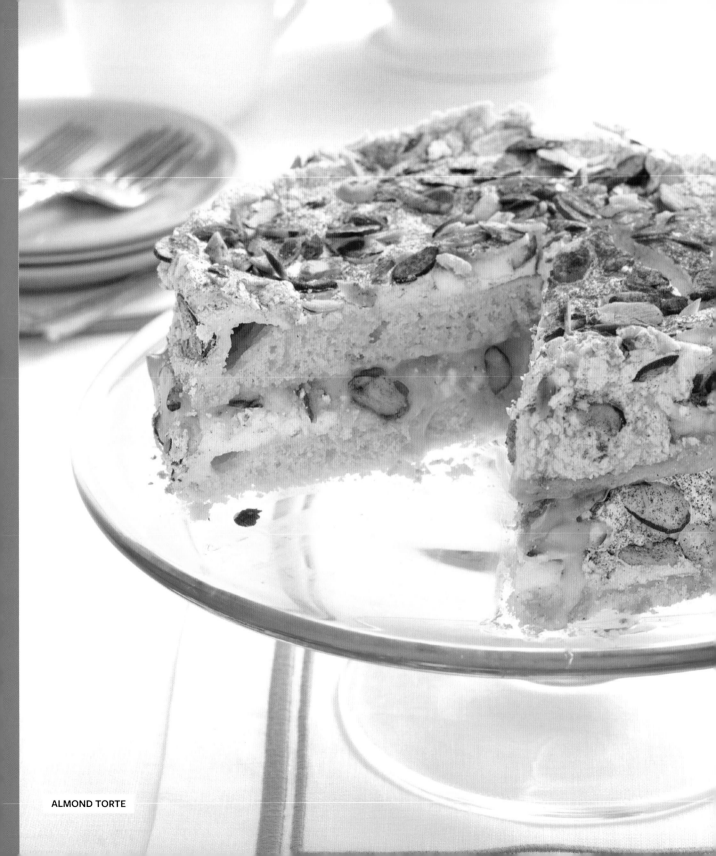

ALMOND TORTE

Almond Torte

Reduced-fat sour cream, egg whites and applesauce lighten up this gorgeous torte.
—**KATHY OLSEN** MARLBOROUGH, NH

PREP: 45 MIN. + CHILLING
BAKE: 25 MIN. + COOLING
MAKES: 16 SERVINGS

- ⅓ **cup sugar**
- 1 **tablespoon cornstarch**
- ½ **cup reduced-fat sour cream**
- 3 **egg yolks**
- 1 **tablespoon butter**
- 1 **teaspoon vanilla extract**
- ½ **teaspoon almond extract**

CAKE

- 4 **egg whites**
- ⅓ **cup butter, softened**
- 1½ **cups sugar, divided**
- 2 **egg yolks**
- ⅓ **cup fat-free milk**
- ¼ **cup unsweetened applesauce**
- 1 **teaspoon vanilla extract**
- 1 **cup cake flour**
- 1 **teaspoon baking powder**
- ⅛ **teaspoon salt**
- ½ **cup sliced almonds**
- ½ **teaspoon ground cinnamon**

1. In a double boiler or metal bowl over simmering water, constantly whisk the sugar, cornstarch, sour cream and egg yolks until mixture reaches 160° or is thick enough to coat the back of a spoon.

2. Remove from the heat; stir in butter and extracts until blended. Press waxed paper onto surface of custard. Refrigerate for several hours or overnight.

3. Place egg whites in a large bowl; let stand at room temperature for 30 minutes. Line two 8-in. round baking pans with waxed paper. Coat sides and paper with cooking spray; sprinkle with flour and set aside.

4. In a large bowl, beat butter and ½ cup sugar until blended, about 2 minutes. Add egg yolks; mix well. Beat in the milk, applesauce and vanilla (mixture may appear curdled). Combine the flour, baking powder and salt; add to butter mixture. Transfer to prepared pans; set aside.

5. Using clean beaters, beat egg whites on medium speed until soft peaks form. Gradually beat in remaining sugar, 2 tablespoons at a time, on high until stiff glossy peaks form and sugar is dissolved. Spread evenly over batter; sprinkle with almonds and cinnamon.

6. Bake at 350° for 25-30 minutes or until meringue is lightly browned. Cool in pans on wire racks for 10 minutes (meringue will crack). Loosen edges of cakes from pans with a knife. Using two large spatulas, carefully remove one cake to a serving plate, meringue side up; remove remaining cake to a wire rack, meringue side up. Cool cakes completely.

7. Carefully spread custard over cake on serving plate; top with remaining cake. Store in the refrigerator.

PER SERVING *1 slice equals 215 cal., 8 g fat (4 g sat. fat), 79 mg chol., 99 mg sodium, 32 g carb., 1 g fiber, 4 g pro.* **Diabetic Exchanges:** *2 starch, 1 fat.*

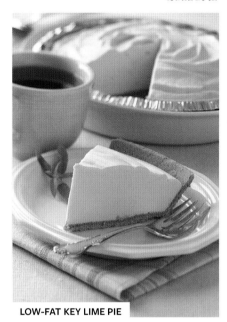

LOW-FAT KEY LIME PIE

Low-Fat Key Lime Pie

For a taste of paradise, try this creamy confection. It's low in fat, sugar and fuss. Dessert doesn't get any better than that!
—**FRANCES VANFOSSAN** WARREN, MI

PREP: 20 MIN. + CHILLING
MAKES: 8 SERVINGS

- 1 **package (.3 ounce) sugar-free lime gelatin**
- ¼ **cup boiling water**
- 2 **cartons (6 ounces each) Key lime yogurt**
- 1 **carton (8 ounces) frozen fat-free whipped topping, thawed**
- 1 **reduced-fat graham cracker crust (8 inches)**

1. In a large bowl, dissolve gelatin in boiling water. Whisk in yogurt. Fold in whipped topping. Pour into crust.

2. Cover and refrigerate for at least 2 hours or until set.

PER SERVING *1 piece equals 194 cal., 3 g fat (1 g sat. fat), 2 mg chol., 159 mg sodium, 33 g carb., 0 fiber, 3 g pro.* **Diabetic Exchanges:** *2 starch, ½ fat.*

top tip

How to Get Soft Peaks

To reach soft peaks stage, beat egg whites on medium speed until you can lift the beater from the whites and the points of the peaks slightly curl over.

Mini Raspberry Mousse Parfaits

Skip the stress when you're expecting guests—these tiny parfaits can be refrigerated ahead of time.

—TASTE OF HOME TEST KITCHEN

PREP: 30 MIN. + CHILLING
MAKES: 4 SERVINGS

- 1¾ cups fresh or frozen unsweetened raspberries, thawed
- 3 tablespoons sugar
- 2 teaspoons cornstarch
- 2 teaspoons orange juice
- 1⅓ cups whipped topping
- 12 cubes angel food cake (½-inch cubes)

1. Press raspberries through a strainer and discard seeds and pulp. In a small saucepan, combine sugar and cornstarch; stir in raspberry juice. Bring to a boil; cook and stir for 2 minutes or until thickened. Refrigerate until chilled.

2. Divide raspberry mixture in half. Stir orange juice into one portion; set aside. Place remaining mixture in a small bowl; fold in whipped topping.

3. Divide angel food cake among four small cocktail glasses or dessert dishes. Layer each with a scant tablespoon of reserved raspberry-orange mixture and ⅓ cup creamy mixture. Refrigerate until serving.

PER SERVING *143 cal., 4 g fat (4 g sat. fat), 0 chol., 29 mg sodium, 24 g carb., 1 g fiber, 1 g pro. Diabetic Exchanges: 1 starch, 1 fat, ½ fruit.*

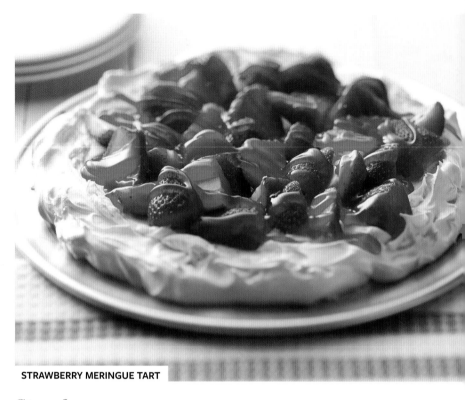

STRAWBERRY MERINGUE TART

Strawberry Meringue Tart

A friend shared this recipe with me and I made a few minor changes to make it less fattening. It will charm your guests!

—KAREN GRANT TULARE, CA

PREP: 25 MIN. • **BAKE:** 55 MIN. + STANDING
MAKES: 8 SERVINGS

- 3 egg whites
- ⅛ teaspoon cream of tartar
- ¾ cup sugar

FILLING

- 1 package (8 ounces) reduced-fat cream cheese
- ⅓ cup confectioners' sugar
- ½ cup marshmallow creme
- 1 cup reduced-fat whipped topping
- 5 cups fresh strawberries, halved
- ¼ cup strawberry glaze

1. Line a large pizza pan with parchment paper; set aside. In a large bowl, beat egg whites and cream of tartar on medium speed until soft peaks form. Gradually add sugar, 1 tablespoon at a time, beating on high until stiff glossy peaks form and the sugar is dissolved.

2. Spread into a 10-in. circle on prepared pan, forming a shallow well in the center. Bake at 225° for 45-55 minutes or until set and lightly browned. Turn oven off; leave meringue in oven for 1 to 1¼ hours.

3. For filling, in a large bowl, beat cream cheese and confectioners' sugar until smooth. Beat in marshmallow creme. Fold in whipped topping. Cover and refrigerate for at least 1 hour.

4. Just before serving, spread filling into meringue shell. Top with the strawberries. Drizzle with glaze.

PER SERVING *1 slice equals 196 cal., 6 g fat (4 g sat. fat), 16 mg chol., 123 mg sodium, 32 g carb., 2 g fiber, 4 g pro. Diabetic Exchanges: 1½ starch, 1 fat, ½ fruit.*

Yummy Chocolate Cake

When you're trying to eat better but still crave sweets, this chocolaty cake is the scrumptious solution!

—LADONNA REED PONCA CITY, OK

PREP: 20 MIN. • **BAKE:** 15 MIN. + COOLING
MAKES: 16 SERVINGS

- 1 **package chocolate cake mix (regular size)**
- 1 **package (2.1 ounces) sugar-free instant chocolate pudding mix**
- 1¾ **cups water**
- 3 **egg whites**

FROSTING

- 1¼ **cups cold fat-free milk**
- ¼ **teaspoon almond extract**
- 1 **package (1.4 ounces) sugar-free instant chocolate pudding mix**
- 1 **carton (8 ounces) frozen reduced-fat whipped topping, thawed Chocolate curls, optional**

1. In a large bowl, combine the cake mix, pudding mix, water and egg whites. Beat on low speed for 1 minute; beat on medium for 2 minutes.

2. Pour into a 15x10x 1-in. baking pan coated with cooking spray. Bake at 350° for 12-18 minutes or until a toothpick inserted near the center comes out clean. Cool on a wire rack.

3. For frosting, place milk and extract in a large bowl. Sprinkle with a third of the pudding mix; let stand for 1 minute. Whisk pudding into milk. Repeat twice with remaining pudding mix. Whisk pudding 2 minutes longer. Let stand for 15 minutes. Fold in whipped topping. Frost cake. Garnish with chocolate curls if desired.

PER SERVING *1 piece (calculated without chocolate curls) equals 197 cal., 5 g fat (3 g sat. fat), trace chol., 409 mg sodium, 35 g carb., 1 g fiber, 3 g pro.* **Diabetic Exchanges:** *2 starch, ½ fat.*

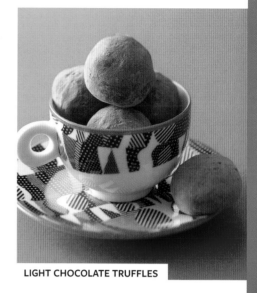

LIGHT CHOCOLATE TRUFFLES

Light Chocolate Truffles

I made these for my husband on Valentine's Day, and later for Christmas gifts. Everyone loves them!

—DONNI WORTHEN BRANSON, MO

PREP: 25 MIN. + CHILLING
MAKES: ABOUT 1½ DOZEN

- ⅓ **cup semisweet chocolate chips**
- 4 **ounces reduced-fat cream cheese**
- ⅓ **cup plus 2 teaspoons baking cocoa, divided**
- 1¼ **cups plus 2 teaspoons confectioners' sugar, divided**

1. In a microwave, melt chocolate chips; stir until smooth. Set aside.

2. In a small bowl, beat cream cheese until fluffy. Beat in ⅓ cup cocoa and melted chocolate. Gradually beat in 1¼ cups confectioners' sugar. Lightly coat hands with confectioners' sugar; roll chocolate mixture into 1-in. balls. Roll in the remaining cocoa or confectioners' sugar. Cover and refrigerate for at least 1 hour.

PER SERVING *1 truffle equals 62 cal., 2 g fat (1 g sat. fat), 4 mg chol., 24 mg sodium, 11 g carb., trace fiber, 1 g pro.* **Diabetic Exchanges:** *½ starch, ½ fat.*

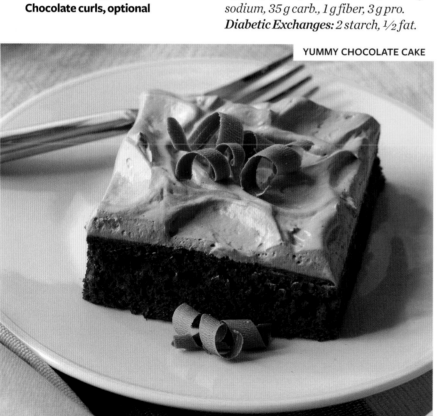

YUMMY CHOCOLATE CAKE

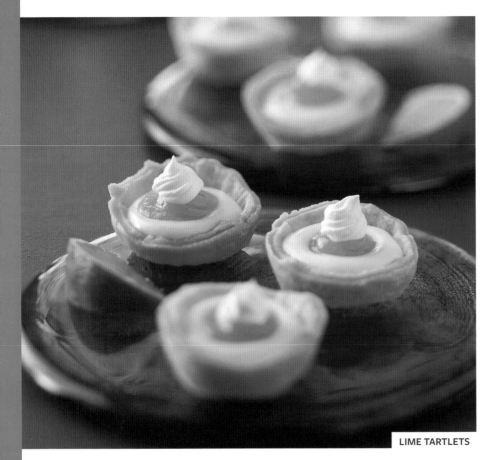

Chocolate Cream Dessert

Our daughter and her boyfriend are both on restricted diets, but serving this at birthday parties allows them to enjoy dessert, too.

—**RONALD SCORSE** SNOWFLAKE, AZ

PREP: 15 MIN. + COOLING
BAKE: 15 MIN. + COOLING
MAKES: 15 SERVINGS

- ¼ cup cold butter, cubed
- 1 cup all-purpose flour
- 1 package (8 ounces) reduced-fat cream cheese, softened
  Artificial sweetener equivalent to 2 tablespoons sugar
- 1 carton (8 ounces) frozen reduced-fat whipped topping, thawed, divided
- 1½ cups cold fat-free milk
- 1 package (¼ ounces) instant sugar-free chocolate pudding mix

1. In a small bowl, cut butter into flour until crumbly. Press into an 11-in. x 7-in. baking dish coated with cooking spray. Bake at 350° for 15-18 minutes or until lightly browned. Cool completely.
2. In a large bowl, beat cream cheese and sweetener until smooth. Fold in half of the whipped topping. Carefully spread over the crust.
3. In another large bowl, combine milk and pudding mix. Beat on low speed for 2 minutes. Let stand for 2 minutes or until soft-set. Spread over the cream cheese. Top with the remaining whipped topping.
PER SERVING *134 cal., 184 mg sodium, 6 mg chol., 14 g carb., 4 g pro, 6 g fat. Diabetic Exchanges: 1½ fat, 1 starch.*

Lime Tartlets

Made with refrigerated pie pastry, these dainty tartlets are party-perfect. I like to serve them with a slice of melon.

—**BILLIE MOSS** WALNUT CREEK, CA

PREP: 30 MIN.
BAKE: 10 MIN./BATCH + COOLING
MAKES: 4 DOZEN

- 2 packages (15 ounces each) refrigerated pie pastry
- 1 package (8 ounces) cream cheese, softened
- 1 cup (8 ounces) plain yogurt
- 3 tablespoons confectioners' sugar
- 1 jar (10 ounces) lime curd, divided
  Whipped cream and lime slices, optional

1. Preheat oven to 450°. Roll out each pastry on a lightly floured surface. Using a 2½-in. round cookie cutter, cut out 12 circles from each pastry. Press rounds onto the bottoms and up the sides of greased miniature muffin cups. Prick bottoms with a fork.
2. Bake 8-10 minutes or until golden brown. Cool 5 minutes before removing from pans to wire racks.
3. In a large bowl, beat cream cheese, yogurt and confectioners' sugar until smooth. Stir in ½ cup lime curd. Spoon into tart shells; top with remaining lime curd. Garnish with whipped cream and lime slices if desired.
PER SERVING *1 tartlet equals 121 cal., 7 g fat (3 g sat. fat), 14 mg chol., 86 mg sodium, 13 g carb., 0 fiber, 1 g pro. Diabetic Exchanges: 1 starch, 1 fat.*

Butterscotch Bliss Layered Dessert

Take this lovely treat to a gathering, and I bet you'll bring home an empty dish!
—**JANICE VERNON** LAS CRUCES, NM

PREP: 20 MIN. + CHILLING
MAKES: 24 SERVINGS

- 1½ **cups graham cracker crumbs**
  Sugar substitute equivalent to ½ cup sugar, divided
- 6 **tablespoons butter, melted**
- 2 **packages (8 ounces each) reduced-fat cream cheese**
- 3 **cups cold fat-free milk, divided**
- 2 **packages (1 ounce each) sugar-free instant butterscotch pudding mix**
- 1 **carton (8 ounces) frozen reduced-fat whipped topping, thawed**
- ½ **teaspoon rum extract**

1. In a small bowl, combine the cracker crumbs, ¼ cup sugar substitute and butter. Press into a 13-in. x 9-in. dish coated with cooking spray.

2. In a small bowl, beat the cream cheese, ¼ cup milk and remaining sugar substitute until smooth. Spread over crust.

3. In another bowl, whisk remaining milk with the pudding mix for 2 minutes. Let stand for 2 minutes or until soft-set. Gently spread over cream cheese layer. Combine whipped topping and extract; spread over the top. Refrigerate for at least 4 hours.
NOTE *This recipe was tested with Splenda no-calorie sweetener.*
PER SERVING *1 piece equals 136 cal., 8 g fat (6 g sat. fat), 21 mg chol., 245 mg sodium, 12 g carb., trace fiber, 3 g pro.* **Diabetic Exchanges:** *1 starch, 1 fat.*

Cookies 'n' Cream Berry Desserts

This sweet and colorful berry medley makes a pretty final course, especially in warm-weather months when the fruit is in season. With a whipped cream topping and a sprinkling of miniature meringue cookies, it's a winning dish.
—**LILY JULOW** LAWRENCEVILLE, GA

PREP: 10 MIN. + STANDING
MAKES: 6 SERVINGS

- 2 **cups quartered fresh strawberries**
- 1¼ **cups fresh raspberries**
- 1¼ **cups fresh blackberries**
- ⅔ **cup fresh blueberries**
- 4 **tablespoons sugar, divided**
- 2 **teaspoons lemon juice**
- 4 **ounces reduced-fat cream cheese**
- 1½ **cups fat-free whipped topping**
  Dash ground cinnamon
- 12 **miniature meringue cookies, quartered**

1. In a large bowl, combine the berries, 2 tablespoons sugar and lemon juice; let stand at room temperature for 30 minutes.

2. In a small bowl, beat cream cheese until smooth. Beat in the whipped topping, cinnamon and remaining sugar until combined. Just before serving, divide the berry mixture among six dessert dishes. Dollop with topping and sprinkle with cookies.
PER SERVING *⅔ cup berries with 3 tablespoons topping and 2 cookies equals 179 cal., 4 g fat (3 g sat. fat), 13 mg chol., 94 mg sodium, 32 g carb., 5 g fiber, 3 g pro.* **Diabetic Exchanges:** *1 starch, 1 fruit, 1 fat.*

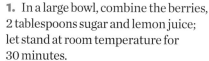

BUTTERSCOTCH BLISS LAYERED DESSERT

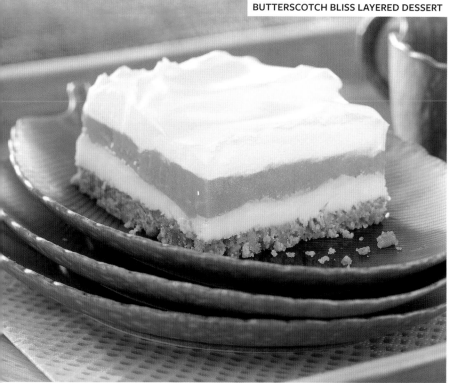

English Trifle

Impress guests with this layered dessert. It feeds a crowd!

—ALDAH BOTHMANN-POWELL

SAN ANTONIO, TX

PREP: 45 MIN. + CHILLING
MAKES: 12 SERVINGS

- 1 package (.3 ounce) sugar-free strawberry gelatin
- 1 cup boiling water
- 1 cup cold water
- 1 cup mashed strawberries
- 1 teaspoon sugar
- 1 can (8 ounces) unsweetened pineapple chunks
- 1 cup sliced firm bananas
- 1 prepared angel food cake (8 to 10 ounces), cut into 1-inch cubes
- 2 cups sliced fresh strawberries
- 2 cups cold fat-free milk
- 1 package (1 ounce) sugar-free instant vanilla pudding mix
- 1 carton (8 ounces) frozen fat-free whipped topping, thawed
- ¼ cup slivered almonds, toasted

1. In a small bowl, dissolve gelatin powder in boiling water. Stir in cold water. Transfer half of the gelatin mixture to a small bowl; cover and refrigerate for 1 hour or until slightly thickened. Reserve remaining gelatin mixture; let stand at room temperature.

2. In a small bowl, combine mashed strawberries and sugar; set aside. Drain pineapple, reserving ¼ cup juice; cut pineapple chunks in half and set aside. Toss banana slices with reserved pineapple juice; set aside.

3. In a 3-qt. trifle bowl, layer half of each of the following: cake cubes, mashed strawberries, pineapple, banana mixture and sliced strawberries. Pour the refrigerated gelatin over top. Set aside remaining cake and fruit. Place trifle and reserved gelatin in refrigerator for 20 minutes or until gelatin is slightly thickened.

4. In a small bowl, whisk milk and pudding mix for 2 minutes. Let stand for 2 minutes or until soft-set. Spread half over trifle. Repeat layers with remaining cake, fruit, reserved gelatin and pudding. Top with whipped topping. Cover and refrigerate. Just before serving, sprinkle with almonds.

PER SERVING *1 cup equals 155 cal., 2 g fat (trace sat. fat), 1 mg chol., 274 mg sodium, 32 g carb., 2 g fiber, 4 g pro.* ***Diabetic Exchanges:*** *1½ starch, ½ fruit.*

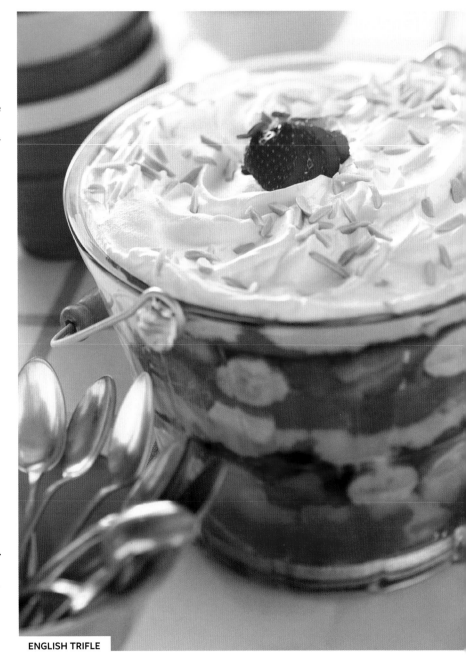

ENGLISH TRIFLE

Frozen Peach Yogurt

Pack in some calcium while also relaxing with a creamy, cool dessert.

—GAUDREY TASTEOFHOME.COM

PREP: 20 MIN.
PROCESS: 20 MIN. + FREEZING
MAKES: 6 CUPS

- 4 **medium peaches, peeled and sliced**
- 1 **envelope unflavored gelatin**
- 1 **cup fat-free milk**
- ½ **cup sugar**
  Dash salt
- 2½ **cups vanilla yogurt**
- 2 **teaspoons vanilla extract**

1. Place peaches in a blender. Cover and process until blended; set aside. In a small saucepan, sprinkle gelatin over milk; let stand for 1 minute. Heat over low heat, stirring until the gelatin is completely dissolved. Remove from the heat; stir in sugar and salt until sugar dissolves. Add the yogurt, vanilla and reserved peaches.
2. Fill cylinder of ice cream freezer two-thirds full; freeze according to the manufacturer's directions. When yogurt is frozen, transfer to a freezer container; freeze for 2-4 hours before serving.
PER SERVING *¾ cup equals 149 cal., 1 g fat (1 g sat. fat), 4 mg chol., 83 mg sodium, 29 g carb., 1 g fiber, 6 g pro. Diabetic Exchanges: 1 starch, ½ fruit, ½ reduced-fat milk.*

top tip
Peachy Peeling
After putting peaches in boiling, then ice water, use a paring knife to peel off the skin. Repeat the process for a few seconds if the skin doesn't easily come off.

Chocolate Peanut Butter Bombes

Kids of all ages are sure to love these delicious frozen bombes with the peanut butter surprise inside.

—TASTE OF HOME TEST KITCHEN

PREP: 25 MIN. + FREEZING
MAKES: 8 SERVINGS

- 1 **package (8 ounces) fat-free cream cheese**
- 3 **tablespoons chocolate syrup**
- ½ **cup confectioners' sugar**
- 1 **carton (12 ounces) frozen reduced-fat whipped topping, thawed**
- 8 **miniature peanut butter cups**
- ½ **cup fat-free hot fudge ice cream topping, warmed**
- 2 **tablespoons chopped salted peanuts**

1. Line eight 6-oz. ramekins or custard cups with plastic wrap; set aside. In a large bowl, beat cream cheese and chocolate syrup until smooth. Beat in the confectioners' sugar; fold in whipped topping.
2. Spoon into prepared cups; insert a peanut butter cup into the center of each. Cover and freeze for 4-5 hours or until firm.
3. Invert bombes into dessert dishes; removing plastic wrap and cups. Drizzle with hot fudge topping and sprinkle with peanuts.
PER SERVING *1 bombe equals 270 cal., 8 g fat (6 g sat. fat), 3 mg chol., 224 mg sodium, 40 g carb., 1 g fiber, 7 g pro. Diabetic Exchanges: 3 starch, 1 fat.*

CHOCOLATE PEANUT BUTTER BOMBES

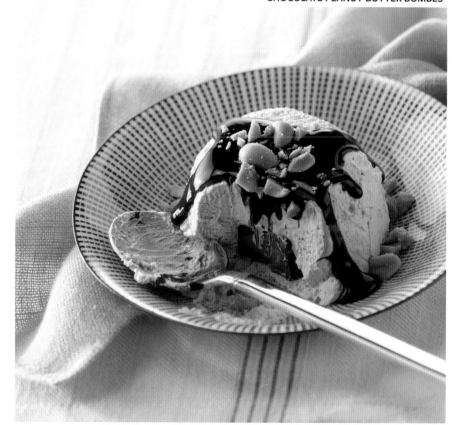

Raspberry Angel Cake

Virtually fat-free and without any cholesterol, this cake is also guilt-free.

—SHERI ERICKSON MONTROSE, IA

PREP: 15 MIN. • **BAKE:** 45 MIN. + COOLING
MAKES: 12 SERVINGS

- 1 package (16 ounces) angel food cake mix
- ½ teaspoon almond extract
- ½ teaspoon vanilla extract
- 1 package (.3 ounce) sugar-free raspberry gelatin
- 1 package (12 ounces) frozen unsweetened raspberries, thawed
- 1 tablespoon sugar

1. Prepare cake batter according to package directions. Fold in extracts. Spoon two-thirds of the batter into an ungreased 10-in. tube pan. Add gelatin powder to remaining batter; drop by tablespoonfuls over batter in pan. Cut through with a knife to swirl.

2. Bake according to package directions. Immediately invert pan onto a wire rack; cool completely, about 1 hour. Carefully run a knife around the sides of pan to remove cake. Cut into slices.

3. Combine raspberries and sugar; serve over cake.

PER SERVING *1 slice with 2 tablespoons sauce equals 155 cal., trace fat (0 sat. fat), 0 chol., 224 mg sodium, 35 g carb., 1 g fiber, 4 g pro.* **Diabetic Exchange:** *2 starch.*

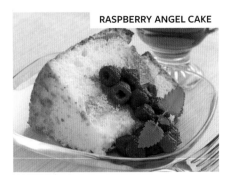
RASPBERRY ANGEL CAKE

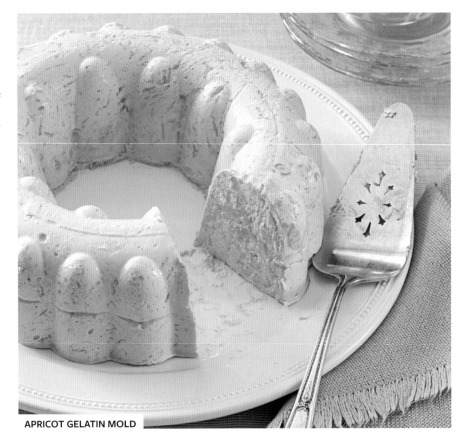
APRICOT GELATIN MOLD

Apricot Gelatin Mold

When my husband and I were dating, he fell in love with this dish from my mother, so I just had to get the recipe from her. You can substitute peach or orange gelatin if you prefer.

—SUZANNE HOLCOMB ST. JOHNSVILLE, NY

PREP: 25 MIN. • **COOK:** 10 MIN. + CHILLING
MAKES: 12 SERVINGS

- 1 can (8 ounces) unsweetened crushed pineapple
- 2 packages (3 ounces each) apricot or peach gelatin
- 1 package (8 ounces) reduced-fat cream cheese
- ¾ cup grated carrots
- 1 carton (8 ounces) frozen fat-free whipped topping, thawed

1. Drain pineapple, reserving juice in a 2-cup measuring cup; add enough water to measure 2 cups. Set pineapple aside. Pour juice mixture into a small saucepan. Bring to a boil; remove from heat. Dissolve gelatin in juice mixture. Cool for 10 minutes.

2. In a large bowl, beat cream cheese until creamy. Gradually add gelatin mixture, beating until smooth. Refrigerate for 30-40 minutes or until slightly thickened.

3. Fold in pineapple and carrots, then whipped topping. Transfer to an 8-cup ring mold coated with cooking spray. Refrigerate until set. Unmold onto a serving platter.

PER SERVING *1/2 cup equals 144 cal., 4 g fat (3 g sat. fat), 13 mg chol., 128 mg sodium, 23 g carb., trace fiber, 3 g pro.* **Diabetic Exchanges:** *1 1/2 starch, 1 fat.*

Banana Split Dessert

My father-in-law is diabetic, but this pudding dessert is one treat he can definitely have. It boasts all the flavors of a true banana split—without the mess!

—ANN JANSEN DEPERE, WI

PREP: 25 MIN. + CHILLING
MAKES: 15 SERVINGS

- 2 cups reduced-fat graham cracker crumbs (about 10 whole crackers)
- 5 tablespoons reduced-fat margarine, melted
- 1 can (12 ounces) cold reduced-fat evaporated milk
- ¾ cup cold fat-free milk
- 2 packages (1 ounce each) sugar-free instant vanilla pudding mix
- 2 medium firm bananas, sliced
- 1 can (20 ounces) unsweetened crushed pineapple, drained
- 1 carton (8 ounces) frozen reduced-fat whipped topping, thawed
- 3 tablespoons chopped walnuts
- 2 tablespoons chocolate syrup
- 5 maraschino cherries, quartered

1. Combine cracker crumbs and margarine; press into a 13-in. x 9-in. dish coated with cooking spray.
2. In a large bowl, whisk the evaporated milk, fat-free milk and pudding mixes for 2 minutes (mixture will be thick).
3. Spread pudding evenly over crust. Layer with bananas, pineapple and whipped topping. Sprinkle with nuts; drizzle with chocolate syrup. Top with cherries. Refrigerate for at least 1 hour before cutting.
NOTE *This recipe was tested with Parkay Light stick margarine.*
PER SERVING *1 piece equals 194 cal., 6 g fat (3 g sat. fat), 4 mg chol., 312 mg sodium, 33 g carb., 1 g fiber, 3 g pro.* ***Diabetic Exchanges:*** *1½ starch, 1 fat, ½ fruit.*

BANANA SPLIT DESSERT

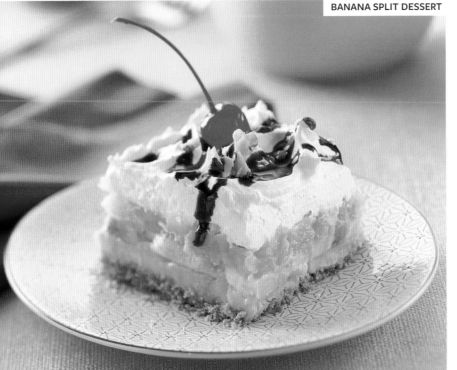

Chocolate Peanut Butter Parfaits

When a friend gave me this recipe I knew it was a keeper. You will not believe that this dessert is light.

—PAT SOLOMAN CASPER, WY

PREP: 20 MIN. + CHILLING
MAKES: 6 SERVINGS

- 2 tablespoons reduced-fat chunky peanut butter
- 2 tablespoons plus 2 cups cold fat-free milk, divided
- 1 cup plus 6 tablespoons reduced-fat whipped topping, divided
- 1 package (1.4 ounces) sugar-free instant chocolate fudge pudding mix
- 3 tablespoons finely chopped salted peanuts

1. In a small bowl, combine peanut butter and 2 tablespoons milk. Fold in 1 cup whipped topping; set aside. In another small bowl, whisk remaining milk with pudding mix for 2 minutes. Let stand for 2 minutes or until soft-set.
2. Spoon half of the pudding into six parfait glasses or dessert dishes. Layer with reserved peanut butter mixture and remaining pudding. Refrigerate for at least 1 hour. Refrigerate remaining whipped topping.
3. Just before serving, garnish each parfait with 1 tablespoon whipped topping and 1½ teaspoons peanuts.
PER SERVING *1 parfait equals 146 cal., 6 g fat (3 g sat. fat), 2 mg chol., 300 mg sodium, 16 g carb., 1 g fiber, 6 g pro.* ***Diabetic Exchanges:*** *1 fat, ½ starch, ½ fat-free milk.*

Swedish Apple Pie

Folks will think you bought this at the store, but you'll wow them when you announce it's homemade! The blend of whole wheat and all-purpose flours offers more fiber and less fat than a traditional pie crust.

—SARAH KLIER ADA, MI

PREP: 15 MIN. • **BAKE:** 25 MIN.
MAKES: 8 SERVINGS

- ½ cup sugar
- ¼ cup whole wheat flour
- ¼ cup all-purpose flour
- 1 teaspoon baking powder
- ½ teaspoon salt
- ½ teaspoon ground cinnamon
- 1 egg
- ¼ teaspoon vanilla extract
- 2 medium tart apples, chopped
- ¾ cup chopped walnuts or pecans, toasted
  Confectioners' sugar, optional

1. In a large bowl, combine the sugar, flours, baking powder, salt and cinnamon. In a small bowl, whisk egg and vanilla. Stir into dry ingredients just until moistened. Fold in apples and walnuts.

2. Transfer to a 9-in. pie plate coated with cooking spray. Bake at 350° for 25-30 minutes or until a toothpick inserted near the center comes out clean. Sprinkle with confectioners' sugar if desired. Serve warm.

PER SERVING *1 piece equals 174 cal., 7 g fat (1 g sat. fat), 26 mg chol., 207 mg sodium, 25 g carb., 2 g fiber, 5 g pro.* **Diabetic Exchanges:** *1½ starch, 1 fat.*

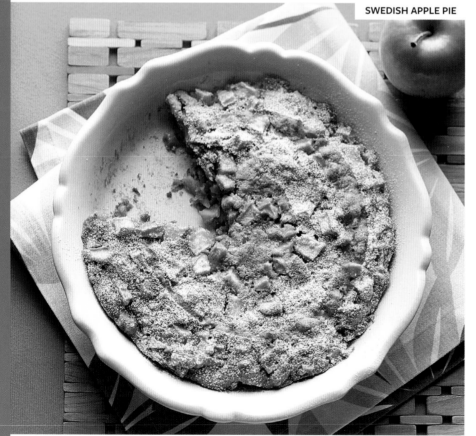

SWEDISH APPLE PIE

Blueberry Raspberry Gelatin

With chopped pecans and plenty of fresh blueberries, this gelatin is ready for a party or potluck.

—JUDY SCOTT FORTUNA, CA

PREP: 20 MIN. + CHILLING
MAKES: 6 SERVINGS

- 1 package (.3 ounce) sugar-free raspberry gelatin
- 1 cup boiling water
- ¾ cup cold water
- 1 cup fresh or frozen unsweetened blueberries, thawed

TOPPING

- 2 ounces reduced-fat cream cheese
- ¼ cup fat-free sour cream
  Sugar substitute equivalent to 2 teaspoons sugar
- ½ teaspoon vanilla extract
- 2 tablespoons chopped pecans, toasted

1. In a small bowl, dissolve gelatin in boiling water. Stir in cold water. Cover and refrigerate until partially set. Fold in blueberries. Transfer to an 8-in. x 4-in. loaf pan coated with cooking spray. Cover and refrigerate for 1 hour or until set.

2. For topping, in a small bowl, beat the cream cheese and sour cream until smooth. Stir in the sugar substitute and vanilla. Unmold gelatin; cut into six slices. Top each slice with the topping and pecans.

NOTE *This recipe was tested with Splenda no-calorie sweetener.*

PER SERVING *⅓ cup equals 72 cal., 4 g fat (2 g sat. fat), 8 mg chol., 80 mg sodium, 6 g carb., 1 g fiber, 3 g pro.* **Diabetic Exchanges:** *1 fat, ½ starch.*

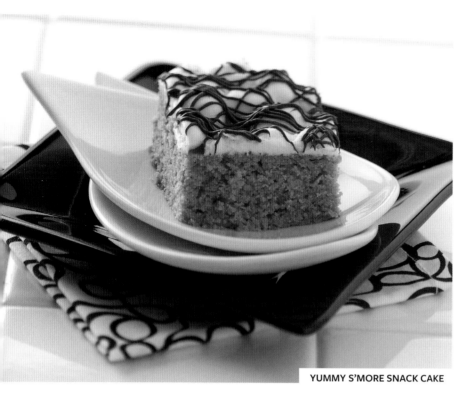

YUMMY S'MORE SNACK CAKE

Chocolate Cream Delight

This dreamy dessert satisfies our chocolate cravings and is easy to double for guests.

—WANDA BENDA JACKSON, MN

PREP: 30 MIN. + CHILLING
MAKES: 9 SERVINGS

- 1 cup chocolate wafer crumbs
- 1 tablespoon sugar
- 2 tablespoons butter, melted
- 2 packages (1.3 ounces each) sugar-free cook-and-serve chocolate pudding mix
- 3½ cups fat-free milk
- 3 ounces reduced-fat cream cheese, cubed
- 2 cups reduced-fat whipped topping
- 2 tablespoons chopped pecans

1. In a small bowl, combine the wafer crumbs, sugar and butter; press onto the bottom of an 8-in. square dish coated with cooking spray. Cover and refrigerate.
2. In a large saucepan, combine the pudding mixes and milk until smooth. Bring to a boil, stirring constantly. Remove from the heat; cool slightly.
3. Spread half of the pudding over crust. Stir cream cheese into remaining pudding until smooth; gently spread over pudding layer. Cover and refrigerate for at least 2 hours or until set.
4. Spread whipped topping over the dessert. Sprinkle with the pecans. Cut into squares.
PER SERVING *1 piece equals 211 cal., 10 g fat (6 g sat. fat), 16 mg chol., 276 mg sodium, 25 g carb., 1 g fiber, 6 g pro. Diabetic Exchanges: 2 fat, 1½ starch.*

Yummy S'more Snack Cake

This cake is the next best thing to s'mores by the campfire. Adjust the amount of marshmallows and chocolate chips to make it as ooey-gooey as you desire.

—DEBORAH WILLIAMS PEORIA, AZ

PREP: 20 MIN. • **BAKE:** 20 MIN. + COOLING
MAKES: 20 SERVINGS

- 2½ cups reduced-fat graham cracker crumbs (about 15 whole crackers)
- ½ cup sugar
- ⅓ cup cake flour
- ⅓ cup whole wheat flour
- 2 teaspoons baking powder
- ¼ teaspoon salt
- 3 egg whites
- 1 cup light soy milk
- ¼ cup unsweetened applesauce
- ¼ cup canola oil
- 2 cups miniature marshmallows
- 1 cup (6 ounces) semisweet chocolate chips

1. In a large bowl, combine the first six ingredients. In a small bowl, whisk the egg whites, soy milk, applesauce and oil. Stir into dry ingredients just until moistened. Transfer to a 13-in. x 9-in. baking pan coated with cooking spray.
2. Bake at 350° for 12-15 minutes or until a toothpick inserted near the center comes out clean. Sprinkle with marshmallows. Bake 4-6 minutes longer or until the marshmallows are softened. Cool on a wire rack for 10 minutes.
3. In a microwave, melt chocolate chips; stir until smooth. Drizzle over cake. Cool completely on a wire rack.
PER SERVING *1 piece equals 168 cal., 6 g fat (2 g sat. fat), 0 chol., 159 mg sodium, 28 g carb., 2 g fiber, 3 g pro. Diabetic Exchanges: 2 starch, 1 fat.*

Lemon Fluff Dessert

Get this mouthwatering dessert started with just a can of evaporated milk and graham crackers. You can also make it a day ahead and refrigerate for convenience.

—**LEOLA MCKINNEY** MORGANTOWN, WV

PREP: 25 MIN. + CHILLING
MAKES: 12 SERVINGS

1	**can (12 ounces) evaporated milk**
1	**package (3 ounces) lemon gelatin**
1	**cup sugar**
1⅓	**cups boiling water**
¼	**cup lemon juice**
1¾	**cups graham cracker crumbs**
5	**tablespoons butter, melted**

1. Pour milk into a small metal bowl; place mixer beaters in the bowl. Cover and refrigerate for at least 2 hours.
2. Meanwhile, in a large bowl, dissolve gelatin and sugar in boiling water. Stir in lemon juice. Cover and refrigerate until syrupy, about 1½ hours.
3. In a small bowl, combine crumbs and butter; set aside 2 tablespoons for garnish. Press remaining crumbs onto the bottom of a 13-in. x 9-in. dish. Beat chilled milk until soft peaks form. Beat gelatin until tiny bubbles form. Fold milk into gelatin. Pour over prepared crust. Sprinkle with the reserved crumbs. Cover and refrigerate until set. Cut into squares.

ORANGE FLUFF DESSERT *Substitute orange gelatin and juice for the lemon gelatin and juice.*

LIME FLUFF DESSERT *Substitute lime gelatin and juice for the lemon gelatin and juice.*

PER SERVING *1 piece equals 221 cal., 8 g fat (5 g sat. fat), 22 mg chol., 151 mg sodium, 35 g carb., trace fiber, 3 g pro. Diabetic Exchanges: 2 starch, 1 fat.*

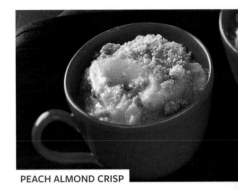

PEACH ALMOND CRISP

Peach Almond Crisp

Any stone fruit (peaches, cherries, apricots, plums) tastes great in this crisp.

—**LILY JULOW** LAWRENCEVILLE, GA

PREP: 15 MIN. • **BAKE:** 20 MIN.
MAKES: 8 SERVINGS

⅔	**cup sliced almonds**
½	**cup all-purpose flour**
¼	**cup packed dark brown sugar**
3	**tablespoons cold butter**
1	**tablespoon sugar**
¼	**teaspoon ground cinnamon**
	Dash ground nutmeg
8	**medium peaches, peeled and sliced**
3	**tablespoons thawed orange juice concentrate**
	Reduced-fat vanilla ice cream, optional

1. In a food processor, combine the first seven ingredients. Cover and process until crumbly; set aside.
2. Place peaches in an 11-in. x 7-in. baking dish coated with cooking spray; drizzle with orange juice concentrate. Sprinkle with almond mixture. Bake at 400° for 20-25 minutes or until topping is golden brown. Serve warm with ice cream if desired.

PER SERVING *¾ cup (calculated without ice cream) equals 193 cal., 9 g fat (3 g sat. fat), 11 mg chol., 33 mg sodium, 28 g carb., 3 g fiber, 4 g pro. Diabetic Exchanges: 2 fat, 1 fruit, ½ starch.*

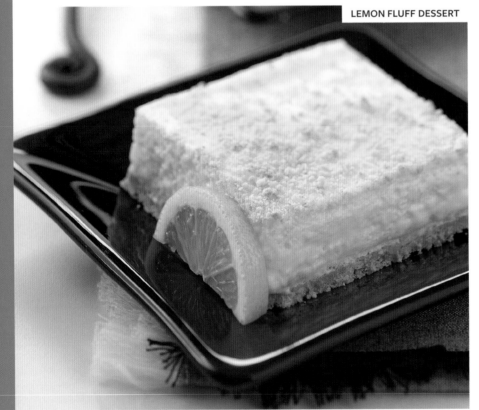

LEMON FLUFF DESSERT

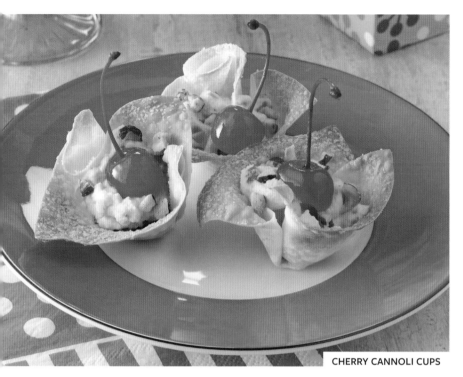

CHERRY CANNOLI CUPS

Pineapple Pudding Cake

My mother used to love making this simple dessert in the summertime. It never lasts very long!

—**KATHLEEN WORDEN** NORTH ANDOVER, MA

PREP: 25 MIN. • **BAKE:** 15 MIN. + CHILLING
MAKES: 20 SERVINGS

- 1 package (9 ounces) yellow cake mix
- 1½ cups cold fat-free milk
- 1 package (1 ounce) sugar-free instant vanilla pudding mix
- 1 package (8 ounces) fat-free cream cheese
- 1 can (20 ounces) unsweetened crushed pineapple, well drained
- 1 carton (8 ounces) frozen fat-free whipped topping, thawed
- ¼ cup chopped walnuts, toasted
- 20 maraschino cherries, well drained

1. Prepare the cake mix batter according to package directions; pour into a 13-in. x 9-in. baking pan coated with cooking spray.
2. Bake at 350° for 15-20 minutes or until a toothpick inserted near the center comes out clean. Cool completely on a wire rack.
3. In a large bowl, whisk milk and pudding mix for 2 minutes. Let stand for 2 minutes or until soft-set.
4. In a small bowl, beat cream cheese until smooth. Beat in pudding mixture until blended. Spread evenly over cake. Sprinkle with pineapple; spread with whipped topping. Sprinkle with walnuts and garnish with cherries. Refrigerate until serving.
PER SERVING *1 piece equals 131 cal., 2 g fat (1 g sat. fat), 1 mg chol., 217 mg sodium, 24 g carb., 1 g fiber, 3 g pro.* **Diabetic Exchange:** *1½ starch.*

Cherry Cannoli Cups

Try an Italian favorite without a lot of fuss. These cute little cups, filled with a rich cherry-cheese filling, are easy to assemble using wonton wrappers.

—**MARIE SHEPPARD** CHICAGO, IL

PREP: 35 MIN. • **COOK:** 5 MIN./BATCH
MAKES: 4 DOZEN

- 48 wonton wrappers
- ¼ cup butter, melted
- ¼ cup sugar
- 2 cups chopped hazelnuts, divided
- 1 carton (15 ounces) part-skim ricotta cheese
- 4 ounces cream cheese, softened
- 3 tablespoons confectioners' sugar
- 1 tablespoon hazelnut liqueur, optional
- 1 teaspoon vanilla extract
- 2 jars (one 16 ounces, one 10 ounces) maraschino cherries, drained

1. Place wonton wrappers on a work surface; brush with melted butter.
Sprinkle with sugar. Press into greased miniature muffin cups. Sprinkle each wonton cup with 1 teaspoon hazelnuts.
2. Bake at 350° for 5-7 minutes or until lightly browned. Remove to a wire rack to cool completely.
3. In a large bowl, beat the ricotta, cream cheese, confectioners' sugar, liqueur if desired and vanilla until smooth. Cut 24 cherries in half and set aside. Chop remaining cherries; fold into cheese mixture.
4. Spoon 1 tablespoon filling into each wonton cup. Sprinkle with remaining hazelnuts. Top each with a reserved cherry half.
TO MAKE AHEAD *Wonton cups and ricotta filling can be made a day in advance. Store cooled wonton cups in an airtight container. Cover and refrigerate ricotta filling.*
PER SERVING *1 cannoli cup equals 109 cal., 6 g fat (2 g sat. fat), 9 mg chol., 71 mg sodium, 13 g carb., 1 g fiber, 3 g pro.* **Diabetic Exchanges:** *1 starch, 1 fat.*

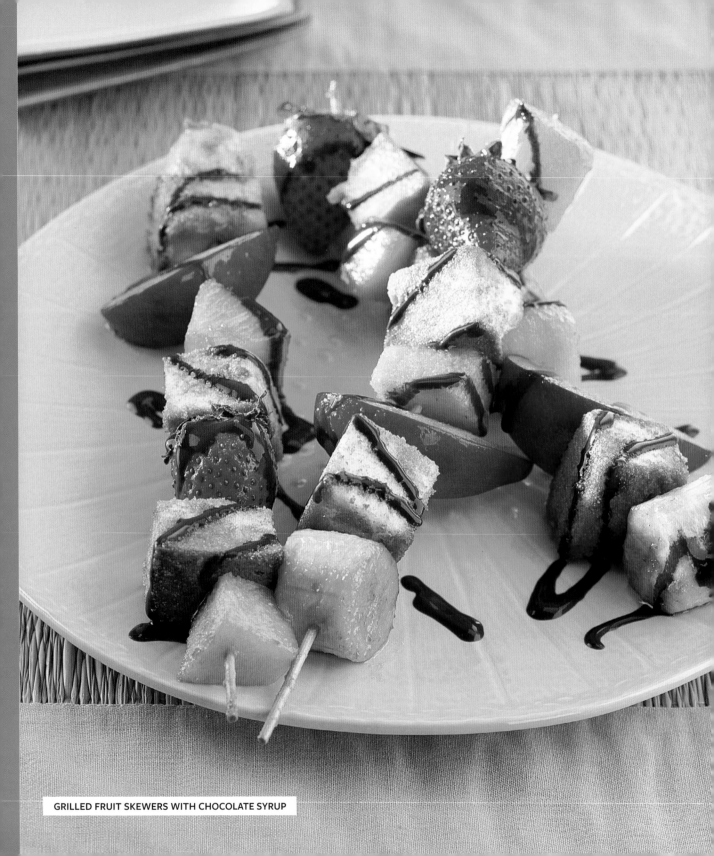

GRILLED FRUIT SKEWERS WITH CHOCOLATE SYRUP

Grilled Fruit Skewers with Chocolate Syrup

With toasted angel food cake and chocolate syrup, this recipe makes fruit seem especially decadent. And it's fun to grill out for dessert!

—MELISSA HASS GILBERT, SC

START TO FINISH: 25 MIN.
MAKES: 8 SERVINGS

- 2 cups cubed angel food cake
- 1 cup fresh strawberries
- 1 cup cubed fresh pineapple
- 1 cup cubed cantaloupe
- 1 large banana, cut into 1-inch slices
- 2 medium plums, pitted and quartered
  Butter-flavored cooking spray
- ½ cup packed brown sugar
- 8 teaspoons chocolate syrup

1. On eight metal or soaked wooden skewers, alternately thread the cake cubes and fruits. Spritz each skewer with butter-flavored spray and roll in brown sugar.

2. Place skewers on a piece of heavy-duty foil. Place foil on grill rack. Grill, covered, over medium heat for 4-5 minutes on each side or until fruits are tender, turning once. Drizzle each skewer with 1 teaspoon chocolate syrup.

PER SERVING *1 skewer equals 131 cal., 1 g fat (trace sat. fat), 0 chol., 93 mg sodium, 30 g carb., 2 g fiber, 2 g pro. Diabetic Exchanges: 1 starch, 1 fruit.*

Raspberry Swirl Frozen Dessert

It may take a little longer to prepare this luscious sweet, but it will be so worth it.

—KAREN SUDERMAN SUGAR LAND, TX

PREP: 45 MIN. • **COOK:** 20 MIN. + FREEZING
MAKES: 12 SERVINGS

- ⅔ cup graham cracker crumbs
- 2 tablespoons butter, melted
- 5 teaspoons sugar

FILLING

- 3 eggs, separated
- ¼ cup plus 1 tablespoon water, divided
- 1 cup sugar, divided
- ⅛ teaspoon salt
- ⅛ teaspoon cream of tartar
- 1 package (8 ounces) reduced-fat cream cheese
- 1½ cups reduced-fat whipped topping
- 1 package (10 ounces) frozen sweetened raspberries, thawed

1. In a small bowl, combine the cracker crumbs, butter and sugar. Press into an 11-in. x 7-in. dish coated with cooking spray. Cover and refrigerate for at least 15 minutes.

2. Meanwhile, for filling, in a small heavy saucepan, combine the egg yolks, ¼ cup water, ½ cup sugar and salt. Cook and stir over low heat until mixture reaches 160° or is thick enough to coat the back of a metal spoon. Cool quickly by placing pan in a bowl of ice water; stir for 2 minutes. Set aside.

3. In a small heavy saucepan over low heat, combine the egg whites, cream of tartar and remaining water and sugar.

With a portable mixer, beat on low speed until mixture reaches 160°. Transfer to a small bowl; beat on high until soft peaks form.

4. In a large bowl, beat cream cheese until smooth. Gradually beat in egg yolk mixture. Fold in whipped topping, then egg white mixture. Drain raspberries, reserving 3 tablespoons juice. In a small bowl, crush half of the berries with 1 tablespoon juice. Set remaining berries and juice aside.

5. Spread a third of cream cheese mixture over crust; spoon half of crushed berry mixture over the top. Repeat layers. Cut through with a knife to swirl raspberries.

6. Top with remaining cream cheese mixture. Sprinkle with reserved berries and drizzle with remaining juice. Cover and freeze for 5 hours or until firm. Remove from the freezer 15 minutes before cutting.

PER SERVING *1 piece equals 217 cal., 9 g fat (5 g sat. fat), 71 mg chol., 164 mg sodium, 32 g carb., 1 g fiber, 4 g pro. Diabetic Exchanges: 2 starch, 1½ fat.*

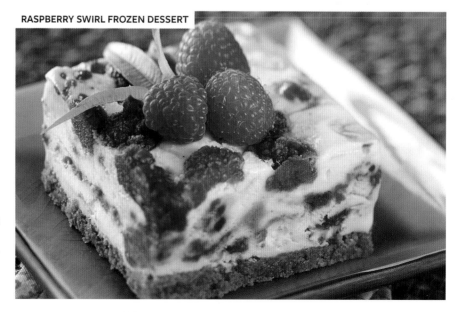

RASPBERRY SWIRL FROZEN DESSERT

cookies, bars & more

Indulge that sweet tooth. Share these goodies with loved ones, and go ahead—**grab one for yourself.** Enjoy ooey-gooey bars and chocolaty cookies, really!

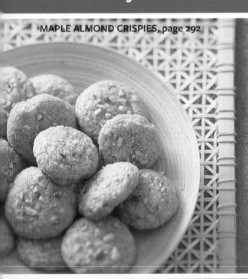
MAPLE ALMOND CRISPIES, page 292

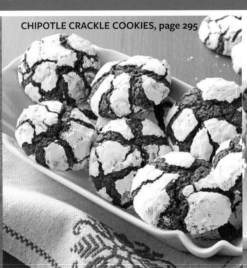
CHIPOTLE CRACKLE COOKIES, page 295

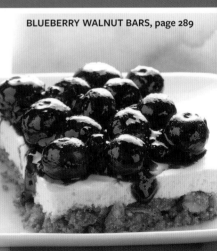
BLUEBERRY WALNUT BARS, page 289

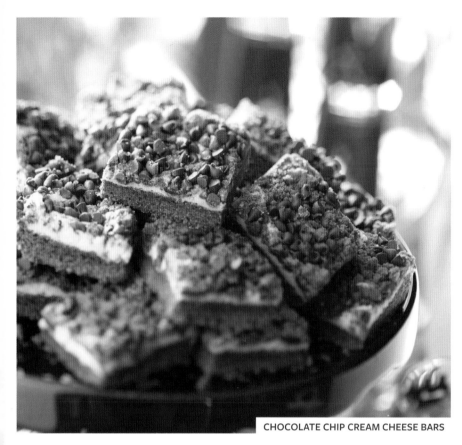

CHOCOLATE CHIP CREAM CHEESE BARS

Lemon Shortbread Cookies

I received this recipe from my cousin after she re-created the cookies she loved from a restaurant. The recipe ended up in the cookbook she made for my family.

—**LORIE MINER** KAMAS, UT

PREP: 25 MIN.
BAKE: 15 MIN./BATCH + COOLING
MAKES: 2 DOZEN

- ½ **cup butter, softened**
- ⅓ **cup sugar**
- 4 **teaspoons grated lemon peel**
- 1 **teaspoon vanilla extract**
- 1 **cup all-purpose flour**
- 2 **tablespoons plus 1½ teaspoons cornstarch**
- ¼ **teaspoon ground nutmeg**
- ⅛ **teaspoon salt**

DRIZZLE
- ½ **cup confectioners' sugar**
- 2 **to 3 teaspoons lemon juice**

1. In a small bowl, cream butter and sugar until light and fluffy. Beat in lemon peel and vanilla. Combine the flour, cornstarch, nutmeg, and salt; gradually add to creamed mixture and mix well. (Dough will be crumbly.) Shape into a ball.
2. On a lightly floured surface, press dough to ½-in. thickness. Cut with a floured 1-in. fluted cookie cutter; place 1 in. apart on ungreased baking sheets. Prick cookies with a fork. Reroll scraps if desired.
3. Bake at 350° for 12-15 minutes or until firm. Cool for 2 minutes before carefully removing to wire racks to cool completely.
4. Combine confectioners' sugar and lemon juice; drizzle over cookies. Store in an airtight container.
PER SERVING *77 cal., 4 g fat (2 g sat. fat), 10 mg chol., 39 mg sodium, 10 g carb., trace fiber, 1 g pro.* **Diabetic Exchanges:** *1 fat, ½ starch.*

Chocolate Chip Cream Cheese Bars

Lower in fat and calories than you might ever guess, these sweet bars couldn't be easier to whip up!

—**JENNIFER RAFFERTY** MILFORD, OH

PREP: 20 MIN. • **BAKE:** 20 MIN. + COOLING
MAKES: 2 DOZEN

- 1 **package German chocolate cake mix (regular size)**
- ⅓ **cup canola oil**
- 1 **egg**

FILLING
- 1 **package (8 ounces) reduced-fat cream cheese**
- ⅓ **cup sugar**
- 1 **egg**
- 1 **cup miniature semisweet chocolate chips**

1. In a large bowl, combine the cake mix, oil and egg. Set aside 1 cup for topping. Press remaining crumb mixture into a 13x9-in. baking pan coated with cooking spray. Bake at 350° for 10-12 minutes or until set.
2. For filling, in a large bowl, beat cream cheese and sugar until smooth. Add egg; beat well. Spread over crust. Sprinkle with chocolate chips and reserved crumb mixture.
3. Bake for 18-20 minutes or until set. Cool on a wire rack. Cut into bars. Store in the refrigerator.
PER SERVING *1 bar equals 187 cal., 9 g fat (3 g sat. fat), 24 mg chol., 207 mg sodium, 25 g carb., trace fiber, 3 g pro.* **Diabetic Exchanges:** *1½ starch, 1½ fat.*

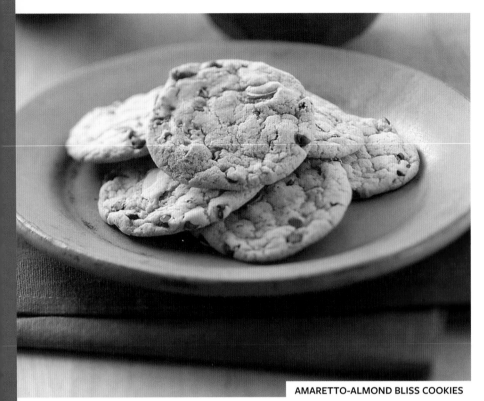
AMARETTO-ALMOND BLISS COOKIES

White Chocolate Cranberry Granola Bars

I created these chewy granola bars while searching for a healthful, portable snack for my family. I often get recipe requests when I bring them to our kids' athletic events and school bake sales.

—**JANIS LOOMIS** MADISON, VA

PREP: 10 MIN. • **BAKE:** 20 MIN. + COOLING
MAKES: 2 DOZEN

- ¼ **cup sugar**
- ¼ **cup honey**
- ¼ **cup maple syrup**
- 2 **tablespoons reduced-fat peanut butter**
- 1 **egg white**
- 1 **tablespoon fat-free evaporated milk**
- 1 **teaspoon vanilla extract**
- 1 **cup whole wheat flour**
- ½ **teaspoon baking soda**
- ½ **teaspoon ground cinnamon**
- ¼ **teaspoon ground allspice**
- 2 **cups old-fashioned oats**
- 1½ **cups crisp rice cereal**
- ⅓ **cup vanilla or white chips**
- ¼ **cup dried cranberries**
- ¼ **cup chopped walnuts**

1. In a large bowl, combine the first seven ingredients. Combine the flour, baking soda, cinnamon and allspice; stir into sugar mixture. Stir in the oats, cereal, chips, cranberries and walnuts.
2. Press into a 13-in. x 9-in. baking pan coated with cooking spray. Bake at 350° for 18-20 minutes or until golden brown. Cool on a wire rack. Cut into bars. Store in an airtight container.
PER SERVING *109 cal., 3 g fat (1 g sat. fat), 1 mg chol., 57 mg sodium, 20 g carb., 2 g fiber, 3 g pro.* **Diabetic Exchanges:** *1½ starch, ½ fat.*

Amaretto-Almond Bliss Cookies

After lightening up these cookies, they're now as guilt-free as they are delicious!

—**VERA DECKER** WINDSOR, NY

PREP: 20 MIN. • **BAKE:** 10 MIN. /BATCH
MAKES: 2½ DOZEN

- ⅓ **cup butter, softened**
- ½ **cup sugar**
- ⅓ **cup packed brown sugar**
- 1 **egg**
- 2 **tablespoons amaretto**
- ½ **teaspoon almond extract**
- 1 **cup all-purpose flour**
- 1 **cup oat flour**
- 1 **teaspoon baking powder**
- 1 **teaspoon baking soda**
- ¼ **teaspoon salt**
- ¾ **cup miniature semisweet chocolate chips**
- ⅔ **cup sliced almonds, toasted**

1. In a large bowl, beat butter and sugars until crumbly, about 2 minutes. Add egg; mix well. Stir in amaretto and almond extract. Combine the flours, baking powder, baking soda and salt; gradually add to the butter mixture and mix well. Stir in chocolate chips and almonds.
2. With lightly floured hands, shape into 1-in. balls. Place 2 in. apart on baking sheets coated with cooking spray. Flatten slightly with a glass coated with cooking spray.
3. Bake at 350° for 7-9 minutes or until tops are cracked and bottoms are lightly browned. Remove to wire racks.
NOTE *As a substitute for 1 cup oat flour, process 1¼ cups quick-cooking or old-fashioned oats until finely ground.*
PER SERVING *106 cal., 5 g fat (2 g sat. fat), 12 mg chol., 93 mg sodium, 15 g carb., 1 g fiber, 2 g pro.* **Diabetic Exchanges:** *1 starch, 1 fat.*

Blueberry Walnut Bars

With power-packing oats, walnuts and blueberries, this treat will please kids and adults alike.

—DAWN ONUFFER CRESTVIEW, FL

PREP: 20 MIN. • **BAKE:** 10 MIN. + COOLING
MAKES: 12 SERVINGS

- ⅔ cup ground walnuts
- ½ cup graham cracker crumbs
- 2 tablespoons plus ⅓ cup sugar, divided
- ⅓ cup old-fashioned oats
- 3 tablespoons reduced-fat butter, melted
- 1 package (8 ounces) reduced-fat cream cheese
- 1 tablespoon orange juice
- ½ teaspoon vanilla extract
- ½ cup reduced-fat whipped topping
- 2 tablespoons blueberry preserves
- 1½ cups fresh blueberries

1. In a small bowl, combine the walnuts, cracker crumbs, 2 tablespoons sugar, oats and butter. Press onto the bottom of an 8-in. square baking dish coated with cooking spray.

2. Bake at 350° for 9-11 minutes or until set and edges are lightly browned. Cool on a wire rack.

3. In a large bowl, beat cream cheese and remaining sugar until smooth. Beat in orange juice and vanilla. Fold in whipped topping. Spread over crust.

4. In a microwave-safe bowl, heat preserves on high for 15-20 seconds or until warmed; gently stir in the blueberries. Spoon over filling. Refrigerate until serving.

NOTE *This recipe was tested with Land O'Lakes light stick butter.*

PER SERVING *1 bar equals 167 cal., 9 g fat (4 g sat. fat), 17 mg chol., 125 mg sodium, 19 g carb., 1 g fiber, 3 g pro. Diabetic Exchanges: 2 fat, 1 starch.*

BLUEBERRY WALNUT BARS

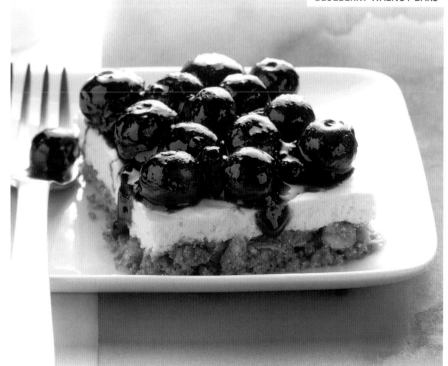

Spiced Cranberry Oatmeal Cookies

These delicious cookies are filled with pecans, dried cranberries and chocolate chips. Every bite is packed with sweetness and crunch.

—KARIE SAXTON SOUTH BOARDMAN, MI

PREP: 30 MIN. • **BAKE:** 10 MIN./BATCH
MAKES: 5½ DOZEN

- ½ cup butter, softened
- ¾ cup packed brown sugar
- ¼ cup sugar blend
- ¾ cup unsweetened applesauce
- 1 egg
- 1 teaspoon vanilla extract
- 3 cups old-fashioned oats
- 1¾ cups all-purpose flour
- 1½ teaspoons ground cinnamon
- 1 teaspoon baking powder
- ½ teaspoon salt
- ½ teaspoon ground nutmeg
- 1 cup dried cranberries
- ½ cup miniature semisweet chocolate chips
- ½ cup chopped pecans

1. In a large bowl, beat the butter, brown sugar and sugar blend until well blended. Beat in the applesauce, egg and vanilla (mixture will appear curdled). Combine the oats, flour, cinnamon, baking powder, salt and nutmeg; gradually add to the butter mixture and mix well. Stir in the cranberries, chocolate chips and the pecans.

2. Drop by tablespoonfuls 2 in. apart onto ungreased baking sheets; flatten slightly. Bake at 350° for 10-12 minutes or until edges are lightly browned. Remove to wire racks.

NOTE *This recipe was tested with Splenda sugar blend.*

PER SERVING *1 cookie equals 71 cal., 3 g fat (1 g sat. fat), 7 mg chol., 36 mg sodium, 11 g carb., 1 g fiber, 1 g pro. Diabetic Exchanges: 1 starch, ½ fat.*

Small Batch Brownies

If you want to make your brownies stand out, dust them with a layer of powdered sugar. It makes them more festive, too!

—TASTE OF HOME TEST KITCHEN

PREP: 15 MIN. • **BAKE:** 15 MIN. + COOLING
MAKES: 6 SERVINGS

- 2 **tablespoons butter**
- ½ **ounce unsweetened chocolate**
- 1 **egg**
- ¼ **teaspoon vanilla extract**
- ⅔ **cup sugar**
- ⅓ **cup all-purpose flour**
- ¼ **cup baking cocoa**
- ¼ **teaspoon salt**
- ¼ **teaspoon confectioners' sugar, optional**

1. In a microwave, melt butter and chocolate; stir until smooth. Cool slightly.

2. In a small bowl, whisk egg and vanilla; gradually whisk in sugar. Stir in chocolate mixture. Combine the flour, cocoa and salt; gradually add to chocolate mixture.

3. Transfer to a 9-in. x 5-in. loaf pan coated with cooking spray. Bake at 350° for 12-16 minutes or until a toothpick inserted near the center comes out clean. Cool on a wire rack. Cut into bars. Dust with the confectioners' sugar if desired.

PER SERVING *1 brownie equals 179 cal., 6 g fat (3 g sat. fat), 45 mg chol., 138 mg sodium, 30 g carb., 1 g fiber, 3 g pro.* **Diabetic Exchanges:** *2 starch, 1 fat.*

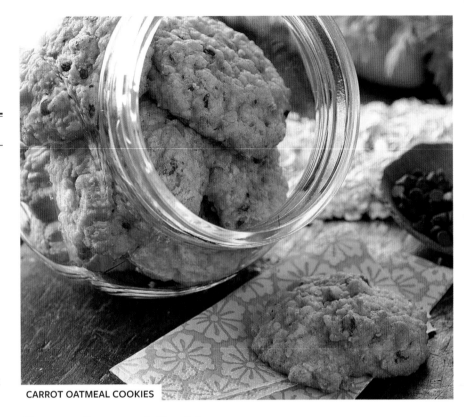

CARROT OATMEAL COOKIES

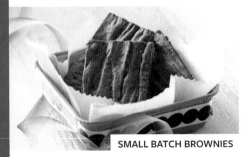

SMALL BATCH BROWNIES

Carrot Oatmeal Cookies

These carrot-flecked cookies my mom made when I was growing up now get a thumbs-up from my own kids.

—CANDACE ZAUGG EAGAR, AZ

PREP: 30 MIN. + CHILLING
BAKE: 10 MIN./BATCH
MAKES: 6 DOZEN

- 1 **cup butter, softened**
- 1 **cup shortening**
- 1½ **cups sugar**
- 1½ **cups packed brown sugar**
- 4 **eggs**
- 2 **teaspoons vanilla extract**
- 2 **cups shredded carrots**
- 4 **cups quick-cooking oats**
- 3½ **cups all-purpose flour**
- 2 **teaspoons baking soda**
- 2 **teaspoons salt**
- 1 **cup chopped walnuts**
- 1 **cup miniature semisweet chocolate chips**

1. In a large bowl, cream the butter, shortening and sugars until light and fluffy. Beat in eggs and vanilla. Beat in carrots. Combine the oats, flour, baking soda and salt; gradually add to creamed mixture and mix well. Stir in walnuts and chocolate chips. Cover and refrigerate for at least 4 hours.

2. Drop by rounded tablespoonfuls 3 in. apart onto baking sheets coated with cooking spray. Bake at 375° for 10-13 minutes or until lightly browned. Cool for 2 minutes before removing to wire racks.

PER SERVING *1 cookie equals 147 cal., 8 g fat (3 g sat. fat), 19 mg chol., 133 mg sodium, 18 g carb., 1 g fiber, 2 g pro.* **Diabetic Exchanges:** *1½ fat, 1 starch.*

Breezy Lemon-Berry Dessert

I love the combination of berries and lemon, and wanted to come up with a light, refreshing dessert that used them both.

— **ANNA GINSBERG** AUSTIN, TX

PREP: 30 MIN. + CHILLING
MAKES: 12 SERVINGS

- **2 envelopes unflavored gelatin**
- **½ cup cold water**
- **1 package (3 ounces) ladyfingers, split**
- **1½ cups fat-free milk**
- **½ cup refrigerated French vanilla nondairy creamer**
- **1 package (3.4 ounces) instant lemon pudding mix**
- **1 carton (12 ounces) frozen reduced-fat whipped topping, thawed, divided**

1. In a small saucepan, sprinkle gelatin over cold water; let stand for 1 minute. Cook over low heat, stirring until gelatin is completely dissolved. Remove from the heat and set aside.

2. Cut ladyfingers in half widthwise; arrange cut side down around the sides of an ungreased 9-in. springform pan. Place remaining ladyfingers in the bottom of the pan (bottom will not be completely covered).

3. In a large bowl, whisk milk, creamer and pudding mix for 2 minutes. Let stand for 2 minutes or until soft-set. Stir in gelatin mixture. Fold in 3 cups of the whipped topping.

4. Spread 2 cups of filling evenly into prepared pan; top with mixed berries. Spread with remaining filling (filling will be higher than ladyfinger border). Cover and refrigerate for 5 hours or until set. Garnish with remaining whipped topping and the strawberries.

NOTE *This recipe was tested with Parkay Light stick margarine.*

PER SERVING *1 slice equals 183 cal., 5 g fat (3 g sat. fat), 26 mg chol., 129 mg sodium, 29 g carb., 2 g fiber, 3 g pro.* **Diabetic Exchanges:** *2 starch, 1 fat.*

BREEZY LEMON-BERRY DESSERT

Sugar-Free Maple Cookies

Mom experimented with so many batches of cookies until she came up with this recipe to satisfy my diabetic brother's sweet tooth. The rest of our family eats them up, too.

—**BRENDA WILE** WINESBURG, OH

PREP: 10 MIN. • **BAKE:** 10 MIN./BATCH
MAKES: 42 COOKIES

- **½ cup reduced-fat margarine, softened**
- **½ cup sour cream**
- **1 cup shredded peeled tart apple**
- **2 eggs**
- **1 teaspoon maple flavoring**
- **½ teaspoon vanilla extract**
- **2 cups all-purpose flour**
  Artificial brown sugar sweetener equivalent to ⅓ cup brown sugar
- **½ teaspoon baking soda**
- **½ teaspoon baking powder**

1. In a bowl, combine margarine, sour cream, apple, eggs, maple flavoring and vanilla. Combine flour, sweetener, baking soda and baking powder; add to apple mixture and mix well.

2. Drop by heaping tablespoonfuls onto baking sheets coated with cooking spray. Bake at 375° for 9-10 minutes or until lightly browned. Cool on wire racks. Store in airtight container.

PER SERVING *1 cookie equals 44 cal., 2 g fat (0 sat. fat), 11 mg chol., 51 mg sodium, 5 g carb., 0 fiber, 1 g pro.* **Diabetic Exchanges:** *½ starch, ½ fat.*

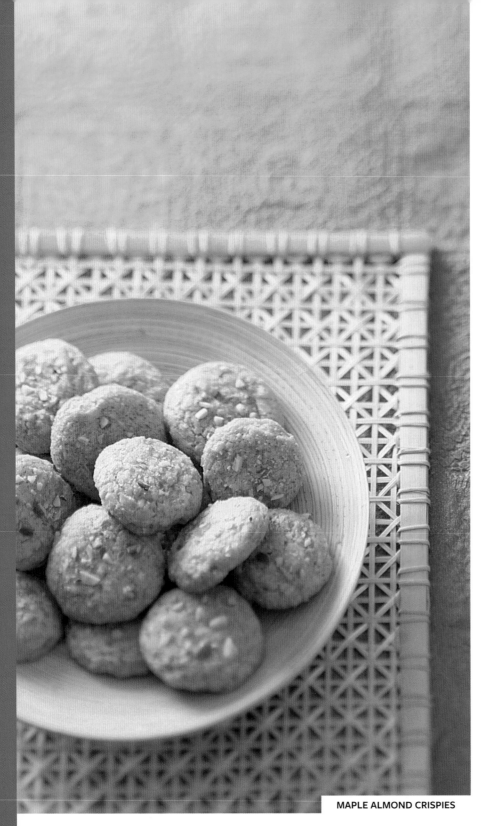

Maple Almond Crispies

Every bite of these cookies contains cinnamon and maple. Your whole family will love them.

—**JEAN ECOS** HARTLAND, WI

PREP: 20 MIN. • **BAKE:** 10 MIN./BATCH
MAKES: ABOUT 3 DOZEN

- ⅓ cup maple syrup
- ¼ cup canola oil
- 1 tablespoon water
- 1 teaspoon almond extract
- 1 cup brown rice flour
- ½ cup almond flour
- ¼ cup sugar
- 1 teaspoon baking powder
- 1 teaspoon ground cinnamon
- ⅛ teaspoon salt
- ½ cup finely chopped almonds

1. In a small bowl, beat the syrup, oil, water and extract until well blended. Combine the flours, sugar, baking powder, cinnamon and salt; gradually beat into syrup mixture until blended. Stir in almonds.

2. Drop by rounded teaspoonfuls onto parchment paper-lined baking sheets; flatten slightly. Bake at 350° for 10-12 minutes or until bottoms are lightly browned. Cool for 1 minute before removing from pans to wire racks.

NOTE *Read all ingredient labels for possible gluten content prior to use. Ingredient formulas can change, and production facilities vary among brands. If you're concerned that your brand may contain gluten, contact the company.*

PER SERVING *54 cal., 3 g fat (trace sat. fat), 0 chol., 18 mg sodium, 6 g carb., 1 g fiber, 1 g pro.* **Diabetic Exchanges:** *½ starch, ½ fat.*

MAPLE ALMOND CRISPIES

Apricot Date Squares

Memories of my mom's fruity date bars inspired me to come up with this wonderful treat. Occasionally I replace the apricot jam with orange marmalade.

—SHANNON KOENE BLACKSBURG, VA

PREP: 45 MIN. • **BAKE:** 20 MIN. + COOLING
MAKES: 3 DOZEN

- 1 **cup water**
- 1 **cup sugar**
- 1 **cup chopped dates**
- ½ **cup 100% apricot spreadable fruit or jam**
- 1¾ **cups old-fashioned oats**
- 1½ **cups all-purpose flour**
- 1 **cup flaked coconut**
- 1 **cup packed brown sugar**
- 1 **teaspoon ground cinnamon**
- ¼ **teaspoon salt**
- ¾ **cup cold butter, cubed**

1. In a small saucepan, combine the water, sugar and dates. Bring to a boil.

Reduce heat; simmer, uncovered, for 30-35 minutes or until mixture is reduced to 1⅓ cups and is slightly thickened, stirring occasionally.
2. Remove from the heat. Stir in spreadable fruit until blended; set aside. In a food processor, combine the oats, flour, coconut, brown sugar, cinnamon and salt. Add butter; cover and process until mixture resembles coarse crumbs.
3. Press 3 cups of crumb mixture into a 13-in. x 9-in. baking dish coated with cooking spray. Spread the date mixture to within ½ in. of edges. Sprinkle with the remaining crumb mixture; press down gently.
4. Bake at 350° for 20-25 minutes or until edges are lightly browned. Cool on a wire rack. Cut into squares.
PER SERVING *1 bar equals 147 cal., 5 g fat (3 g sat. fat), 10 mg chol., 65 mg sodium, 25 g carb., 1 g fiber, 1 g pro.* **Diabetic Exchanges:** *1½ starch, 1 fat.*

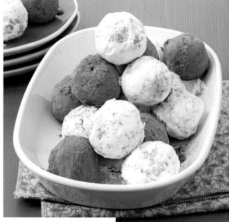

MOCHA PECAN BALLS

Mocha Pecan Balls

Dusted in either confectioners' sugar or cocoa, this 6-ingredient dough rolls up into truffle-like treats. Best part of all, there's no baking required!

—LORRAINE DAROCHA MOUNTAIN CITY, TN

START TO FINISH: 25 MIN.
MAKES: 4 DOZEN

- 2½ **cups crushed vanilla wafers (about 65 wafers)**
- 2 **cups plus ¼ cup confectioners' sugar, divided**
- ⅔ **cup finely chopped pecans, toasted**
- 2 **tablespoons baking cocoa**
- ¼ **cup reduced-fat evaporated milk**
- ¼ **cup cold strong brewed coffee**
  Additional baking cocoa, optional

1. In a large bowl, combine the wafer crumbs, 2 cups confectioners' sugar, pecans and cocoa. Stir in milk and coffee (mixture will be sticky).
2. With hands dusted in confectioners' sugar, shape dough into ¾-in. balls; roll in remaining confectioner's sugar or additional baking cocoa if desired. Store in an airtight container.
PER SERVING *1 cookie equals 61 cal., 2 g fat (trace sat. fat), 1 mg chol., 20 mg sodium, 10 g carb., trace fiber, trace pro.* **Diabetic Exchange:** *1 starch.*

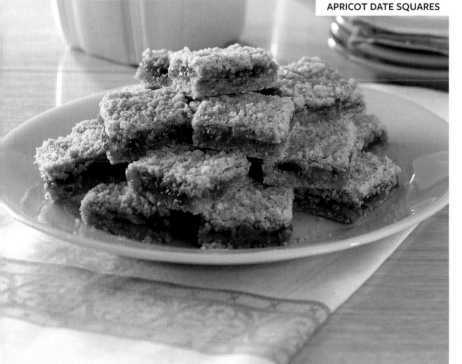

APRICOT DATE SQUARES

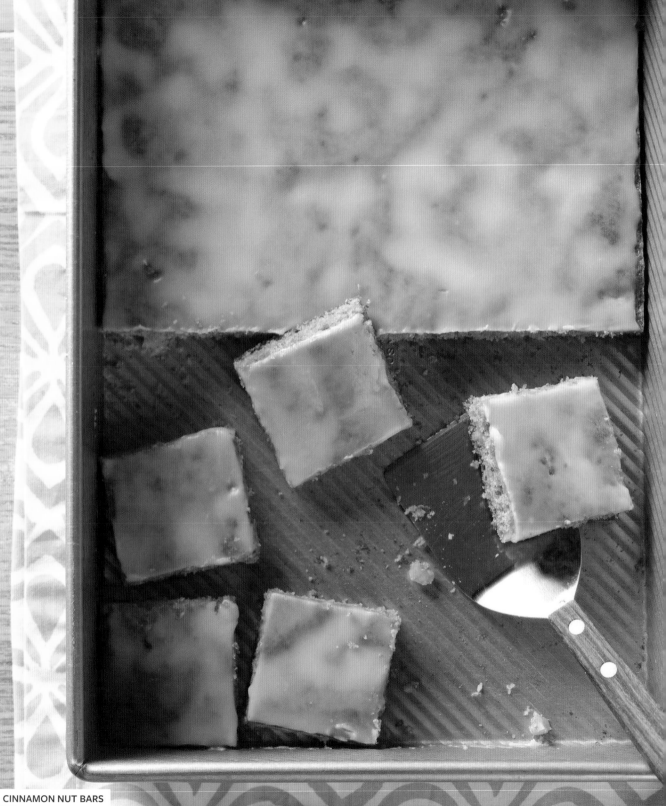

CINNAMON NUT BARS

Cinnamon Nut Bars

Classic bar meets good-for-you ingredients in this updated recipe. If you have the patience, store the bars in a tin for a day to allow the flavors to meld. Be sure to let the bars cool before you pack them up!

—**HEIDI LINDSEY** PRAIRIE DU SAC, WI

PREP: 20 MIN. • **BAKE:** 15 MIN. + COOLING
MAKES: 2 DOZEN

- ½ cup whole wheat flour
- ½ cup all-purpose flour
- ½ cup sugar
- 1½ teaspoons ground cinnamon
- 1¼ teaspoons baking powder
- ¼ teaspoon baking soda
- 1 egg, beaten
- ⅓ cup canola oil
- ¼ cup unsweetened applesauce
- ¼ cup honey
- 1 cup chopped walnuts

ICING

- 1 cup confectioners' sugar
- 2 tablespoons butter, melted
- 1 teaspoon vanilla extract
- 1 tablespoon water
- 2 tablespoons honey

1. In a large bowl, combine the flours, sugar, cinnamon, baking powder and baking soda. In another bowl, combine the egg, oil, applesauce and honey. Stir into the dry ingredients just until moistened. Fold in walnuts.

2. Spread batter into a 13-in. x 9-in. baking pan coated with cooking spray. Bake at 350° for 15-20 minutes or until a toothpick inserted near the center comes out clean.

3. Combine icing ingredients; spread over warm bars. Cool completely before cutting into bars.

PER SERVING *1 bar equals 142 cal., 7 g fat (1 g sat. fat), 11 mg chol., 44 mg sodium, 18 g carb., 1 g fiber, 2 g pro.* ***Diabetic Exchanges:*** *1 starch, 1 fat.*

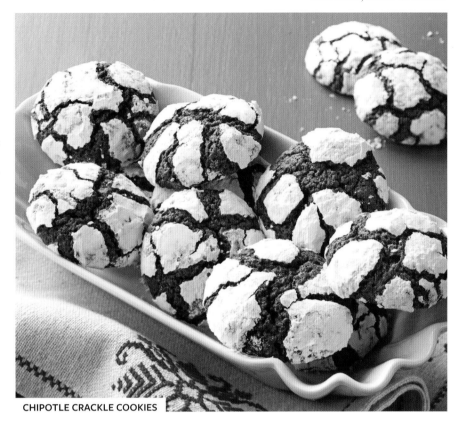

CHIPOTLE CRACKLE COOKIES

Chipotle Crackle Cookies

I bake these special cookies for birthdays, the holidays and more! The addition of ground chipotle chili pepper gives them a little zing. The dough is sometimes sticky, so I dust my hands with confectioners' sugar for easier handling.

—**GLORIA BRADLEY** NAPERVILLE, IL

PREP: 25 MIN. + CHILLING
BAKE: 10 MIN./BATCH
MAKES: 2½ DOZEN

- 2 eggs
- 1 cup sugar
- ¼ cup canola oil
- 2 teaspoons vanilla extract
- 2 ounces unsweetened chocolate, melted and cooled
- 1 cup all-purpose flour
- 1 tablespoon toasted wheat germ
- ¾ teaspoon baking powder
- ¼ teaspoon salt
- ⅛ teaspoon ground chipotle pepper
- ¼ cup miniature semisweet chocolate chips
- ⅓ cup confectioners' sugar

1. In a large bowl, beat the eggs, sugar, oil and vanilla until combined. Add melted chocolate. Combine the flour, wheat germ, baking powder, salt and chipotle pepper. Gradually add to egg mixture and mix well. Fold in chocolate chips. Cover and refrigerate for 2 hours.

2. Place confectioners' sugar in a small bowl. Shape dough into 1-in. balls; roll in confectioners' sugar. Place 2 in. apart on baking sheets coated with cooking spray. Bake at 350° for 8-10 minutes or until set. Remove to wire racks to cool.

PER SERVING *1 cookie equals 85 cal., 4 g fat (1 g sat. fat), 14 mg chol., 35 mg sodium, 13 g carb., 1 g fiber, 1 g pro.* ***Diabetic Exchanges:*** *1 starch, ½ fat.*

Cream Cheese Slice-and-Bake Cookies

Once you make the batter, let it chill in the refrigerator for a few hours, then just slice and bake!

—TASTE OF HOME TEST KITCHEN

PREP: 25 MIN. + CHILLING
BAKE: 15 MIN./BATCH
MAKES: ABOUT 5½ DOZEN

- 1 **cup butter, softened**
- 1 **package (3 ounces) cream cheese, softened**
- 1 **cup sugar**
- 1 **egg**
- ½ **teaspoon rum extract**
- ¼ **teaspoon vanilla extract**
- 3 **cups all-purpose flour**
- ½ **teaspoon salt**
- ½ **teaspoon baking powder**
- ¼ **teaspoon baking soda**
- ½ **teaspoon ground nutmeg**
- 1 **cup finely chopped almonds**

1. In a large bowl, cream the butter, cream cheese and sugar until light and fluffy. Beat in the egg and extracts. Combine the flour, salt, baking powder, baking soda and nutmeg; gradually add to creamed mixture and mix well.
2. Shape into two 9-in. rolls. Roll each in almonds; wrap in plastic wrap. Refrigerate for 2 hours or until firm.
3. Cut into ¼-in. slices. Place 2 in. apart on parchment paper-lined baking sheets. Bake at 375° for 11-13 minutes or until bottoms are lightly browned. Cool for 1 minute before removing from pans to wire racks.
TO MAKE AHEAD *Dough can be made 2 days in advance. Cookies can be baked 1 week ahead of time and stored in an airtight container at room temperature or frozen for up to 1 month.*
PER SERVING *1 cookie equals 74 cal., 4 g fat (2 g sat. fat), 12 mg chol., 50 mg sodium, 8 g carb., trace fiber, 1 g pro.*
Diabetic Exchanges: *1 fat, ½ starch.*

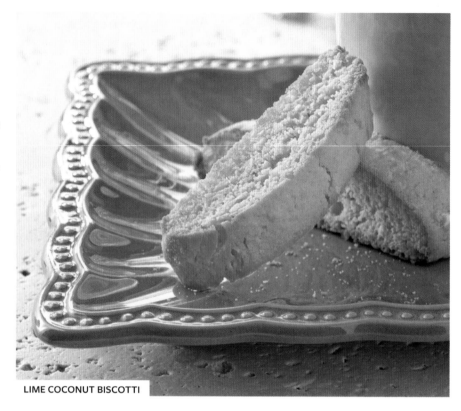

LIME COCONUT BISCOTTI

Lime Coconut Biscotti

Dunk this biscotti into your morning cup of coffee or enjoy as an afternoon snack or after-dinner dessert.

—DIANA BURRINK CRETE, IL

PREP: 25 MIN. • **BAKE:** 30 MIN.
MAKES: 32 COOKIES

- ¾ **cup sugar**
- ¼ **cup canola oil**
- 2 **eggs**
- ¼ **cup lime juice**
- 1 **teaspoon vanilla extract**
- ¼ **teaspoon coconut extract**
- 1¾ **cups all-purpose flour**
- ⅔ **cup cornmeal**
- 1½ **teaspoons baking powder**
- ¼ **teaspoon salt**
- 1 **cup flaked coconut**
- 1 **teaspoon grated lime peel**

1. In a small bowl, beat sugar and oil until blended. Beat in the eggs, lime juice, vanilla and coconut extracts. Combine the flour, cornmeal, baking powder and salt; gradually add to sugar mixture and mix well (dough will be sticky). Stir in coconut and lime peel.
2. Divide dough in half. With lightly floured hands, shape each half into a 12-in. x 2-in. rectangle on a parchment paper-lined baking sheet. Bake at 350° for 20-25 minutes or until set.
3. Place pan on a wire rack. When cool enough to handle, transfer to a cutting board; cut diagonally with a serrated knife into ¾-in. slices. Place cut side down on ungreased baking sheets. Bake for 5-6 minutes on each side or until golden brown. Remove to wire racks to cool. Store in an airtight container.
PER SERVING *1 cookie equals 89 cal., 3 g fat (1 g sat. fat), 13 mg chol., 49 mg sodium, 14 g carb., 1 g fiber, 1 g pro.*
Diabetic Exchanges: *1 starch, ½ fat.*

Cherry-Chocolate Coconut Meringues

Making meringue cookies doesn't have to be difficult! These are also a great dessert option for those on gluten-free diets.

—MARY SHIVERS ADA, OK

PREP: 15 MIN.
BAKE: 25 MIN./BATCH + COOLING
MAKES: 3 DOZEN

  3 **egg whites**
  ½ **teaspoon almond extract**
     Dash salt
  ⅓ **cup sugar**
  ⅔ **cup confectioners' sugar**
  ¼ **cup baking cocoa**
  1¼ **cups finely shredded unsweetened coconut**
  ½ **cup dried cherries, finely chopped**

1. Place egg whites in a large bowl; let stand at room temperature for 30 minutes.

2. Add extract and salt; beat on medium speed until soft peaks form. Gradually add sugar, 1 tablespoon at a time, beating on high until stiff glossy peaks form and sugar is dissolved. Combine confectioners' sugar and cocoa; beat into egg white mixture. Fold in coconut and cherries.

3. Drop by rounded tablespoonfuls 2 in. apart onto baking sheets coated with cooking spray. Bake at 325° for 25-28 minutes or until firm to the touch. Cool completely on pans on wire racks. Store in an airtight container.

NOTE *Look for unsweetened coconut in the baking or health food section.*

PER SERVING *1 cookie equals 42 cal., 2 g fat (1 g sat. fat), 0 chol., 10 mg sodium, 6 g carb., 1 g fiber, 1 g pro.* **Diabetic Exchange:** *½ starch.*

CHERRY-CHOCOLATE COCONUT MERINGUES

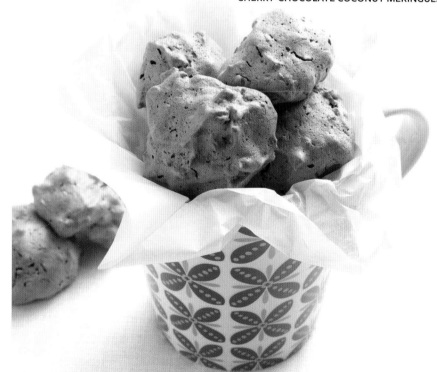

White Chip Cranberry Blondies

Replacing some oil with applesauce keeps the batter moist without sacrificing flavor.
—TASTE OF HOME TEST KITCHEN

PREP: 15 MIN. • **BAKE:** 15 MIN. + COOLING
MAKES: 20 BARS

  2 **eggs**
  ¼ **cup canola oil**
  ¼ **cup unsweetened applesauce**
  1½ **teaspoons vanilla extract**
  1⅓ **cups all-purpose flour**
  ⅔ **cup packed brown sugar**
  1 **teaspoon baking powder**
  ½ **teaspoon salt**
  1 **cup dried cranberries, divided**
  ½ **cup white baking chips**
  ½ **cup chopped pecans**

1. In a large bowl, beat the eggs, oil, applesauce and vanilla. Combine flour, brown sugar, baking powder and salt; stir into egg mixture until blended. Stir in ½ cup cranberries (batter will be thick).

2. Spread into a 13-in. x 9-in. baking pan coated with cooking spray. Top with the chips, pecans and remaining cranberries; gently press the toppings down.

3. Bake at 350° for 15-20 minutes or until a toothpick inserted near the center comes out clean. Cool on a wire rack. Cut into bars.

PER SERVING *1 bar equals 154 cal., 7 g fat (1 g sat. fat), 22 mg chol., 92 mg sodium, 22 g carb., 1 g fiber, 2 g pro.* **Diabetic Exchanges:** *1½ starch, 1 fat.*

top tip

Dress Up Bars

I place individual bars in muffin cup liners for an easy, pretty presentation.
—RENEE Z. TACOMA, WA

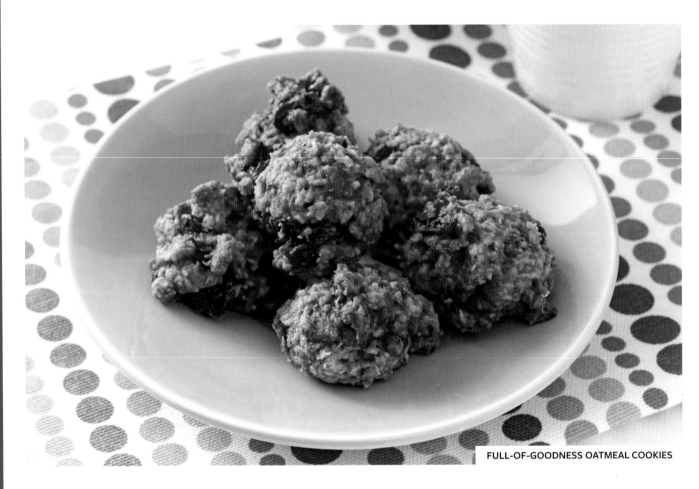

Full-of-Goodness Oatmeal Cookies

I love to bake goodies for my co-workers, so I created this healthier version of the classic oatmeal cookie. This way, I don't get blamed for ruining any diets!

—**SHARON BALESTRA** BLOOMFIELD, NY

PREP: 35 MIN. • **BAKE:** 10 MIN./BATCH
MAKES: 6 DOZEN

- 2 **tablespoons hot water**
- 1 **tablespoon ground flaxseed**
- 1 **cup pitted dried plums, chopped**
- 1 **cup chopped dates**
- ½ **cup raisins**
- ⅓ **cup butter, softened**
- ¾ **cup packed brown sugar**
- 1 **egg**
- 2 **teaspoons vanilla extract**
- ½ **cup unsweetened applesauce**
- ¼ **cup maple syrup**
- 1 **tablespoon grated orange peel**
- 3 **cups quick-cooking oats**
- 1 **cup all-purpose flour**
- ½ **cup whole wheat flour**
- 1 **teaspoon baking soda**
- 1 **teaspoon ground cinnamon**
- ½ **teaspoon salt**
- ¼ **teaspoon ground nutmeg**
- ¼ **teaspoon ground cloves**

1. In a small bowl, combine water and flaxseed. In a large bowl, combine the plums, dates and raisins. Cover with boiling water. Let flaxseed and plum mixtures stand for 10 minutes.

2. Meanwhile, in a large bowl, cream butter and brown sugar until light and fluffy. Beat in egg and vanilla. Beat in the applesauce, maple syrup and orange peel. Combine the oats, flours, baking soda, cinnamon, salt, nutmeg and cloves; gradually add to creamed mixture and mix well. Drain plum mixture; stir plum mixture and flaxseed into the dough.

3. Drop by rounded teaspoonfuls 2 in. apart onto lightly greased baking sheets. Bake at 350° for 8-11 minutes or until set. Cool for 2 minutes before removing from pans to wire racks.

PER SERVING *1 cookie equals 56 cal., 1 g fat (1 g sat. fat), 5 mg chol., 40 mg sodium, 11 g carb., 1 g fiber, 1 g pro.* ***Diabetic Exchange:*** *1 starch.*

Harvest Snack Cake

Ginger, cinnamon and nutmeg give this dessert a familiar spice-cake flavor, and raisins and shredded carrots help to keep it nice and moist.

—HILARY CARROLL DEARBORN, MI

PREP: 15 MIN. • **BAKE:** 30 MIN.
MAKES: 15 SERVINGS

- **2 cups whole wheat flour**
- **1¼ cups packed brown sugar**
- **2 teaspoons baking soda**
- **¾ teaspoon ground cinnamon**
- **½ teaspoon ground nutmeg**
- **⅛ to ¼ teaspoon ground ginger**
- **2 eggs**
- **½ cup unsweetened applesauce**
- **1 teaspoon vanilla extract**
- **1½ cups shredded carrots**
- **1 cup raisins**

1. In a large bowl, combine the flour, brown sugar, baking soda, cinnamon, nutmeg and ginger. Combine the eggs, applesauce and vanilla; stir into dry ingredients just until moistened. Fold in the carrots and raisins (the batter will be thick).

2. Spread evenly in a 13-in. x 9-in. baking pan coated with cooking spray. Bake at 350° for 30-35 minutes or until a toothpick inserted near the center comes out clean. Cool on a wire rack.

PER SERVING *1 piece equals 170 cal., 1 g fat (0.55 g sat. fat), 28 mg chol., 191 mg sodium, 39 g carb., 3 g fiber, 3 g pro.* ***Diabetic Exchanges:*** *2 starch, ½ fruit.*

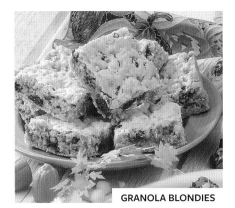

GRANOLA BLONDIES

Granola Blondies

You won't be able to pass up these treats. I often welcome guests with them.

—JANET FARLEY SNELLVILLE, GA

PREP: 15 MIN. • **BAKE:** 25 MIN.
MAKES: 1 DOZEN

- **1 egg**
- **1 egg white**
- **1¼ cups packed brown sugar**
- **¼ cup canola oil**
- **1 cup all-purpose flour**
- **1 teaspoon baking powder**
- **½ teaspoon salt**
- **2 cups reduced-fat granola with raisins**
- **1 cup dried cranberries or cherries**

1. In a large bowl, beat the egg, egg white, brown sugar and oil until blended. Combine the flour, baking powder and salt; gradually stir into sugar mixture just until blended. Stir in the granola and cranberries (batter will be thick).

2. Spread into a 9-in. square baking pan coated with cooking spray. Bake at 350° for 25-30 minutes or until golden brown and set. Cool on a wire rack. Cut into bars.

PER SERVING *1 brownie equals 256 cal., 6 g fat (1 g sat. fat), 18 mg chol., 173 mg sodium, 49 g carb., 2 g fiber, 3 g pro.* ***Diabetic Exchanges:*** *3 starch, ½ fat.*

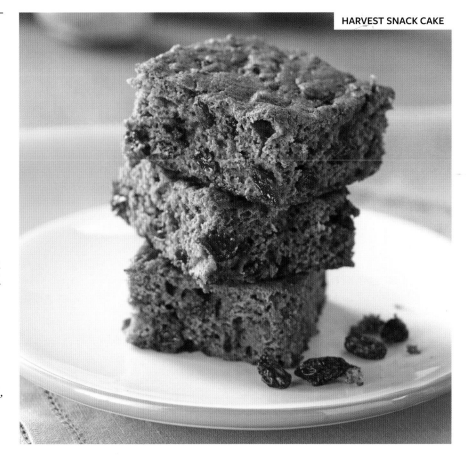

HARVEST SNACK CAKE

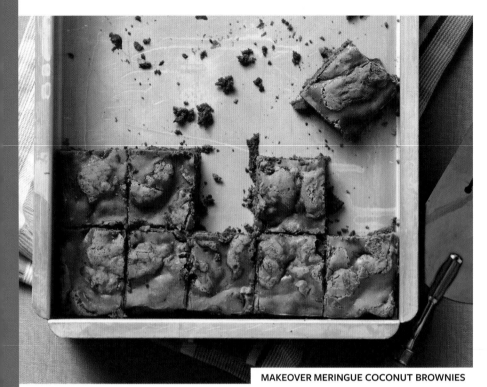

MAKEOVER MERINGUE COCONUT BROWNIES

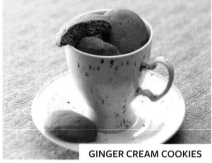

GINGER CREAM COOKIES

Makeover Meringue Coconut Brownies

A chocolate lover's dream, these bars will definitely satisfy a craving!

—**ELLEN AHO** SOUTH PARIS, ME

PREP: 30 MIN. • **BAKE:** 30 MIN. + COOLING
MAKES: 2 DOZEN

- ⅓ cup butter, softened
- ⅓ cup plus ¾ cup packed brown sugar, divided
- ⅓ cup sugar
- 1 teaspoon vanilla extract
- 2 cups all-purpose flour
- ½ teaspoon baking soda
- ¼ teaspoon salt
- ⅓ cup fat-free milk
- 1 cup (6 ounces) semisweet chocolate chips
- 1 cup flaked coconut
- ½ cup chopped walnuts
- 3 egg whites
- ¼ teaspoon cream of tartar

1. In a small bowl, cream the butter, ⅓ cup brown sugar and sugar until light and fluffy. Beat in vanilla. Combine the flour, baking soda and salt; add to the creamed mixture alternately with milk, beating well after each addition. Press into a 13-in. x 9-in. baking pan coated with cooking spray. Sprinkle with chocolate chips, coconut and walnuts.

2. In a large bowl, beat egg whites and cream of tartar until soft peaks form. Gradually beat in remaining brown sugar, 1 tablespoon at a time. Beat until stiff peaks form. Spread over the top. Bake at 350° for 30-35 minutes or until a toothpick inserted near the center comes out clean (do not overbake).

3. Cool on a wire rack. Cut into bars. Store in the refrigerator.

PER SERVING *1 brownie equals 181 cal., 8 g fat (4 g sat. fat), 7 mg chol., 92 mg sodium, 27 g carb., 1 g fiber, 2 g pro.* ***Diabetic Exchanges:*** *2 starch, 1 fat.*

Ginger Cream Cookies

These cookies are cakelike in texture and the spices really blend together well.

—**SUVILLA JORDAN** BUTLER, PA

PREP: 25 MIN. • **BAKE:** 10 MIN./BATCH
MAKES: 3 DOZEN

- ½ cup molasses
- ¼ cup sugar blend
- ¼ cup canola oil
- 1 egg
- 1 teaspoon vanilla extract
- 2 cups all-purpose flour
- 1½ teaspoons ground cinnamon
- 1 teaspoon baking soda
- 1 teaspoon ground ginger
- ¾ teaspoon ground cloves
- ¾ teaspoon ground nutmeg

1. In a large bowl, beat the molasses, sugar blend, oil, egg and vanilla until well blended. Combine the remaining ingredients; gradually add to molasses mixture and mix well.

2. Drop by rounded teaspoonfuls 2 in. apart onto baking sheets lightly coated with cooking spray.

3. Bake at 350° for 8-10 minutes or until the edges are lightly browned. Remove to wire racks to cool.

NOTE *This recipe was tested with Splenda sugar blend.*

PER SERVING *1 cookie equals 60 cal., 2 g fat (trace sat. fat), 6 mg chol., 39 mg sodium, 10 g carb., trace fiber, 1 g pro.* ***Diabetic Exchanges:*** *½ starch, ½ fat.*

Makeover Cream Cheese Streusel Bars

With an oh-so-chocolaty crust, crispy topping and soft cream cheese filling, these delectable bars are still diet-friendly!

—**JANET COOPS** DUARTE, CA

PREP: 20 MIN. • **BAKE:** 30 MIN. + COOLING
MAKES: 15 SERVINGS

- 1¼ cups confectioners' sugar
- 1 cup all-purpose flour
- ⅓ cup baking cocoa
- ¼ teaspoon salt
- ½ cup cold butter
- 1 package (8 ounces) reduced-fat cream cheese
- 1 can (14 ounces) fat-free sweetened condensed milk
- 1 egg, lightly beaten
- 2 teaspoons vanilla extract

1. In a large bowl, combine the confectioners' sugar, flour, cocoa and salt; cut in butter until crumbly. Set aside ½ cup for topping; press the remaining crumb mixture into an 11-in. x 7-in. baking pan coated with cooking spray. Bake at 325° for 8-12 minutes or until set.

2. In a small bowl, beat the cream cheese, milk, egg and vanilla until blended. Pour over crust. Bake for 15 minutes. Top with reserved crumb mixture; bake 5-10 minutes longer or until filling is set. Cool on a wire rack. Store in the refrigerator.

PER SERVING *1 bar equals 245 cal., 10 g fat (6 g sat. fat), 43 mg chol., 197 mg sodium, 34 g carb., 1 g fiber, 6 g pro. Diabetic Exchanges: 2 starch, 2 fat.*

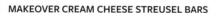

MAKEOVER CREAM CHEESE STREUSEL BARS

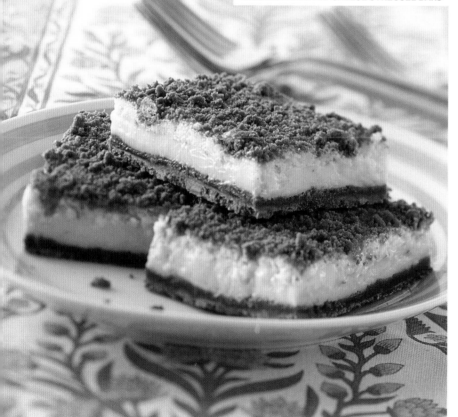

Almond Crispies

A triple almond punch (almond extract, ground almonds and blanched almonds) and cinnamon sugar make these cookies extra-good. The dough freezes well when made ahead. I sometimes make a batch with toasted pecans, and place a pecan half in the center of each cookie.

—**TRISHA KRUSE** EAGLE, ID

PREP: 20 MIN. + CHILLING
BAKE: 20 MIN./BATCH • **MAKES:** 3 DOZEN

- 3 tablespoons plus 1 cup sugar, divided
- ⅛ teaspoon ground cinnamon
- ⅓ cup butter, softened
- 1 egg
- ¼ cup fat-free milk
- ½ teaspoon almond extract
- ½ teaspoon vanilla extract
- 2½ cups all-purpose flour
- ¼ cup ground almonds
- ⅛ teaspoon salt
- 36 blanched almonds

1. In a small bowl, combine 3 tablespoons sugar and cinnamon; set aside.

2. In a large bowl, beat butter and remaining sugar until crumbly. Beat in the egg, milk and extracts. Combine the flour, ground almonds and salt; add to the creamed mixture and mix well. Cover and refrigerate for at least 1 hour.

3. Roll into 1-in. balls. Place 2 in. apart on ungreased baking sheets. Coat bottom of glass with cooking spray, then dip in cinnamon-sugar mixture. Flatten cookies with prepared glass, redipping in cinnamon-sugar mixture as needed. Top each cookie with an almond.

4. Bake at 325° for 16-18 minutes or until lightly browned. Remove cookies to wire racks.

PER SERVING *1 cookie equals 86 cal., 3 g fat (1 g sat. fat), 10 mg chol., 23 mg sodium, 14 g carb., trace fiber, 2 g pro. Diabetic Exchanges: 1 starch, 1 fat.*

Chocolate-Glazed Almond Bars

The moist almond filling and flaky golden crust these bars offer is something special.

—ROBIN HART NORTH BRUNSWICK, NJ

PREP: 25 MIN. • **BAKE:** 20 MIN. + COOLING
MAKES: 40 BARS

- 2 cups all-purpose flour
- ½ cup packed brown sugar
- ½ teaspoon salt
- ¾ cup cold butter, cubed
- 3 egg whites
- 1 cup sugar
- 1 can (12½ ounces) almond cake and pastry filling
- 2 cups sliced almonds
- 4 ounces bittersweet chocolate, chopped

1. In a large bowl, combine the flour, brown sugar and salt. Cut in butter until mixture resembles coarse crumbs. Pat into a 13-in. x 9-in. baking pan coated with cooking spray. Bake at 350° for 18-22 minutes or until edges are lightly browned.

2. Meanwhile, in a large bowl, whisk the egg whites, sugar and almond filling until blended. Stir in the almonds. Pour over crust. Bake for 20-25 minutes or until set. Cool completely on a wire rack.

3. In a microwave, melt chocolate; stir until smooth. Drizzle over top. Let stand until set. Cut into bars. Store in an airtight container in the refrigerator.

NOTE *This recipe was tested with Solo brand cake and pastry filling. Look for it in the baking aisle.*

PER SERVING *1 bar equals 156 cal., 8 g fat (3 g sat. fat), 9 mg chol., 70 mg sodium, 21 g carb., 1 g fiber, 2 g pro.*
Diabetic Exchanges: 1½ fat, 1 starch.

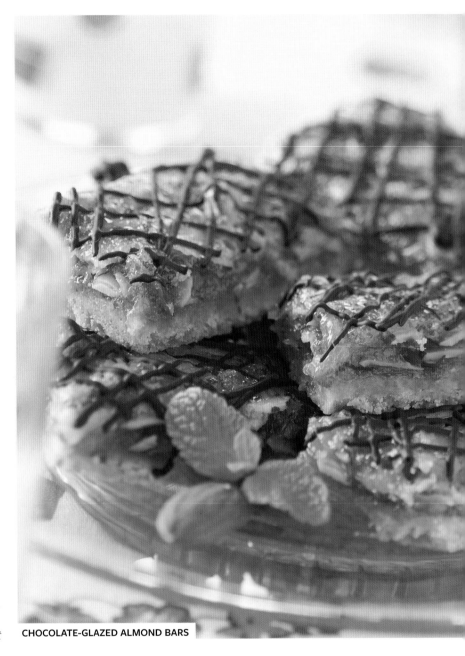

CHOCOLATE-GLAZED ALMOND BARS

top tip

Separating Whites & Yolks

It's easiest to separate egg whites from the yolks when the eggs are cold. Buying an egg separator can also make the job a breeze.

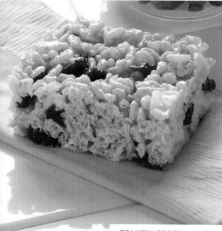

FRUITY CEREAL BARS

Fruity Cereal Bars

With dried apple and cranberries, these cereal bars are perfect for snacks or brown-bag lunches.

—GIOVANNA KRANENBERG CAMBRIDGE, MN

START TO FINISH: 30 MIN.
MAKES: 20 SERVINGS

- 3 **tablespoons butter**
- 1 **package (10 ounces) large marshmallows**
- 6 **cups crisp rice cereal**
- ½ **cup chopped dried apple**
- ½ **cup dried cranberries**

1. In a large saucepan, combine butter and marshmallows. Cook and stir over medium-low heat until melted. Remove from the heat; stir in the cereal, apples and cranberries.

2. Pat into a 13-in. x 9-in. pan coated with cooking spray; cool. Cut into squares.

PER SERVING *1 bar equals 105 cal., 2 g fat (1 g sat. fat), 5 mg chol., 102 mg sodium, 22 g carb., trace fiber, 1 g pro. Diabetic Exchanges: 1½ starch, ½ fat.*

Chunky Peanut Butter Cookies

My husband really liked this cookie recipe, but I wanted it to be lower in fat. Thanks to the *Taste of Home* Test Kitchen, the recipe now has 31% less fat than the original!

—TASTE OF HOME TEST KITCHEN

PREP: 25 MIN. • **BAKE:** 15 MIN./BATCH
MAKES: 5 DOZEN

- ⅓ **cup butter, softened**
- ⅓ **cup reduced-fat butter, softened**
- 1 **cup packed brown sugar**
- ½ **cup sugar blend**
- 1 **cup reduced-fat chunky peanut butter**
- 2 **eggs**
- 2 **cups all-purpose flour**
- 1½ **cups quick-cooking oats**
- 1 **teaspoon baking powder**
- 1 **teaspoon salt**
- ½ **teaspoon baking soda**
- 1 **cup raisins**
- ¾ **cup flaked coconut**
- ½ **cup miniature semisweet chocolate chips**

CHUNKY PEANUT BUTTER COOKIES

1. In a large bowl, cream the butters, brown sugar and sugar substitute until light and fluffy. Beat in peanut butter. Add eggs, one at a time, beating well after each addition. Combine the flour, oats, baking powder, salt and baking soda; gradually add to creamed mixture and mix well. Stir in the raisins, coconut and chocolate chips.

2. Drop by rounded tablespoonfuls onto ungreased baking sheets. Bake at 350° for 12-14 minutes or until golden brown. Cool for 2 minutes before removing to wire racks.

NOTE *This recipe was tested with Land O'Lakes light stick butter and Splenda sugar blend.*

PER SERVING *1 cookie equals 104 cal., 4 g fat (2 g sat. fat), 11 mg chol., 109 mg sodium, 15 g carb., 1 g fiber, 2 g pro. Diabetic Exchanges: 1 starch, 1 fat.*

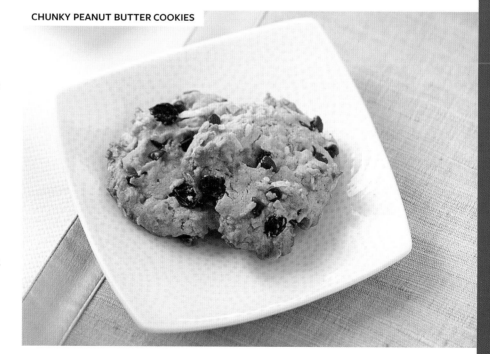

General Index

Alphabetical Index